Table of Contents

T0384475

Metabolic Revolution: Shifting the Nutritional Paradigm

Why This Book Has to Exist:

As we progress deeper into the 21st century, the health of our population is declining at an unprecedented rate. Despite the various dietary guidelines, health campaigns, and the constant influx of advice from doctors, dietitians, and the media, the facts are clear: our nation is sicker than ever. Chronic diseases like heart disease, diabetes, cancer, and obesity are on the rise, and the average person's quality of life is deteriorating. This raises a serious question—how is it possible that, with all the advances in medicine and nutrition, we are facing such a profound health crisis?

The answer lies in the very system we trust to keep us healthy. We are bombarded with information from so-called authorities who often fail to address the root causes of our declining health. The problem isn't just personal choices; it's systemic. People trust the guidance of the medical establishment and public health authorities without realizing that these institutions are often influenced by industries like Big Food and Big Pharma, whose priorities may not align with long-term health and well-being. Unless we question these narratives and examine the evidence for ourselves, we will continue on this destructive path.

It's also worth noting that, as a relatively young nation, we are facing a unique health crisis. Unlike other nations that have existed for thousands of years, our modern industrialized food system has developed rapidly, and we are now paying the price. With technology's rise and convenience at the forefront of our daily lives, we are surrounded by processed foods, sugar-laden diets, and medications that treat symptoms but ignore the root causes of disease.

This book is a product of years of research; mine and others—who challenge the conventional wisdom surrounding health and nutrition. Science isn't static; it evolves, and the evidence we have today points to one undeniable fact: our mainstream dietary recommendations are broken. Through this book, I will show you *why* the system promotes these outdated and harmful messages and *how* we can break free from them. I believe that with the right information, we can empower ourselves to create a healthier future for the next generation—one free from the debilitating diseases that plague our current society. We need to wake up and realize what is happening. Nobody said it will be easy, but we have to take action and realize who the good guys are, and who the bad guys are. Together, we can shift the nutritional paradigm, and this book is the first step toward making that change.

As generations progress, we need to recognize the genetic impact our diets are having on us. Juices are served in schools and hospitals, processed foods are everywhere, and we're led to believe that even moderate carbohydrate consumption is normal. While we've been conditioned to accept this, we owe it to ourselves and future generations to understand the biological consequences of consuming these altered 'foods.' Diabetes, cancer, mental health issues, depression, anxiety, auto-immune issues, obesity, heart disease, among others. There is a reason that heart disease is STILL our NUMBER ONE killer. Our children—and their children—deserve better.

One thing we must do is be completely aware of the situation and realize what you need to do to make your life better. If you can benefit your life and the lives of your family, that is a huge leap in the right direction.

We must realize the myths and systemic lies that propel the crisis of health and make decisions based on informed truths. We must understand cholesterol

Join me as we journey through the world of health as we know it, and let's work together to create meaningful change. We find ourselves in this deep hole because our understanding of nutrition has been skewed for generations.

Introduction: Let's Distinguish the Perception of Metabolism vs. What Metabolism Actually Is

The concept of metabolism is commonly misunderstood. You've probably heard someone say, "Oh, my metabolism is slow," linking it to a struggle with weight loss. This has become a cultural shorthand for metabolism, associating it solely with how quickly or slowly we burn calories. But metabolism is far more intricate and foundational to our overall health.

When I was brainstorming titles for this book, I chose *Metabolic Revolution: The Nutritional Paradigm* and searched to ensure the title was unique. I was met with countless books focused on weight loss, proving just how prevalent this narrow perception of metabolism is. For most people, metabolism simply equates to a "fast" or "slow" rate of burning calories—either a gift of youth or a struggle of aging.

In reality, metabolism encompasses every biochemical reaction happening within us to sustain life. It's not just about burning calories but about the efficient transformation and distribution of energy at a cellular level. From maintaining our body temperature and repairing cells to breaking down nutrients and removing waste, metabolism is a complex, multi-layered process essential to our survival and vitality.

Let's dive deeper to fully understand what metabolism really entails and why redefining it matters for our approach to nutrition and overall health.

"No Amount of Evidence Will Ever Convince an Idiot"

-Mark Twain

My Story and Why I wrote this book

I never imagined that I would find myself deeply immersed in the world of nutrition. As a child, I had no interest in the health or medical industry—I wanted to become a police officer like my older brother. But life has a way of steering us in unexpected directions. My journey into nutrition and health began with my family's history of health issues. When my mother had a heart attack at the age of 57, everything changed. She lived until she was 72, but her final years were filled with misery. She endured a quintuple bypass surgery, followed by a triple bypass, and eventually passed away from multiple complications related to heart disease.

My father's story wasn't much different, though he didn't experience an early heart attack. Instead, he developed type 2 diabetes, which eventually progressed to type 1—a rare but possible occurrence. His health continued to decline over the years. Looking back, I often wonder if I could have made a difference had I started my nutritional journey earlier. Of course, much of the research surrounding heart disease and nutrition is relatively new, but I was there to witness firsthand the impact of outdated medical advice. Tragically, my father passed away during what was supposed to be a "routine" atherectomy—a procedure in which a rotating device scrapes away plaque from arterial walls. The doctor accidentally tore an artery wall, causing my father to go into cardiac arrest. Although they stabilized him and continued the procedure, a second cardiac arrest took his life.

I still remember the recommendations the doctors gave to my mother: eat low-fat foods, avoid cholesterol, consume more whole grains, and eat plenty of fruits and vegetables. Despite following these guidelines, her condition only worsened. She eventually ended up on dialysis due to renal failure, and her heart grew weaker with every passing day. Cholesterol was the focal point of her treatment, but nothing they recommended helped.

My father, too, developed heart disease after years of uncontrolled type 2 diabetes, following the same advice: eat more fruits and vegetables, oatmeal, and cereals touted as "heart healthy." There was always a box of Cheerios in the pantry, proudly endorsed by the American Heart Association. He was told to eat margarine and avoid saturated fats. In hindsight, these recommendations were not only misleading, but they were also downright harmful.

Around 2020, during the global pandemic lockdown, while I was traveling to San Jose for a meeting with my wife Yesenia, I received results from a blood test that shook me to my core. My triglycerides were in the 700s, my fasting glucose was at 350, my A1c was a staggering 14.9, and my cholesterol was "high" (more on that later). I was hit with the sudden reality that if I didn't make a change, I might not have much time left. The image I had in my head were all my kids who were all young at the time, the youngest being my daughter Hideko, who was only 5 years old. I couldn't put myself in a position to leave this world before watching them all grow up.

I started small, cutting out sugars, but as I dove deeper into research and the science of health, I uncovered a world of information that I had never known. I became obsessed with the physiology of health, diabetes, dyslipidemia, and metabolic disorders.

For several reasons, I earned several nutrition certificates and began educating myself. I began self-experiments and became a guinea pig for science. Through my research, I realized that most people trust doctors implicitly, believing them to be the ultimate authority on health. But many doctors, including cardiologists, nephrologists, and general practitioners, said to me that they receive little to no training in nutrition science during medical school. And what they do learn is often outdated, or completely irrelevant to the benefit of the patient. Doctors for the most part are well intentioned. I don't believe they are trying to mislead you, but the world works a bit differently that most of us believe.

This is where my dilemma lies. I have so much to share, so much to convey, but *who will listen*? I'm not a doctor, and my background wasn't even in health—yet I've made it my life's mission, and now it IS my background. I started taking Inflammation and Diabetes courses through Harvard Medical School and Arizona State University to earn credibility in nutritional science, but in truth, it's just for credibility. Much of what I've "learned" in those courses doesn't align with the research I've uncovered (which I will cite and explain throughout this book). While most of the science is correct, the human body is so complex that we are still discovering more of its' functions to this day. I will go over some of the more important developments. By the way, some are intentionally suppressed. I will go over that as well.

So here I am, looking back and realizing that I am on a journey to uncover the truth—truth that is free from bias, free from corporate interests, and free from the influence of pharmaceutical companies. My struggle is that most people will believe what they want to believe, whether it's their grandmother's home remedies or advice from a doctor funded by Big Pharma, pushing the latest drug. My hope is that this book will reach enough people to help stop the lies, halt the decline in public health, and shift the world's nutritional paradigm. After all, even our schools and hospitals, institutions where health should be a priority, are serving some of the worst, most nutritionally void foods. I want the future generations to have a chance at thriving. I want my kids to avoid "genetically" related disorders and live as happy and healthy as possible. This is my key, that I offer to the future, for a better life.

Please keep in mind that though I have made every attempt to provide information that is accurate and complete, but this book is not intended as a substitute for professional medical advice. This book is not meant to be used, nor should it be used, to diagnose or treat any medical or psychological condition.

Chapter 1: The State of the World's Health — A Focus on the U.S.

First, we must understand. Understand the root causes of our decline. This understanding includes how we've arrived at our current state and what changes can set future generations on a healthier path. According to recent CDC data, approximately **50%** of Americans are classified as *obese*. This staggering figure is hard to fathom when you consider that, in the 1980s, obesity affected only about 13.4% of the population. The acceleration has been exponential, and the consequences are becoming more visible with each passing year.

Obesity as a New Normal

One of the biggest challenges we face is that obesity has become normalized. I have seen celebrities calling for the normalization of obesity. Social messaging often frames obesity as inclusivity, while sentiments like "My metabolism is slowing down because I'm getting older" perpetuate misconceptions and worsen health outcomes. I recall seeing ads promoting the idea that most people don't resemble the slim models in magazines. But here's the reality: while body diversity exists, the epidemic levels of obesity we see today are symptomatic of a society that has lost sight of balanced eating and optimal health. Yes folks, we ARE supposed to look like that. Unlike our ancestors who ate to survive, we eat for convenience and pleasure, very much at the expense of our health. Obesity most of the time is also a symptom of something wrong. If we don't recognize it as such, we set ourselves up for certain disaster.

Rising Health Crises: Obesity and Chronic Disease

With obesity at an all-time high and on track to characterize the majority of the population, chronic disease is following close behind. Heart disease remains the leading cause of death in the United States, taking more than 700,000 lives each year—not just cases, but deaths. Obesity often signals deeper systemic health issues, including insulin resistance, inflammation, and hormonal imbalances. Each of these factors plays a critical role in our country's health crisis, especially as they converge within metabolic syndrome, a significant driver of heart disease.

The Impact on Children's Health (This is What Really Matters)

The health crisis doesn't only affect adults. Childhood obesity now affects 20% of American children, compared to just 5% in the 1970s. For many of these children, obesity foreshadows a future burdened with chronic illness, cardiovascular risks, and a reduced quality of life. In addition to physical health concerns, these children face psychological challenges, with increased rates of depression, anxiety, and social stigmatization. Dietary choices are a major contributor; many children consume government-subsidized school meals that are nutritionally inadequate, while food marketing campaigns promote sugary cereals, snacks, and drinks. As a result, children are being primed for metabolic issues from an early age.

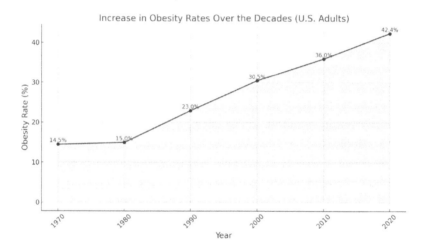

Processed Foods and Nutritional Misinformation

A central factor in this health decline is the overwhelming presence of processed foods and nutritional disinformation. The food industry has carefully crafted a public perception that foods like "whole grain" cereals, "low-fat" snacks, and sugary drinks marketed as "healthy" are beneficial. In reality, these products are often loaded with sugars, refined grains, and unhealthy fats that contribute to metabolic disease. For example, the "heart-healthy" seal on certain processed foods, often endorsed by organizations funded by food companies, creates a false sense of security. Sugary cereals and low-fat yogurts laden with high-fructose corn syrup are marketed as healthy, despite evidence linking refined carbs and sugars to metabolic syndrome, diabetes, and obesity.

Fructose and Non-Alcoholic Fatty Liver Disease (NAFLD): A Silent Crisis

Among the most silent yet prevalent consequences of our diet is non-alcoholic fatty liver disease (NAFLD), which now affects more than 25% of the global population, with alarming rates in the U.S. Once considered rare, NAFLD has become one of the most common liver disorders, particularly in children and adolescents. The condition arises when excess fructose and refined carbs overload the liver, causing fat to accumulate. Fructose, found in high-fructose corn syrup and sugar-laden processed foods, is metabolized specifically by the liver. Unlike glucose, which is used by all cells, fructose overwhelms the liver, leading to fat deposits and inflammation. Shockingly, these foods are still heavily marketed to children and regularly served in school lunches and hospital meals, contributing to the rise in NAFLD and overall metabolic dysfunction. Dr. Robert Lustig observed a significant rise in non-alcoholic fatty liver disease (NAFLD) among children, leading him to question why it's so prevalent today. In his book *Metabolical*, which I highly recommend, Lustig highlights how NAFLD has become a principal driver of childhood obesity. He argues that modern diets—particularly those high in processed foods and fructose-laden sugars—are the root causes. Unlike in previous generations, children today are frequently exposed to high-fructose corn syrup in everything from sodas to seemingly "healthy" options like fruit-flavored yogurts and cereals. This fructose overwhelms the liver, causing fat accumulation and setting the stage for metabolic disorders.

Lustig's insights underscore a major shift in childhood health: diseases once associated with adults, like NAFLD, are now striking children due to the dietary landscape shaped by processed food industries. This trend points to the urgent need for rethinking children's diets to combat the rise in metabolic dysfunction.

The Financial Cost of Chronic Disease

The economic burden of chronic disease is staggering. The U.S. spends more on healthcare than any other nation, with a significant portion directed at managing chronic, preventable conditions. For example, the annual cost of treating diabetes in the U.S. exceeds $327 billion, while heart disease costs nearly $229 billion, and obesity-related healthcare expenses range between $147 billion to $210 billion each year. This reactive approach to healthcare focuses on managing symptoms rather than addressing root causes. Medical institutions are rarely incentivized to promote true preventive health, relying instead on medications to manage blood pressure, cholesterol, and blood sugar without addressing the dietary and lifestyle factors driving these conditions.

A Necessary Shift: From Symptom Management to Health Creation

Breaking this cycle requires a fundamental shift in how we view food, lifestyle, and health. Our current model emphasizes treating symptoms instead of preventing disease. We must move towards a holistic, root-cause approach to health—one that understands the importance of whole, unprocessed foods, prioritizes metabolic health, and emphasizes the impact of lifestyle choices. Statistics only tell part of the story. Behind the numbers are real people whose lives are affected not due to a lack of medical intervention but because they lack accurate information and practical guidance. Our healthcare system has become reactionary, focusing on treatment rather than prevention, and it is failing to keep Americans healthy.

Reframing the Solution: Embracing Nutritional Basics

Growing research supports the benefits of diets that align with human evolution, emphasizing whole foods, high-quality animal proteins, healthy fats, and minimal processed foods. Unlike the low-fat, high-carbohydrate diets promoted for decades, a balanced intake of nutrient-dense foods supports metabolic health, reduces inflammation, and mitigates the risk of chronic disease. This chapter will lay the foundation for understanding why metabolic health matters, how far we've strayed from it, and why reversing these trends is essential. We must critically examine the standard American diet, government-backed dietary guidelines, and the influence of food corporations that prioritize profit over health.

Key Health Statistics in the U.S.

- **Obesity Rate:** Nearly 50% of U.S. adults are classified as obese, a stark increase from 13.4% in the 1980s.
- **Diabetes and Prediabetes:** Over 37 million Americans have diabetes, with another 96 million classified as pre-diabetic. (Keep in mind that prediabetes is the same as diabetes more on that in the following chapters)
- **NAFLD (Non-Alcoholic Fatty Liver Disease):** Now the most common liver disease in the world, affecting roughly 25% of the global population.

Top Causes of Death in the United States

1. Heart Disease
2. Cancer
3. COVID-19 (recent years)
4. Unintentional Injuries
5. Chronic Lower Respiratory Diseases
6. Stroke
7. Alzheimer's Disease
8. Diabetes
9. Kidney Disease
10. Suicide

The Progression of Metabolic Diseases

Diabetes: Since the mid-20th century, diabetes rates have surged, affecting millions of Americans and leaving millions more at risk.

Metabolic Syndrome: This syndrome now impacts approximately 1 in 3 U.S. adults, encompassing high blood pressure, abdominal obesity, and insulin resistance, which collectively raise the risk of heart disease, stroke, and diabetes.

NAFLD: Once rare, this liver disease now impacts up to 25% of the global population and is closely associated with processed foods, high fructose intake, and sedentary lifestyles.

These statistics serve as a wake-up call. In this chapter, we'll dive deeper into these topics, examining how we got here, the full impact of metabolic syndrome, and the steps we must take to shift the trajectory for future generations. Together, let's work to disrupt this cycle of preventable disease and pave the way for a healthier and more sustainable future.

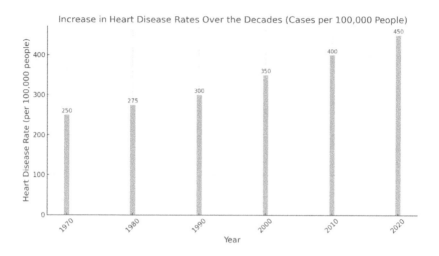

Increase in Heart Disease Rates Over the Decades (Cases per 100,000 People)

By the Numbers

In the scope of human history, heart disease and metabolic disorders are relatively new. For thousands of years, humans evolved on diets and lifestyles that promoted metabolic health, with minimal incidence of diseases like coronary artery disease, hypertension, and type 2 diabetes. However, over the last century—particularly since the industrial and agricultural revolutions—heart disease has transformed from a rare ailment to one of the most prevalent causes of death worldwide. The rapid increase in cardiovascular issues coincides with a shift in human lifestyle, diet, and environmental factors, which together have contributed to a significant decline in public health.

A Brief History: Rare Heart Disease and the Early Cardiologists

At the dawn of the 20th century, heart disease was virtually unheard of, and few specialists existed to treat cardiovascular issues. In fact, it's reported that there were only a handful of cardiologists in the United States around the year 1900. According to records, there were only around 3 or 4 known cardiologists in the U.S. at the turn of the century—a stark contrast to the tens of thousands practicing today. At that time, heart attacks and strokes were so rare that they were barely documented in medical literature. Can you step back and think about that for a second? See how much heart disease has progressed in such a short time? If you don't recognize this, then there clearly is a bigger problem.

The 20th Century: A Health Decline Fueled by Diet and Lifestyle Changes

The shift from rural, agrarian lifestyles to urban, industrialized ones brought dramatic changes in daily routines, diet, and overall health. Processed foods, refined sugars, and trans fats became staples in the average diet, while physical activity decreased as more people moved from manual labor jobs to sedentary ones. This lifestyle change not only led to a rise in metabolic disorders but also increased chronic stress levels, which further compounded the risk of heart disease.

As early as the 1950s, researchers began noticing the rise in cardiovascular issues and obesity. The Framingham Heart Study, which began in 1948, provided one of the first long-term analyses of heart disease risk factors. The study tracked generations of participants and revealed that factors like high blood pressure, high cholesterol, and obesity increased the risk of heart disease. However, while the study linked these factors to heart disease, it also coincided with the rise of processed foods, artificial fats, and high-carbohydrate diets—all of which exacerbated the growing heart disease epidemic.

Generational Health Decline: The Impact of Industrialization and Processed Foods

Over the past century, the shift toward industrialized food production has had devastating effects on health. Before processed foods became common, people ate diets rich in natural fats, proteins, and whole foods. The introduction of refined carbohydrates, artificial ingredients, and preservatives disrupted this balance, leading to a range of metabolic issues.

The American diet, now heavily centered around refined grains, sugars, and processed oils is vastly different from the diets of our ancestors. Processed food consumption has increased from around 30% in the early 20th century to over 60% today. This dietary shift has led to an increase in conditions like obesity, diabetes, and hypertension, all of which are significant risk factors for heart disease. Additionally, as food production became more industrialized, the quality of food has declined, with nutrient-dense foods being replaced by calorie-dense, nutrient-poor options.

The Rise of Cardiovascular Specialists: A Symptom of Growing Health Problems

The number of cardiologists has surged alongside the rise in cardiovascular disease. According to the American College of Cardiology, there were about 18,000 practicing cardiologists in the United States as of 2020, compared to just a few at the turn of the century. This increase reflects the drastic rise in cardiovascular health issues, which have necessitated a larger workforce of specialists. Heart disease now accounts for about 32% of all deaths globally, making it the leading cause of death worldwide.

Statistics show that the rates of cardiovascular disease have grown nearly 10-fold since the early 1900s, and about 48% of U.S. adults are affected by some form of cardiovascular disease today. The rise in cardiologists is both a response to and a reflection of this alarming trend in public health.

Statistics Highlighting the Decline in Health Over the Past 100 Years

Numerous health statistics demonstrate the sharp decline in metabolic and cardiovascular health over the past century. Here are a few that illustrate this trend:

Heart Disease Mortality Rates: In 1900, heart disease was responsible for fewer than 10% of all deaths in the United States. By the mid-20th century, this figure had risen to 30%, and today, it's the leading cause of death, responsible for approximately 1 in 4 deaths.

Obesity Rates: At the start of the 20th century, less than 5% of the U.S. population was considered obese. Today, over 42% of adults in the U.S. are classified as obese, with an additional 30% classified as overweight.

Diabetes Incidence: Type 2 diabetes, once known as adult-onset diabetes, was extremely rare at the beginning of the 20th century. Today, nearly 10% of the U.S. population has diabetes, with an additional 33% experiencing prediabetes or insulin resistance.

Processed Food Consumption: Processed and convenience foods now comprise over 60% of the average American diet. In the early 1900s, diets were composed almost entirely of whole foods, with minimal processed ingredients.

These numbers show a troubling pattern: as industrialization, sedentary lifestyles, and processed foods have increased, so too have chronic health issues. This shift toward metabolic dysfunction has become so widespread that conditions like obesity, diabetes, and heart disease are now seen as normal parts of aging, rather than preventable ailments.

Metabolic Dysfunction: The Foundation of Chronic Disease

One of the most significant factors behind the rise in heart disease is metabolic dysfunction. Poor diet and lifestyle habits have led to widespread insulin resistance, which is now recognized as a major risk factor for cardiovascular disease, diabetes, and even some cancers. Insulin resistance disrupts the body's ability to process glucose effectively, leading to chronic inflammation, oxidative stress, and high blood pressure—all of which contribute to the development of heart disease.

Interestingly, indigenous and isolated populations with diets centered on natural, unprocessed foods have much lower rates of heart disease and metabolic disorders. Studies have shown that groups like the Inuit, Maasai, and Hadza have minimal incidence of heart disease and diabetes. However, as Western diets have been introduced to these populations, rates of these conditions have sharply increased, underscoring the impact of diet on metabolic health.

Breaking the Cycle: Awareness and Prevention

Understanding the historical context of heart disease and its modern-day prevalence can help us make better choices. Returning to diets and lifestyles that promote metabolic health—such as those high in whole foods, healthy fats, and limited in sugar—may help reduce the prevalence of cardiovascular disease in future generations. Additionally, physical activity, stress management, and regular health monitoring are essential to maintaining a strong heart and healthy metabolism.

Preventative measures, such as reducing sugar and processed food intake, can help reverse metabolic dysfunction before it progresses to chronic disease. Public health efforts focusing on educating the public about healthy food choices and lifestyle habits are key to reducing the burden of heart disease and improving overall quality of life.

A Call for Change in Health Perception and Practices

The rise of heart disease is not just a consequence of individual choices; it's a reflection of the systemic issues embedded in modern society. To combat this, we must rethink our approach to health and nutrition, recognizing that what is "normal" today is not necessarily healthy. By understanding the factors that have led to the health decline of modern generations, we can work to create a future where heart disease and metabolic disorders are once again rare, not inevitable.

A Profit-Driven Food Industry and the Decline in Food Quality

The quality of the food we consume today is a far cry from what our ancestors ate just a few centuries ago. In the pursuit of profit, the food industry has transformed the very nature of our diets, replacing nutrient-dense, whole foods with genetically modified organisms (GMOs), artificial additives, and heavily processed options. This shift has been driven largely by the prioritization of efficiency, scalability, and, ultimately, profitability over human health. The result is a society plagued by chronic diseases, metabolic disorders, and declining overall health.

For generations, our diets were based on whole, natural foods that aligned with our biological needs. However, as the demand for cheaper, more accessible food grew, so did the drive to increase production speed and shelf life. With this came an array of modifications—genetic engineering, chemical preservatives, and synthetic flavors—transforming food into a product optimized for profit rather than health.

Genetically Modified Organisms (GMOs)

GMOs have become a cornerstone of modern agriculture, designed to enhance crop yields, resist pests, and tolerate herbicides. While these innovations have helped feed a growing global population, they've also introduced significant health concerns and contributed to the decline in food quality. The genetic manipulation of crops has altered not only their natural properties but also the nutritional value they once provided.

Genetic modification has also affected the quality of fruits and vegetables, with many varieties bred for size, sweetness, and resistance to bruising, rather than nutrient density. The result is produce that may look appealing but lacks the nutrient profile that our bodies evolved to need. By prioritizing aesthetic appeal and shelf life over quality, we've sacrificed the health benefits that natural, whole foods were once known to provide.

The Rise of Additives and Artificial Ingredients: Cheap but Dangerous

In addition to GMOs, the food industry has increasingly relied on artificial additives, preservatives, and flavor enhancers to make food more appealing and longer lasting. These substances were introduced to maximize profit by extending shelf life, improving taste, and creating highly palatable products that keep consumers coming back for more.

Additives like high-fructose corn syrup, artificial sweeteners, trans fats, and synthetic flavorings are now pervasive in processed foods. While they may make foods taste better or last longer, they also pose risks to health. High-fructose corn syrup, for instance, has been linked to obesity, insulin resistance, and non-alcoholic fatty liver disease (NAFLD). Trans fats, though now banned in many countries, were once a staple in processed foods, contributing to inflammation, heart disease, and other chronic conditions.

The food industry's reliance on these cheap ingredients has created a diet that's calorie-dense but nutrient-poor, contributing to malnutrition even in affluent societies. Many people today consume more calories than ever before, yet they're often deficient in essential vitamins and minerals, a phenomenon known as "hidden hunger." This paradox of overfed but undernourished individuals highlights the dangers of prioritizing profit over proper nutrition.

The Shift Away from the "Proper Human Diet"

Historically, humans thrived on diets rich in whole foods—meat, fish, eggs, fruits, vegetables, nuts, and seeds. This "proper human diet" supported metabolic health, longevity, and overall well-being. However, the industrialization of food production has led to a drastic shift away from these traditional, nutrient-dense foods in favor of refined grains, sugars, and processed oils.

For instance, prior to the industrial era, most of the fats in our diets came from animal sources, which are rich in nutrients like omega-3 fatty acids, vitamin K2, and conjugated linoleic acid (CLA). Today, these healthy fats have been largely replaced by industrial seed oils like soybean, corn, and canola oil. These oils are high in omega-6 fatty acids, which promote inflammation when consumed in excess and have been linked to conditions like obesity, heart disease, and diabetes.

This shift has resulted in a diet that not only lacks essential nutrients but also disrupts our natural metabolic processes. The overconsumption of refined sugars, in particular, has led to a rise in insulin resistance, a condition that underpins many chronic diseases. Unlike the balanced, whole-food diets of our ancestors, today's diet is filled with artificial foods that the body doesn't recognize or process efficiently, leading to metabolic dysfunction and a decline in health.

Profit Over Longevity: The Cost of Cheap, Processed Food

The prioritization of profits over public health has made food more affordable and accessible than ever, but at a significant cost. Today, processed and fast foods are often cheaper and more convenient than whole, natural foods, making them the default choice for many people. This convenience, however, masks the hidden costs of poor health, increased medical expenses, and reduced quality of life.

The marketing tactics used by food companies further reinforce this cycle. Companies spend billions on advertising to promote highly processed, sugar-laden products, often targeting children and low-income families. This constant exposure creates a culture where processed foods are seen as "normal" and even desirable, while nutrient-dense, whole foods are viewed as expensive or inconvenient.

This shift has not only impacted individual health but has also created a public health crisis. Chronic diseases, many of which are diet-related, now account for over 70% of healthcare costs in the United States. Obesity, diabetes, heart disease, and cancer are more prevalent than ever, and the financial burden of these conditions continues to grow. By focusing on short-term profits, the food industry has contributed to a long-term decline in health, with profound consequences for individuals and society as a whole.

The intersection of health and diet with the interests of powerful industries, particularly pharmaceutical and food companies, highlights a complex and often troubling dynamic. In recent decades, we have witnessed a significant rise in chronic diseases such as obesity, diabetes, and heart disease, which have been linked to the consumption of processed and unhealthy foods. The pharmaceutical industry has capitalized on this trend by developing a vast array of medications aimed at managing these chronic conditions. While these medications can provide necessary relief, they often serve to maintain a cycle of dependency, wherein individuals rely on pharmaceuticals to manage symptoms rather than addressing the underlying causes of their health issues. This model prioritizes profit over proactive health management, leading to a healthcare landscape that favors treatment over prevention, as there are fewer financial incentives to promote holistic approaches that encourage healthy eating and lifestyle choices.

In parallel, the food industry plays a critical role in shaping dietary habits through the production and marketing of processed foods that are often high in sugars, unhealthy fats, and additives. These foods are designed to be convenient and appealing, yet they contribute significantly to the increasing rates of chronic illnesses. Major food corporations often prioritize profit margins over public health, creating an environment where unhealthy eating patterns become normalized. The marketing strategies employed by these companies frequently downplay the negative health impacts of their products, which can mislead consumers into making poor dietary choices. This relentless promotion of unhealthy foods creates a paradox where individuals are inundated with options that are both easily accessible and detrimental to their health, further entrenching them in a cycle of poor dietary habits and associated health risks.

Addressing this intertwined relationship between health, diet, and profit motives requires a multifaceted approach. Public awareness campaigns and educational initiatives that emphasize the importance of whole nutrient-dense foods can empower individuals to make informed dietary choices that support their long-term health. Moreover, advocating for policy changes that promote transparency in food marketing and incentivizing the production of healthy food options can help shift the landscape towards better public health outcomes. By recognizing the role of these industries in shaping health behaviors and outcomes, we can work towards a system that prioritizes the well-being of individuals over corporate profits. Only through concerted efforts can we break the cycle of dependency on medications and foster a culture of health that champions preventive care and dietary awareness.

The Way Forward: Returning to Quality and the Proper Human Diet

To reverse these trends, we need to return to a diet based on quality, whole foods—what many nutrition experts refer to as the "proper human diet." This means choosing foods that are as close to their natural state as possible, free from GMOs, artificial additives, and excessive processing. By prioritizing nutrient density over convenience and artificial appeal, we can restore the balance that our bodies need to thrive.

This shift requires a fundamental change in mindset, as well as a willingness to question the current food system. It means supporting local farmers who practice sustainable agriculture, choosing organic or Non-GMO options when possible, and learning to cook with whole ingredients. While these choices may come with a higher price tag, they are an investment in long-term health and well-being, reducing the risk of chronic disease and enhancing quality of life.

Furthermore, individuals can make a difference by advocating for transparency and accountability within the food industry. Demanding clearer labeling, supporting policies that promote sustainable farming, and reducing reliance on processed foods can all contribute to a healthier food system.

Choosing Health Over Profit

The transformation of the food industry over the past century has prioritized profit at the expense of public health. By filling our diets with cheap, processed foods, the industry has contributed to a decline in health that affects every generation. Foods must align with our biological needs and promote lasting health.

Chapter Two: Metabolic Syndrome

Metabolic syndrome is commonly defined by a collection of symptoms, including obesity, high blood pressure, high blood sugar, elevated triglycerides, and low HDL cholesterol. However, there are additional markers that merit attention in defining and understanding metabolic syndrome: We need to pay attention to **high uric acid, elevated fasting insulin levels, and elevated inflammatory markers**. Each of these factors profoundly influences our overall health. In this chapter, we'll examine each component, diving into the science behind how these indicators interact and contribute to metabolic syndrome.

Metabolic Syndrome

- o Obesity (waist to height ratio)
- o High Blood Pressure
- o High Blood Sugar (Fating glucose) or (a1c glycated blood)
- o Elevated Triglycerides
- o Low HDL Cholesterol
- o *Elevated Uric Acid*
- o *Elevated Fasting Insulin*
- o *Elevated Inflammatory Markers*

Obesity and the Role of Insulin

Obesity is one of the most visible signs of metabolic syndrome, yet it stems from underlying biochemical processes. The main driver of obesity within metabolic syndrome is chronically elevated insulin levels, which result from a high intake of carbohydrate-rich foods. Insulin, known as the "fat storage hormone," plays a crucial role in deciding whether the body should store or burn fat. With every meal high in carbohydrates, insulin is released to lower blood sugar, signaling the body to store excess energy as fat.

This mechanism leads to two main types of fat accumulation: **visceral fat** (around internal organs) and **subcutaneous fat** (the visible fat under the skin). While both types of fat impact health, visceral fat is especially dangerous due to its active release of inflammatory molecules. This inflammation is a core factor of metabolic syndrome, setting off a cycle of fat storage, insulin resistance, and metabolic imbalance.

Obesity is a central feature of metabolic syndrome and plays a key role in its progression due to its complex metabolic and hormonal impacts. Metabolic syndrome is characterized by a cluster of conditions that increase the risk of cardiovascular disease, type 2 diabetes, and other serious health issues. Excess body fat, particularly visceral fat around the organs, is strongly associated with insulin resistance—a primary driver of metabolic syndrome. Visceral fat is metabolically active, releasing inflammatory markers and hormones that disrupt normal metabolic processes, including blood sugar regulation and lipid metabolism.

One of the critical ways obesity influences metabolic syndrome is through the excessive release of free fatty acids and pro-inflammatory cytokines, which interfere with insulin's effectiveness. When cells become resistant to insulin, the pancreas compensates by producing more, leading to chronically high insulin levels. This insulin elevation keeps the body in "storage mode," contributing further to fat accumulation, especially in the abdominal area, which only reinforces the cycle of insulin resistance. Understanding this process will help you make better decisions as most people do not know this.

Dietary choices, particularly high carbohydrate and high sugar intake, exacerbate this cycle by continuously spiking insulin, leading to additional fat storage and inflammation. You may remember the advice of "Eat small meals throughout the day to keep your metabolism up". This process reinforces metabolic dysfunction, fueling not only insulin resistance but also high blood pressure, elevated triglycerides, and low HDL cholesterol, all markers of metabolic syndrome. Reducing obesity, particularly visceral fat, through lifestyle modifications like a lower carbohydrate diet, regular exercise, and stress management can improve insulin sensitivity and potentially reverse or mitigate the effects of metabolic syndrome. Addressing obesity is thus crucial for breaking the cycle of metabolic dysfunction and restoring metabolic health. Many disorders and disease stem from poor diet, or less than optimal diet. We should all take a closer look at the damage that everyday food has done and is doing to our bodies. Throughout this book, we will reflect on what is optimal and what is less than desirable for consumption. We need to understand the biochemical effects of food in the system. As you will see, everything is built from the foundation of our diet and how we choose what we eat.

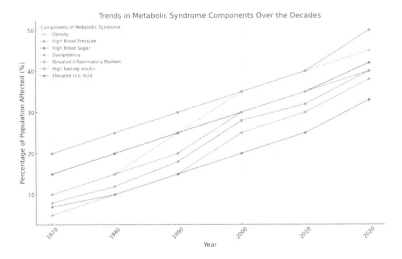

As you can clearly see, they are all on the same path in the same direction. Someone has to wake up and realize how these markers are all tied together, and concurrently causing a health crisis in the world. *Centers for Disease Control and Prevention (CDC)*

Insulin Resistance and Its Impact

Insulin is essential for transporting glucose from the bloodstream into cells for energy. However, with a high intake of refined carbohydrates and sugars, the body's cells can become desensitized to insulin—a state known as **insulin resistance**. The pancreas compensates by producing even more insulin to keep blood sugar levels steady. Over time, however, the pancreas struggles to maintain this balance, and blood glucose begins to rise. This state keeps the body in a constant "storage mode," which prevents the burning of fat for energy and leads to further fat accumulation, primarily around the abdomen.

Key contributors to insulin resistance include:

Refined Carbohydrates and Sugars: Diets high in sugars and refined carbohydrates cause frequent insulin spikes, which over time desensitizes the cells to insulin.

High Fructose Intake: Unlike glucose, which is metabolized throughout the body, fructose is metabolized almost exclusively by the liver. Excessive fructose intake leads to liver fat accumulation and worsens insulin resistance.

Obesity plays a central role in the development of insulin resistance, a condition that often goes undetected by conventional diagnostic methods until it has progressed to type 2 diabetes. Insulin resistance, driven by excess body fat (especially visceral fat) causes the body's cells to become less responsive to insulin. This desensitization forces the pancreas to produce even more insulin to regulate blood sugar levels, leading to consistently high insulin levels long before blood glucose begins to rise.

In standard medical practice, however, diabetes is typically diagnosed when fasting glucose or HbA1c levels become elevated, rather than through earlier indicators like fasting insulin. This approach often results in a delayed diagnosis. By the time blood glucose levels are high enough to indicate diabetes, many years of insulin resistance has already inflicted damage to blood vessels and organs. High insulin levels is the hallmark of metabolic syndrome and obesity, both of which can precede a diabetes diagnosis by years, if not decades. However, because insulin tests are not routinely conducted, these early warning signs are frequently missed.

Doctors tend to focus on glucose levels alone when assessing diabetes risk, which overlooks the upstream issue of insulin resistance caused by chronic obesity. Foods high in sugars and refined carbohydrates cause repetitive spikes in insulin, further worsening insulin resistance and prompting fat storage, particularly in the abdominal area. This cycle reinforces metabolic dysfunction, and without intervention, it may progress undetected until fasting glucose levels are high. Earlier use of fasting insulin tests, coupled with weight management and dietary modifications, could prevent this late-stage diagnosis by identifying and addressing insulin resistance sooner.

Hypertension: A Symptom, Not the Root Problem

Hypertension, while commonly discussed as an isolated condition, is closely intertwined with metabolic syndrome—a cluster of risk factors including high blood pressure, insulin resistance, elevated blood sugar, excess abdominal fat, and abnormal cholesterol levels. Together, these conditions paint a comprehensive picture of metabolic health, and each can exacerbate the effects of the others, creating a cycle of escalating health risks. Hypertension is not only a symptom of metabolic syndrome but also a contributing factor that influences and is influenced by the syndrome's other components.

Hypertension's Role in Metabolic Syndrome

Metabolic syndrome is recognized as a major risk factor for cardiovascular disease and diabetes, and hypertension is often one of the earliest indicators of this condition. Within the context of metabolic syndrome, hypertension does not develop in isolation; it arises in concert with other metabolic imbalances, particularly insulin resistance and chronic inflammation. When these factors exist together, they increase oxidative stress on the cardiovascular system and create conditions that make hypertension harder to control. Over time, this interconnectedness leads to cumulative damage to blood vessels and organs, amplifying the overall risk for heart disease, stroke, and other serious health issues.

Insulin Resistance and Blood Pressure

One of the core issues in metabolic syndrome is insulin resistance, a condition in which cells become less responsive to insulin, the hormone that helps regulate blood glucose levels. When cells resist insulin, the pancreas compensates by producing more, leading to high circulating insulin levels. Insulin plays a role in blood pressure regulation, as it influences sodium retention in the kidneys, which can cause fluid retention and, subsequently, elevate blood pressure. Chronic high insulin levels can, therefore, drive hypertension and contribute to the vascular damage that is typical in metabolic syndrome.

Furthermore, insulin resistance and high blood pressure together create a cycle where each condition exacerbates the other. Elevated blood pressure stresses the cardiovascular system, making it harder

26

for insulin to transport glucose efficiently. This continuous strain can worsen insulin resistance, leading to a harmful feedback loop that accelerates the progression of metabolic syndrome.

Chronic Inflammation as a Link

Another significant contributor to both hypertension and metabolic syndrome is chronic inflammation. In metabolic syndrome, excess fat tissue—especially around the abdomen—releases inflammatory molecules called cytokines. These molecules trigger a persistent low-level inflammatory response throughout the body, which, over time, can lead to arterial stiffness and reduced elasticity in blood vessels. When blood vessels lose flexibility, they become more resistant to blood flow, causing an increase in blood pressure. This vascular stiffness is one of the hallmarks of both metabolic syndrome and hypertension.

Chronic inflammation also damages the endothelium, the delicate lining of blood vessels, impairing its ability to produce nitric oxide, a molecule essential for blood vessel relaxation. Without sufficient nitric oxide, blood vessels remain constricted, further raising blood pressure. Thus, the inflammatory processes within metabolic syndrome directly feed into hypertension, creating conditions that favor its development and make management more challenging.

Abdominal Obesity and Its Impact on Blood Pressure

Central or abdominal obesity is a defining feature of metabolic syndrome and is closely associated with hypertension. Excess abdominal fat places direct pressure on organs, increases blood volume, and amplifies vascular resistance. Beyond these physical impacts, fat cells in abdominal tissue release substances that contribute to insulin resistance and inflammation, as well as hormones like leptin, which affect blood pressure regulation. This cascade of biochemical changes sets the stage for elevated blood pressure as part of the broader metabolic syndrome profile.

Moreover, abdominal fat also promotes the release of angiotensinogen, a precursor to a hormone called angiotensin II, which constricts blood vessels and raises blood pressure. In individuals with metabolic syndrome, this system is often overactive, leading to a state of chronic vasoconstriction and sustained high blood pressure. Thus, abdominal obesity not only contributes to hypertension but also perpetuates other components of metabolic syndrome.

Dyslipidemia and Vascular Health

Dyslipidemia, another key component of metabolic syndrome, refers to abnormal cholesterol levels, particularly elevated triglycerides and low HDL (high-density lipoprotein) cholesterol. This imbalance in blood lipids can further impair vascular health, making blood vessels more susceptible to damage and less efficient at regulating blood flow. Elevated triglycerides, for example, increase the risk of fatty deposits in blood vessels, which narrows the arteries and restricts blood flow. This buildup of plaque in the arteries, known as atherosclerosis, not only worsens hypertension but also raises the risk of cardiovascular events like heart attacks and strokes.

Low levels of HDL cholesterol compound these risks, as HDL is responsible for transporting cholesterol away from the arteries and back to the liver for excretion. When HDL levels are low, as is often the case in metabolic syndrome, the body has a diminished capacity to clear excess cholesterol, which contributes to arterial blockages and increases blood pressure. In this way, dyslipidemia and hypertension are closely linked within the framework of metabolic syndrome, each influencing and exacerbating the effects of the other.

Managing Hypertension in the Context of Metabolic Syndrome

Given the interconnected nature of hypertension and metabolic syndrome, effective management requires a holistic approach that addresses all contributing factors simultaneously. Here are some key strategies for managing hypertension within the context of metabolic syndrome:

Anti-Inflammatory, Nutrient-Rich Diet: To address obesity and insulin resistance, it is essential to adopt a diet that limits processed foods, refined sugars, and unhealthy fats. Instead, prioritize whole, nutrient-dense foods that are rich in vitamins, minerals, and antioxidants. Nutrients like magnesium, potassium, and fiber are key to supporting metabolic health and regulating blood pressure. The Mediterranean-style diet, which emphasizes high-quality proteins, healthy fats (such as olive oil and nuts), whole grains, and a wide array of colorful fruits and vegetables, has been shown to significantly improve insulin sensitivity, reduce inflammation, and promote long-term weight management. While this approach is sustainable for many and offers numerous health benefits, it differs from my initial recommendation of a carnivore diet, which focuses on animal products. Each approach has its merits, depending on individual preferences and health goals. For those seeking a more plant-inclusive, balanced approach, the Mediterranean diet offers a well-rounded and nourishing way to improve metabolic function and overall health.

Regular Physical Activity: Exercise is a powerful tool for combating both hypertension and insulin resistance. Engaging in regular aerobic exercise, resistance training, and flexibility exercises can help lower blood pressure, enhance insulin sensitivity, and aid in weight management. Exercise also helps improve lipid profiles, increase HDL cholesterol, and reduce abdominal fat, addressing multiple aspects of metabolic syndrome.

Weight Management: Maintaining a healthy weight, particularly by reducing abdominal fat, is one of the most effective ways to manage hypertension within the context of metabolic syndrome. Even a modest reduction in weight can lead to significant improvements in blood pressure, insulin sensitivity, and lipid levels.

Stress Reduction and Sleep: Chronic stress and poor sleep quality are both associated with increased blood pressure and worsened metabolic outcomes. Practices such as mindfulness, deep breathing exercises, and regular sleep patterns can help manage stress, supporting both blood pressure and metabolic health.

Natural Supplements and Medications: Certain supplements, such as omega-3 fatty acids, CoQ10, magnesium, and potassium, have shown promise in supporting cardiovascular health and reducing blood pressure. For some individuals, medications may also be necessary, especially when lifestyle modifications alone are insufficient. However, medications should be used as part of a comprehensive management plan, not as a standalone solution.

Reframing the Importance of Metabolic Health

Understanding the relationship between hypertension and metabolic syndrome underscores the importance of addressing metabolic health as a whole rather than targeting blood pressure in isolation. While lowering blood pressure is essential for reducing immediate cardiovascular risks, focusing on comprehensive metabolic health can yield long-term improvements that not only help regulate blood pressure but also address the root causes of insulin resistance, inflammation, and dyslipidemia.

Moreover, taking a holistic approach to hypertension and metabolic syndrome reframes the importance of dietary and lifestyle changes. Rather than viewing these modifications as temporary solutions, they become sustainable strategies for achieving lasting metabolic health. This approach also challenges the misconception that hypertension is inevitable with age or genetics alone; instead, it shows that lifestyle and dietary factors play a significant role in preventing and managing both hypertension and metabolic syndrome.

In conclusion, hypertension is a critical component of metabolic syndrome, and managing it requires a nuanced understanding of how various factors—insulin resistance, inflammation, abdominal obesity, and dyslipidemia—interact to drive health risks. By addressing these factors together, individuals can more effectively control blood pressure, reduce cardiovascular risk, and enhance overall metabolic health. This holistic strategy, rather than a narrow focus on isolated blood pressure management, is essential in today's context of rising rates of metabolic disorders and chronic diseases.

Insulin Resistance as a Driver of Hypertension

Insulin resistance disrupts blood pressure regulation by impairing the body's ability to process glucose. Higher insulin levels signal the kidneys to retain sodium, which increases blood volume and pressure on blood vessel walls. Studies show that about 50% of individuals with hypertension also experience insulin resistance, supporting the concept that high blood pressure often reflects metabolic dysfunction rather than an independent disease.

Chronic Inflammation's Role in Hypertension

Chronic inflammation, often driven by poor diet, stress, and lifestyle, also contributes to high blood pressure. Inflammatory molecules can cause blood vessels to stiffen, restricting blood flow and increasing pressure. Inflammation can also impair endothelial function, reducing the production of nitric oxide, a molecule essential for blood vessel relaxation. A decrease in nitric oxide leads to more rigid blood vessels, further contributing to hypertension. Diet, stress management, and regular physical activity help reduce inflammation, which, in turn, can lower blood pressure.

Inflammation's Role in Metabolic Syndrome: A Focused Analysis

Chronic inflammation has emerged as a significant factor in the development and progression of metabolic syndrome (MetS). It not only contributes to insulin resistance, dyslipidemia, and hypertension but also interacts with elevated uric acid levels to exacerbate metabolic dysfunction. Understanding how inflammation operates at a cellular and molecular level provides insights into potential therapeutic targets for managing MetS.

The Inflammatory Process

Inflammation is a complex biological response of the immune system to harmful stimuli, such as pathogens or tissue injury. It involves the activation of immune cells, the release of inflammatory mediators, and changes in blood flow. Chronic inflammation, characterized by the persistent presence of pro-inflammatory cytokines, can lead to tissue damage and metabolic disturbances.

Key Inflammatory Mediators

Cytokines:

Tumor Necrosis Factor-alpha (TNF-α): A major pro-inflammatory cytokine produced by adipose tissue, TNF-α impairs insulin signaling by promoting serine phosphorylation of insulin receptor substrates, contributing to insulin resistance.

Interleukin-6 (IL-6): Elevated levels of IL-6 are associated with obesity and metabolic syndrome. IL-6 promotes inflammation and has been implicated in insulin resistance and dyslipidemia.

C-Reactive Protein (CRP): CRP is a marker of systemic inflammation and is often elevated in individuals with MetS. High CRP levels correlate with an increased risk of cardiovascular disease.

Adipokines:

Adipose tissue secretes various adipokines, including leptin and resistin. While leptin plays a role in regulating energy balance, high levels of leptin in the context of obesity can promote inflammation. Resistin is also associated with insulin resistance and inflammation, contributing to the metabolic abnormalities seen in MetS.

Chemokines:

Chemokines such as monocyte chemoattractant protein-1 (MCP-1) facilitate the recruitment of immune cells to sites of inflammation, including adipose tissue. This recruitment perpetuates the inflammatory response and exacerbates metabolic dysfunction.

Inflammation and Insulin Resistance

Insulin resistance is a core component of metabolic syndrome, and chronic inflammation is a significant contributor to its development.

Mechanisms of Insulin Resistance Induced by Inflammation

Impaired Insulin Signaling:

Inflammatory cytokines, particularly TNF-α and IL-6, can disrupt insulin signaling pathways. This disruption occurs through the activation of inflammatory pathways that lead to serine phosphorylation of IRS proteins, inhibiting their ability to propagate the insulin signal. Consequently, this impairs glucose uptake in skeletal muscle and adipose tissue.

Role of Macrophages in Adipose Tissue:

In obesity, the infiltration of macrophages into adipose tissue leads to a state of chronic inflammation. These macrophages release pro-inflammatory cytokines, creating an inflammatory microenvironment that further exacerbates insulin resistance. The ratio of M1 (pro-inflammatory) to M2 (anti-inflammatory) macrophages is crucial; a higher ratio favors a pro-inflammatory state, contributing to systemic insulin resistance.

Endoplasmic Reticulum (ER) Stress:

Chronic inflammation can lead to ER stress in insulin-sensitive tissues, further impairing insulin signaling. This stress results in the accumulation of misfolded proteins and activates inflammatory pathways, which collectively contribute to insulin resistance.

Inflammation and Dyslipidemia

Dyslipidemia, characterized by elevated triglycerides and low HDL cholesterol levels, is another key component of metabolic syndrome, and inflammation plays a critical role in its development.

Impact of Inflammation on Lipid Metabolism

Altered Hepatic Lipid Production:

Inflammatory cytokines such as TNF-α can affect hepatic lipid metabolism by increasing triglyceride production and reducing the clearance of VLDL. This dysregulation leads to hypertriglyceridemia, a common feature of metabolic syndrome.

Oxidation of Lipoproteins:

Chronic inflammation is associated with increased oxidative stress, which can modify LDL particles, rendering them more atherogenic. Oxidized LDL (oxLDL) promotes endothelial dysfunction and inflammation, creating a cycle that exacerbates cardiovascular risk.

Adipose Tissue and Lipid Mobilization:

Inflammation can affect the secretion of adipokines that regulate lipid metabolism. For instance, increased levels of resistin can promote lipolysis, releasing free fatty acids into the circulation, further contributing to dyslipidemia and insulin resistance.

Inflammation and Hypertension

Hypertension is another critical aspect of metabolic syndrome that is influenced by inflammation.

Mechanisms Linking Inflammation and Hypertension

Endothelial Dysfunction:

Chronic inflammation leads to endothelial dysfunction, characterized by decreased nitric oxide (NO) availability and increased production of vasoconstrictors. Pro-inflammatory cytokines can enhance the expression of adhesion molecules on endothelial cells, facilitating leukocyte adhesion and vascular inflammation.

Sympathetic Nervous System Activation:

Inflammatory mediators can activate the sympathetic nervous system, leading to increased heart rate and peripheral vascular resistance. This sympathetic activation contributes to the development of hypertension and enhances cardiovascular risk.

Renin-Angiotensin System (RAS):

Inflammation can stimulate the renin-angiotensin system, leading to increased production of angiotensin II, a potent vasoconstrictor. Elevated angiotensin II levels not only increase blood pressure but also promote inflammation and endothelial dysfunction, creating a feedback loop that exacerbates hypertension.

The Role of Uric Acid in Inflammation and Metabolic Syndrome

Uric acid, a byproduct of purine metabolism, has garnered attention for its role in metabolic syndrome, particularly concerning its inflammatory properties.

Mechanisms of Uric Acid-Induced Inflammation

NLRP3 Inflammasome Activation:

Elevated uric acid levels can activate the NLRP3 inflammasome, leading to the release of pro-inflammatory cytokines such as IL-1β. This activation contributes to systemic inflammation and has been linked to insulin resistance and other components of metabolic syndrome.

Link to Insulin Resistance:

High uric acid levels have been associated with decreased insulin sensitivity. The inflammatory response triggered by uric acid may interfere with insulin signaling pathways, further contributing to metabolic dysfunction.

Impact on Vascular Health:

Uric acid can promote endothelial dysfunction, leading to increased blood pressure and cardiovascular risk. The inflammatory response associated with elevated uric acid can exacerbate existing hypertension and contribute to the development of atherosclerosis.

Clinical Implications

Understanding the role of inflammation in metabolic syndrome has significant clinical implications for screening, prevention, and treatment strategies.

1. Screening for Inflammation

Incorporating inflammatory markers into the assessment of metabolic syndrome can enhance screening and diagnostic strategies. Measuring biomarkers such as CRP, IL-6, and uric acid levels can help identify individuals at higher risk for metabolic syndrome and related health issues.

2. Lifestyle Interventions

Effective management of metabolic syndrome requires a multifaceted approach, including lifestyle modifications aimed at reducing inflammation.

Dietary Interventions: Implementing an anti-inflammatory diet rich in whole foods, including fruits, vegetables, whole grains, and healthy fats, can help lower inflammatory markers and improve metabolic health. Foods high in antioxidants, omega-3 fatty acids, and polyphenols can be particularly beneficial.

Physical Activity: Regular exercise has been shown to have anti-inflammatory effects. Engaging in physical activity improves insulin sensitivity, reduces visceral fat, and lowers systemic inflammation. Aim for at least 150 minutes of moderate-intensity exercise per week.

Weight Management: Reducing body weight, especially visceral fat, can significantly decrease inflammation levels and improve metabolic health. Even modest weight loss can lead to substantial improvements in inflammatory markers and metabolic parameters.

3. Pharmacological Approaches

Targeting inflammation pharmacologically may offer new treatment strategies for metabolic syndrome.

Anti-inflammatory Medications: Research is ongoing regarding the use of anti-inflammatory agents to improve metabolic health. Medications that target inflammation may hold promise for managing insulin resistance and other components of metabolic syndrome.

Uric Acid Lowering Agents: Medications such as allopurinol, which lower uric acid levels, may also have beneficial effects on inflammation and metabolic health. Reducing uric acid may improve insulin sensitivity and decrease the risk of cardiovascular complications.

Future Directions and Research

Further exploration of the relationship between inflammation, elevated insulin, and uric acid in metabolic syndrome is warranted. Key areas for future research include:

Biomarker Development: Identifying reliable biomarkers of inflammation and metabolic dysfunction can help predict the risk of developing metabolic syndrome and guide therapeutic interventions.

Mechanistic Studies: Investigating the specific mechanisms by which inflammation contributes to each component of metabolic syndrome can lead to targeted therapies that address the root causes of the syndrome.

Longitudinal Studies: Long-term studies examining the impact of lifestyle interventions on inflammation, insulin sensitivity, and uric acid levels will provide valuable insights into effective prevention and management strategies.

Inflammation plays a central role in the pathophysiology of metabolic syndrome, influencing insulin resistance, dyslipidemia, hypertension, and elevated uric acid levels. Chronic low-grade inflammation is a hallmark of this syndrome, posing significant health risks, including cardiovascular disease and type 2 diabetes. Addressing inflammation through lifestyle modifications and potential pharmacological interventions can significantly improve metabolic health outcomes. As our understanding of the intricate relationship between inflammation and metabolic syndrome continues to evolve, it holds promise for developing more effective prevention and treatment strategies that enhance overall health and well-being.

The Role of the Sympathetic Nervous System and Stress

Chronic stress plays a significant role in hypertension. When stress is prolonged, stress hormones like cortisol and adrenaline are continuously released, constricting blood vessels and increasing heart rate. Effective stress management—through practices like meditation, exercise, or mindfulness—can help regulate blood pressure naturally, targeting underlying causes rather than symptoms alone.

Reevaluating Sodium's Role in Hypertension

While sodium is often blamed for high blood pressure, recent research suggests a more nuanced role. Sodium sensitivity varies among individuals; for those with metabolic dysfunction, high sodium intake can worsen hypertension, but in metabolically healthy individuals, sodium intake might not have as profound an impact. Instead, insulin resistance and metabolic imbalances are more critical contributors to hypertension than sodium alone.

Addressing Hypertension Holistically

Managing hypertension effectively involves looking beyond blood pressure readings to address the underlying causes of metabolic dysfunction. Lifestyle changes—including a nutrient-dense, low-carb diet, regular exercise, and quality sleep—can naturally reduce blood pressure, often reducing the need for medication.

Blood Sugar Dysregulation: Fasting Glucose and Hemoglobin A1c

Fasting glucose and A1c levels are essential indicators of metabolic health, reflecting the body's ability to regulate blood sugar. Elevated levels signify insulin resistance and chronic high blood sugar, which damages blood vessels and increases the risk of cardiovascular disease. High blood glucose levels produce **Advanced Glycation End-products (AGEs)** that lead to oxidative stress, tissue damage, and contribute to metabolic syndrome.

Triglycerides and Their Role in Metabolic Syndrome

Elevated triglycerides often accompany metabolic syndrome and indicate poor fat and carbohydrate metabolism. Triglycerides serve as an energy source, but when levels are elevated, they signal that the body is struggling to process fat and sugar effectively.

Biochemistry of Triglycerides: Triglycerides are composed of three fatty acids attached to a glycerol molecule and are stored in adipose tissue. High triglycerides, particularly when stored as VLDL particles, contribute to plaque buildup and increase cardiovascular disease risk.

Pathophysiological Effects of High Triglycerides

Atherosclerosis: Elevated triglycerides promote plaque formation within arteries, restricting blood flow.

Low HDL and High Triglycerides: This imbalance disrupts HDL's role in clearing cholesterol, exacerbating plaque buildup.

The TG-to-HDL Ratio and Metabolic Health

The TG-to-HDL ratio provides an effective measure of metabolic and cardiovascular health. A high ratio often suggests insulin resistance, inflammation, and increased cardiovascular risk. Ideal ratios are under 2.0, with higher ratios indicating compromised metabolic health and a need for dietary changes.

What the TG-to-HDL Ratio Reveals About Health A high TG-to-HDL ratio often suggests poor lipid metabolism and insulin resistance. Triglycerides represent the body's stored energy, while HDL helps clear cholesterol from the bloodstream. When triglyceride levels are high and HDL levels are low, this balance indicates excessive fat storage and metabolic dysfunction.

Improving the TG-to-HDL Ratio

Improving the TG-to-HDL ratio can be achieved through:

Dietary Changes: Reducing refined carbs and sugars can lower triglycerides.

Exercise: Physical activity, particularly aerobic and strength training, improves insulin sensitivity and lipid levels.

Uric Acid: A New Player in Metabolic Health

Uric acid, often villainized as a sole contributor to gout, is more complex than it seems. This naturally occurring compound in our body has evolved for crucial purposes and is, in fact, a potent antioxidant and anti-inflammatory agent in moderate amounts. Within controlled levels, uric acid plays a protective role, neutralizing oxidative stress and potentially contributing to the body's defense against chronic inflammation. When metabolic health is intact, the body maintains uric acid within these safe, beneficial ranges. The problem, however, arises when the systems responsible for regulating uric acid fall out of balance, as seen in metabolic syndrome.

The Link Between Metabolic Syndrome and Gout

Gout, often characterized by painful joint inflammation, isn't solely a result of elevated uric acid; rather, it's frequently a downstream effect of larger metabolic issues. Metabolic syndrome, defined by markers like abdominal obesity, insulin resistance, hypertension, and dyslipidemia, interferes with the body's ability to excrete uric acid efficiently. The body's decreased capacity to process uric acid under these conditions leads to its build-up, creating an environment ripe for gout.

Inflammation's Role in Disrupting Uric Acid Expulsion

Chronic inflammation, a key component of metabolic syndrome, hampers the body's ability to process and eliminate uric acid. The kidneys, responsible for the majority of uric acid excretion, become less efficient under conditions of inflammation and insulin resistance. When inflammation is high, cellular functions suffer, including the renal processes that manage uric acid levels. Additionally, insulin resistance, common in metabolic syndrome, can directly impede uric acid clearance by the kidneys, further raising levels and increasing gout risk.

Studies show that reducing inflammation and addressing insulin sensitivity may improve the body's ability to handle uric acid. By lowering systemic inflammation, individuals may see improved renal excretion of uric acid, resulting in fewer gout flare-ups. This brings to light that addressing inflammation and other markers of metabolic syndrome, rather than solely targeting uric acid, may be a more comprehensive approach to managing gout.

Uric Acid as an Anti-Inflammatory Agent

Interestingly, uric acid itself has anti-inflammatory properties. In controlled amounts, uric acid acts as an antioxidant, helping to neutralize free radicals and prevent cellular damage. This function is especially relevant in the brain and immune system, where oxidative stress can trigger inflammatory responses. When kept within the right parameters, uric acid's natural antioxidant abilities can be a valuable asset to the body's inflammatory regulation. The irony is that, while uric acid is involved in gout, it's also part of the body's defense mechanism against excessive inflammation.

However, like many other substances in the body, the key lies in moderation. Excessive uric acid, often due to disrupted metabolic pathways, can crystallize and cause the painful symptoms associated with gout. Herein lies the balance: rather than focusing solely on lowering uric acid, it's crucial to focus on restoring balance within the body's inflammatory and metabolic processes.

Parameters for Healthy Uric Acid Levels

In a healthy body, uric acid remains within a range that supports its beneficial roles without causing harm. It's important to understand that endogenous uric acid production—the production our bodies naturally regulate—should be the primary focus, rather than exogenous sources from foods high in purines.

In a metabolically healthy individual, consuming moderate amounts of purine-rich foods, such as certain meats and seafood, typically doesn't elevate uric acid levels to the point of causing gout. It's only when metabolic syndrome factors are present that the body's capacity to handle exogenous purines may falter. By prioritizing metabolic health, including inflammation management, insulin sensitivity, and kidney function, the body can better regulate uric acid, minimizing the risk of gout without needing extreme dietary restrictions on purines.

Exogenous Purines and Their Impact When Metabolic Markers Are Balanced

When the metabolic markers are in a healthy range, exogenous purines (those from food sources) are generally not problematic. Many individuals with a balanced metabolism can consume foods traditionally high in purines, such as organ meats and certain fish, without experiencing gout flare-ups. This is because a healthy metabolic system can manage purines efficiently, ensuring they don't lead to excessive uric acid accumulation.

However, in individuals with metabolic dysfunction, even normal amounts of dietary purines may exacerbate uric acid build-up. This highlights the need to address the root causes of metabolic syndrome, particularly chronic inflammation, so that the body can resume its natural regulation of uric acid, allowing individuals to enjoy a diverse diet without the heightened risk of gout.

A Comprehensive Approach to Curbing Gout Through Metabolic Health

Addressing gout isn't solely a matter of reducing uric acid; it's about restoring metabolic balance. By prioritizing anti-inflammatory practices—such as a diet low in processed sugars and high in nutrient-dense whole foods—alongside managing insulin sensitivity and improving kidney health, individuals can naturally curb gout symptoms. This comprehensive approach not only helps prevent gout but also improves overall metabolic health, which benefits a range of conditions beyond gout itself.

In summary, gout may often be a symptom of deeper metabolic imbalances rather than an isolated issue of high uric acid. By shifting the focus to treating inflammation and improving metabolic health, we can allow the body to regulate uric acid naturally, reducing the frequency and severity of gout flare-ups without resorting to restrictive diets or medication alone.

Fasting Insulin: An Early Indicator of Metabolic Syndrome

The ACTUAL way we should be diagnosing "diabetes". In my opinion, high insulin levels should be the focus initially, whereas insulin resistance, leading to excess serum glucose, is the real villain. Once we all figure this out, including your trusted doctors and dietitians, we will get a better hold on this. The reason diabetes is in quotes, is because I feel "insulin resistance" is the better suited reference to this condition.

Fasting insulin levels are one of the earliest indicators of metabolic dysfunction. High fasting insulin levels signal insulin resistance, often years before blood sugar rises. Despite its predictive power, fasting insulin is rarely tested in routine exams. Elevated fasting insulin is a primary driver of fat storage, making it an essential measure in assessing metabolic health.

Why Fasting Insulin is Overlooked

Fasting insulin is underutilized due to historical guidelines that focus on glucose and HbA1c levels for diagnosing diabetes. Insulin resistance, however, remains an underlying cause of metabolic syndrome, with high fasting insulin levels often indicating insulin resistance long before blood sugar levels rise.

Recommended Guidelines for Fasting Insulin An ideal fasting insulin level is generally below 10 µU/mL, with optimal levels around 2-5 µU/mL. Levels above 10 µU/mL indicate insulin resistance and metabolic dysfunction. Testing fasting insulin allows for earlier detection and intervention.

How Fasting Insulin Impacts Fat Storage Insulin acts as a "fat-storage hormone," promoting lipogenesis, or fat storage in adipose tissue. High insulin levels prevent the body from burning stored fat for energy.

Fasting insulin is emerging as one of the most valuable indicators in understanding metabolic syndrome. Often overlooked in traditional assessments, fasting insulin levels can reveal insulin resistance well before blood glucose levels rise. Metabolic syndrome—a cluster of conditions including high blood pressure, abdominal obesity, high triglycerides, low HDL cholesterol, and high fasting glucose—is driven largely by insulin resistance. This chapter examines the role of fasting insulin in the development of metabolic syndrome, its connection to the foods we eat, and how managing insulin levels can prevent or even reverse many metabolic issues.

The Role of Insulin in Metabolic Syndrome

Insulin is a hormone produced by the pancreas, primarily responsible for regulating blood glucose levels. After eating, the body breaks down carbohydrates into glucose, which enters the bloodstream. Insulin acts like a key, allowing glucose to enter cells for immediate energy use or storage as glycogen in the liver and muscles. When glucose stores are full, insulin directs the body to store excess energy as fat.

For individuals with insulin resistance—a core component of metabolic syndrome—cells become less responsive to insulin's effects. This reduced sensitivity forces the pancreas to release more insulin to maintain normal blood glucose levels, leading to elevated fasting insulin. Over time, chronically high insulin levels contribute to weight gain, particularly around the abdomen, as insulin promotes fat storage. This increase in visceral fat (fat around the organs) is particularly harmful because it is metabolically active, releasing inflammatory compounds that exacerbate insulin resistance, blood pressure, and other metabolic dysfunctions.

Foods That Spike Insulin and Drive Insulin Resistance

The foods we eat have a profound impact on insulin levels. Carbohydrates, particularly refined sugars and starches, cause a rapid increase in blood glucose, prompting the pancreas to release insulin. Repeated consumption of high-carbohydrate foods keeps insulin levels elevated, eventually overwhelming cells and fostering insulin resistance. Key dietary contributors to high insulin levels include:

Refined Carbohydrates: Foods like white bread, pasta, pastries, and sweets break down quickly into glucose, causing an insulin spike. Frequent intake of these foods leads to repeated insulin releases, which over time contribute to insulin resistance.

Sugary Beverages and Fructose: Fructose, a type of sugar found in many processed foods and drinks, is metabolized primarily in the liver. Excess fructose consumption leads to liver fat accumulation, which disrupts insulin signaling and increases insulin resistance. Unlike glucose, fructose does not cause a direct spike in blood glucose but still promotes insulin resistance through its effects on liver metabolism.

Processed Foods: Many processed foods are high in both refined carbs and unhealthy fats, which exacerbate insulin resistance and metabolic syndrome. These foods provide little nutritional value and promote inflammation, which interferes with insulin signaling.

Frequent Snacking: Eating multiple times throughout the day keeps insulin levels elevated. The body has little chance to enter a low-insulin state where it can switch to fat burning, leading to continuous fat storage and contributing to obesity and insulin resistance.

Lowering Insulin: The Key to Addressing Metabolic Syndrome

By focusing on managing insulin levels, many metabolic issues linked to insulin resistance can be addressed or even reversed. Here are some effective strategies to lower fasting insulin levels and improve metabolic health:

Low-Carbohydrate Diets: Reducing carbohydrate intake helps keep insulin levels in check. Low-carb diets, especially those with a focus on whole foods, limit glucose spikes and allow insulin levels to drop. As insulin lowers, the body shifts from glucose to fat as its primary energy source, promoting fat burning and weight loss, particularly in visceral fat stores.

Intermittent Fasting: Intermittent fasting (IF) involves periods of eating and fasting, allowing insulin levels to drop and giving the body time to improve insulin sensitivity. When fasting, insulin decreases, which enables the body to access stored fat for energy. Studies have shown that IF can improve insulin sensitivity, lower fasting insulin levels, and reduce weight, particularly in people with insulin resistance.

High-Fiber, Whole Foods: Foods high in fiber, such as vegetables, nuts, and seeds, slow the digestion and absorption of glucose, leading to a more gradual insulin response. This steady effect helps prevent the spikes in insulin seen with refined carbohydrates, reducing the risk of insulin resistance over time.

Physical Activity: Exercise, particularly resistance training and high-intensity interval training (HIIT), helps to increase insulin sensitivity by improving glucose uptake by muscles. Active muscles absorb glucose independently of insulin, lowering blood glucose and insulin levels post-exercise. Regular physical activity is one of the most effective ways to manage fasting insulin and improve overall metabolic health.

The Benefits of Lowering Insulin on Metabolic Health

Lowering insulin levels not only addresses insulin resistance but can also improve a host of other metabolic factors. By keeping insulin in check, the body can better regulate blood sugar, reduce visceral fat, lower blood pressure, and improve lipid profiles. Elevated insulin levels are associated with inflammation, so reducing insulin also has anti-inflammatory effects that benefit cardiovascular health and reduce the risk of chronic diseases such as Type 2 diabetes, heart disease, and certain cancers.

Additionally, low insulin states promote autophagy—a cellular cleaning process essential for removing damaged cells and reducing oxidative stress. This process is essential for long-term health and prevention of metabolic syndrome and its associated complications.

Challenges in Monitoring Insulin Levels

Despite the importance of fasting insulin as a marker for metabolic health, it is often overlooked in routine blood tests. The medical focus traditionally remains on blood glucose and HbA1c levels, which indicate advanced stages of metabolic dysfunction. Fasting insulin, however, is an early indicator, rising years before glucose dysregulation. Regular testing for fasting insulin could provide critical insights into metabolic health, allowing for earlier interventions and more effective prevention of metabolic syndrome.

Fasting insulin plays a crucial role in metabolic syndrome, providing insights into the body's long-term management of blood glucose and fat storage. By adopting a low-carbohydrate, nutrient-dense diet, engaging in intermittent fasting, and incorporating regular exercise, individuals can reduce fasting insulin levels and address the root causes of metabolic syndrome. These lifestyle changes not only improve insulin sensitivity but also promote a healthier metabolic state, reducing the risk of chronic diseases and enhancing overall well-being. Prioritizing fasting insulin as a key marker in health assessments can pave the way for a more proactive and effective approach to managing metabolic health.

Chapter 3: Diabetes (Insulin Resistance)–Understanding What it is and What Doctors Think

One thing we must "shift our paradigm" on is how we see diabetes. Diabetes is often referred to as "sugar disease," but its reach goes far beyond elevated blood glucose. It comprises three distinct types: Type 1, Type 2, and the emerging Type 3, which links **insulin resistance** to cognitive decline and conditions like Alzheimer's. This chapter seeks to examine the root causes, diagnostic flaws, and treatment issues associated with diabetes, particularly Type 2. Honestly, these "types" of diabetes should not be classified together, as they are completely different from one another. Type 1 is the pancreas inability to make any insulin, Type 2 is your body being overwhelmed with too much insulin and becoming resistant, and Type 3 is a fairly new addition and being related to sugar causing diseases such as dementia and Alzheimer's disease.

While high fasting glucose levels traditionally signal diabetes, they represent the culmination of a much longer process, often a decade or more of metabolic dysfunction. Recognizing Type 2 as an "insulin-first" disorder reveals an underlying issue with chronically elevated insulin levels rather than with glucose alone.

Type 2 Diabetes: Misdiagnosis and Root Causes

Type 2 diabetes, which accounts for 90-95% of cases, is fundamentally tied to insulin resistance. Each time carbohydrates are consumed; they elicit an insulin response. Continuous carbohydrate intake—particularly refined sugars and starches—leads to chronically high insulin levels, causing cells to become desensitized to insulin. To compensate, the pancreas produces even more insulin, resulting in a metabolic overload that ultimately impairs the pancreas and spikes blood glucose levels.

The Misguided Approach to Diabetes Management

Type 2 diabetes is fundamentally characterized by insulin resistance, where the body's cells do not respond effectively to insulin. In the early stages of the disease, the pancreas compensates by producing more insulin to overcome this resistance and keep blood sugar levels stable. However, as the condition progresses, the body can no longer keep up, leading to elevated blood glucose levels.

Why Adding More Insulin is Problematic

When treatment involves administering more insulin to manage blood glucose levels, it addresses the symptom (high blood sugar) but not the root cause (insulin resistance). Over time, this can exacerbate the underlying problem:

Increased Insulin Resistance: The more insulin that is introduced, the more resistant the insulin receptors on cells can become. This creates a cycle where progressively higher doses of insulin are needed to achieve the same blood sugar-lowering effect.

Worsening Metabolic Health: Excess insulin can lead to weight gain, particularly in the abdominal area, which can further increase insulin resistance and inflammation.

Masking the Problem: Treating diabetes with high doses of insulin without addressing lifestyle factors and underlying metabolic dysfunction ignores critical aspects of health management, such as diet, physical activity, and stress management.

The Importance of Addressing the Root Cause

To effectively manage and potentially reverse type 2 diabetes, it's essential to reduce insulin resistance, not just blood glucose levels. This can often be achieved through:

Dietary Changes: Low-carbohydrate and nutrient-dense diets can help lower the body's need for insulin and improve insulin sensitivity.

Physical Activity: Regular exercise helps muscles use glucose more effectively and increases insulin sensitivity.

Weight Management: Losing excess weight can reduce the fat accumulation around organs, improving insulin response.

Resistance Training: Resistance training will help the muscles be much more efficient at getting rid of the glucose in your bloodstream

Reducing Chronic Inflammation: Addressing underlying inflammation helps the body's cells respond better to insulin.

Re-Evaluating Standard Medical Practice

While insulin therapy is sometimes necessary, especially for those with type 1 diabetes or late-stage type 2 diabetes, starting insulin treatment too early or relying solely on insulin for type 2 diabetes management can lead to long-term complications. Effective treatment strategies should aim at improving insulin sensitivity through lifestyle modifications and potentially other medications that target insulin resistance directly.

Key Insight on Insulin-First Focus

Diagnosing diabetes based solely on fasting glucose or A1c measurements captures high blood sugar only at the later stages. This is akin to identifying a car rim issue by examining the tire's puncture—by the time glucose is high, significant metabolic dysfunction has already damaged various organs and systems. Elevated fasting insulin, on the other hand, serves as a proactive marker, identifying insulin resistance earlier and allowing interventions that could prevent full-blown diabetes.

Pathophysiology of Type 2 Diabetes: The Breakdown from Insulin Resistance to Hyperglycemia

Initial Insulin Response
When glucose levels rise post-meal, the pancreas releases insulin to direct glucose into cells for energy or storage. In balanced systems, this process stabilizes blood sugar efficiently.

Onset of Insulin Resistance
Repeated consumption of carbohydrates and continuous insulin production desensitize cells. The body compensates by producing more insulin to manage glucose, but cells progressively "resist" it.

Metabolic Overload and Fat Storage
With insulin resistance, excess glucose converts to fat, accumulating primarily as visceral fat. This type of fat is metabolically active, driving inflammation and worsening insulin resistance.

Pancreatic Beta Cell Exhaustion

The pancreas becomes overtaxed as it struggles to produce insulin. Beta cells begin to lose function, marking the transition to full Type 2 diabetes, often observed with elevated fasting glucose and A1c.

Chronic Hyperglycemia and Organ Damage

Persistent high glucose results in protein glycation, forming advanced glycation end-products (AGEs). AGEs drive oxidative stress and inflammation, leading to cardiovascular disease, neuropathy, retinopathy, and kidney damage.

Differentiating Type 1 from Type 2

Type 1 Diabetes – An autoimmune condition, where immune cells attack pancreatic beta cells, leaving the body without insulin. It is often diagnosed in youth, requiring insulin therapy for survival, unlike Type 2, which stems from lifestyle factors and is often reversible with intervention.

Type 2 Diabetes – Primarily lifestyle-related and often resulting from carbohydrate-rich diets, inactivity, and genetic predisposition. While many can reverse Type 2 diabetes with dietary and lifestyle changes, advanced cases require medical intervention.

Type 3 Diabetes: Brain Health and the Impact of Carbohydrates

Type 3 diabetes, also known as "brain diabetes," underscores the link between insulin resistance and neurodegenerative diseases, particularly Alzheimer's. The brain's unique reliance on glucose and insulin for energy and cellular signaling means that insulin resistance impacts neurons directly. Chronic high-sugar diets can drive brain insulin resistance, impairing cells' access to glucose and impairing cognitive functions. Amyloid plaques and neurofibrillary tangles, associated with Alzheimer's, are worsened by this insulin resistance.

Dietary and lifestyle changes focused on reducing sugar and refined carbs can improve brain insulin sensitivity, potentially slowing cognitive decline and preserving brain function.

The Diabetes Epidemic: Alarming Statistics

In the U.S. – Over 98 million people have Type 2 diabetes, and understand that there really is no difference between diabetes and prediabetes because if your fasting glucose levels are elevated, there is already a problem. This epidemic contributes to kidney failure, blindness, amputations, and other severe complications, costing the U.S. healthcare system over $327 billion annually.

Globally – Diabetes affects over 530 million adults, a number expected to rise to 643 million by 2030. These statistics highlight the urgent need for preventive measures focusing on metabolic health.

Number and Percentage of U.S. Population with Diagnosed Diabetes, 1958-2015

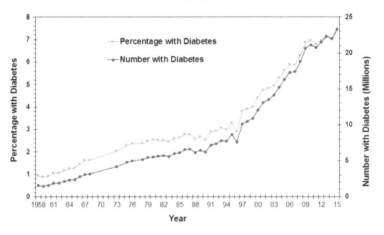

Diagnostic Shortcomings: Why Glucose-Only Testing Misses the Mark

Using glucose levels alone to diagnose diabetes captures only a fraction of metabolic dysfunction. Elevated fasting glucose signals diabetes late in the process. Testing for fasting insulin, however, identifies insulin resistance much earlier, potentially preventing years of silent damage.

Prescription Pitfalls and Dietary Misdirection

Medication Limitations
Many patients are prescribed metformin or insulin for Type 2 diabetes. While these medications can control blood glucose, they often fail to address the root problem of insulin resistance. Statins may also be prescribed but may have extremely limited benefit without addressing dietary and lifestyle factors.

Low-Fat, High-Carb Dietary Misguidance
Common guidelines suggest low-fat, high-carb diets, which exacerbate insulin resistance by increasing the demand for insulin. This dietary pattern keeps patients locked in a cycle of blood sugar spikes and cravings, often making diabetes worse.

Misplaced Focus on Cholesterol and Saturated Fat
The emphasis on lowering cholesterol and avoiding saturated fats overlooks the real problem—refined carbs and sugars. Low-fat diets often inadvertently increase carb consumption, which increases insulin spikes and insulin resistance.

A Root-Cause Approach
Targeting insulin resistance through dietary and lifestyle modifications is essential for managing diabetes. Whole-food, low-carb diets and the inclusion of natural fats promote better insulin sensitivity and metabolic stability.

Turning the System Right-Side Up: A Proactive Framework

Health professionals should shift from treating symptoms to root-cause interventions. This means advocating for dietary recommendations that prioritize metabolic health, reduce reliance on glucose, and stabilize insulin.

Dietary Guidelines for Type 2 Diabetes Management

High-Quality Protein: Opt for nutrient-dense sources like beef, poultry, fish, and eggs. These proteins offer satiety without spiking insulin.

Healthy Fats: Use natural fats—olive oil, butter, ghee, and animal fats. These provide energy and satiety without raising insulin levels.

Low-Carb Vegetables: Leafy greens and cruciferous vegetables offer fiber and micronutrients, supporting metabolic health without raising blood glucose.

Limit Carbohydrates: Avoid refined sugars and carbs, including "healthy" grains. For those including fruits, stick to low-carb options like berries in moderation.

Intermittent Fasting: Allow insulin levels to reset by introducing intermittent fasting, which can improve insulin sensitivity and promote metabolic balance.

Prolonged Fasting: If you can get up to this level, it can do wonders for rebooting your body and immune system. Don't try this without supervision from a *knowledgeable* healthcare provider.

This approach minimizes the need for medications, addressing the root cause and helping individuals restore metabolic health. Further personalization in an individualized diet section will provide guidelines for tailoring diets to unique DNA, genetics, and tolerances, noting that most people may benefit from reducing or eliminating carbohydrates altogether.

Continuous Glucose Monitors (CGMs): A Tool for Real-Time Diabetes Management

A Continuous Glucose Monitor (CGM) is a device that tracks blood glucose levels in real-time, allowing users to see fluctuations throughout the day and night. Unlike traditional glucose meters, which provide a single glucose snapshot, CGMs use a small sensor under the skin to measure glucose every few minutes. This frequent tracking helps identify patterns and responses to various foods, exercise, sleep, and stress, making CGMs especially valuable for those with insulin resistance or Type 2 diabetes.

The Role of CGMs in Insulin Resistance and Metabolic Health

For those managing Type 2 diabetes or at risk of insulin resistance, CGMs offer a proactive way to understand blood glucose behavior. Here's how CGMs contribute:

Immediate Feedback
CGMs provide feedback on how specific foods impact glucose levels, making it easier to adjust dietary choices and avoid foods that spike glucose. This helps patients make real-time decisions to stabilize insulin levels.

Pattern Recognition
Over time, CGMs reveal trends and patterns, such as morning glucose spikes (the "dawn phenomenon") or post-meal blood sugar peaks. This data enables patients to make lifestyle changes based on personal metabolic responses.

Preventing Hypoglycemia and Hyperglycemia

CGMs alert users to dangerous lows or highs, enabling timely interventions to prevent prolonged blood sugar imbalances that can lead to long-term complications.

Improving Diet and Lifestyle Choices

By observing glucose responses to various foods, sleep quality, and exercise routines, patients can personalize their approaches. For instance, discovering that certain carbs or processed foods cause prolonged spikes can motivate a shift to low-carb, nutrient-dense foods.

Expanding Access and Usefulness

While CGMs are primarily used for Type 1 and Type 2 diabetes, they can benefit anyone aiming to monitor and stabilize glucose, such as those seeking to improve metabolic health. Regular CGM use can prevent diabetes by providing an early warning system for insulin resistance, allowing users to implement lifestyle changes long before glucose levels rise to diagnostic thresholds.

CGMs bring a level of self-awareness that empowers users to regain control over metabolic health by reducing reliance on one-time glucose measurements and focusing instead on comprehensive, dynamic glucose tracking.

Today's food environment plays a major role in the rising incidence of diabetes, particularly Type 2. Processed foods, refined carbohydrates, and added sugars dominate many diets and drive chronic blood sugar spikes and excessive insulin release. Foods high in fructose and refined grains contribute to insulin resistance by overwhelming the liver and leading to fat storage, particularly visceral fat. Additionally, the abundance of "low-fat" but high-carb foods has led to an over-reliance on carbohydrates for energy, which keeps insulin levels elevated and exacerbates metabolic dysfunction.

Frequent consumption of such foods promotes a cycle of cravings, further insulin spikes, and gradual development of insulin resistance. This dietary landscape increases the prevalence of metabolic syndrome, a precursor to Type 2 diabetes, and sets the stage for chronic health complications.

One thing that needs to change: doctors STILL commonly prescribe insulin for Type 2 diabetes management, yet this approach is increasingly seen as outdated and even harmful when applied without addressing the underlying issues of insulin resistance and metabolic dysfunction. In Type 2 diabetes, the primary *problem is not insufficient insulin* production but rather an excess of insulin due to the body's inability to utilize it effectively. By prescribing additional insulin, doctors may temporarily lower blood sugar but inadvertently worsen the underlying insulin resistance. Elevated insulin levels, often termed **hyperinsulinemia**, exacerbate metabolic dysfunction by signaling the body to store more energy as fat, further compounding weight gain and promoting visceral fat accumulation, a critical factor in metabolic syndrome.

This practice underscores a gap in understanding the pathophysiology of Type 2 diabetes, where the focus remains heavily on blood glucose control rather than on addressing insulin resistance. Many doctors overlook the significance of dietary and lifestyle interventions that aim to lower endogenous insulin production, leading to a "band-aid" approach with insulin therapy. This approach fails to reverse the condition and, in some cases, can lead to complications like weight gain, increased cardiovascular risk, and continued disease progression.

The current evidence advocates for interventions that focus on reducing insulin demand by emphasizing a low-carbohydrate, high-protein, and healthy fat diet, as well as strategies like intermittent fasting. These methods can improve insulin sensitivity, often reducing or eliminating the need for exogenous insulin altogether. Understanding Type 2 diabetes as an insulin resistance issue, not an insulin deficiency, is critical to promoting metabolic health and preventing long-term complications.

Alcohol's effect on the body

While this doesn't apply directly to diabetes itself, alcohol can have a harrowing effect on the body especially in a compromised state. Metabolic syndrome itself is a disorder that is affected by many things, and alcohol is one of the factors. Let's touch a bit on the role that alcohol can play in your health.

Alcohol's journey through the body begins immediately upon ingestion, with rapid absorption by the stomach and small intestine. Once in the bloodstream, it is carried to the liver, where the real metabolic processing occurs. The liver prioritizes breaking down alcohol over other metabolic functions, given alcohol's toxicity and inability to be stored, which can disrupt other critical metabolic processes.

The primary enzyme responsible for alcohol breakdown is alcohol dehydrogenase (ADH), which converts ethanol into acetaldehyde, a highly reactive and toxic byproduct. Acetaldehyde is short-lived but dangerous, capable of binding with cellular proteins, DNA, and lipids, and initiating oxidative damage and inflammation throughout the body. This harmful substance is further broken down by aldehyde dehydrogenase (ALDH) into acetate, a less harmful compound, which is ultimately converted to water and carbon dioxide. However, acetaldehyde's brief presence in the bloodstream is enough to cause widespread cellular stress and inflammation, especially when alcohol consumption is heavy or chronic.

The liver's prioritization of alcohol metabolism impacts other biochemical pathways, one of which is gluconeogenesis—the liver's process of generating glucose from non-carbohydrate sources. Alcohol suppresses this function, which can lead to hypoglycemia (low blood sugar) in heavy drinkers, particularly risky for individuals with diabetes or metabolic syndrome. This glucose suppression can lead to lightheadedness, fatigue, or more severe consequences if prolonged.

Moreover, alcohol alters lipid metabolism, increasing the liver's tendency to accumulate fat. When the liver is focused on processing ethanol, it shifts energy from breaking down fatty acids (lipid oxidation) to storing them, leading to a buildup of triglycerides within liver cells. Over time, this accumulation contributes to fatty liver disease, which, if unaddressed, can progress to more serious conditions like alcoholic hepatitis and cirrhosis. Excessive fat buildup, combined with the inflammation from acetaldehyde exposure, further damages liver cells and impairs their regenerative capacity, increasing the risk of permanent scarring.

Another key biochemical impact of alcohol consumption is on the body's balance of nicotinamide adenine dinucleotide (NAD+), a coenzyme essential in cellular energy production. The breakdown of alcohol by ADH and ALDH requires large amounts of NAD+, leading to a significant depletion of this coenzyme in liver cells. NAD+ is vital for various metabolic functions, including the oxidation of fatty acids and the production of ATP, the cell's main energy currency. A reduction in NAD+ shifts the liver's balance from lipid oxidation toward fat storage, exacerbating the accumulation of fatty acids within liver cells and hindering overall metabolic function.

Additionally, chronic alcohol consumption elevates the production of reactive oxygen species (ROS), a type of free radical that can damage cell structures, including proteins, lipids, and DNA. Elevated ROS levels can lead to oxidative stress, which is a significant contributor to inflammation and liver damage. As the liver attempts to combat this oxidative stress, it activates inflammatory pathways, leading to a state of chronic inflammation. This inflammation, coupled with direct oxidative damage, creates a cycle of cellular injury, reducing the liver's ability to recover and regenerate over time.

Alcohol also disrupts hormone regulation in the liver, specifically the hormones related to blood pressure, fluid balance, and cholesterol metabolism. This can lead to systemic issues such as increased blood pressure and an imbalanced cholesterol profile, both of which are risk factors for cardiovascular disease. Additionally, alcohol can interfere with the liver's role in processing and removing various toxins and medications, further stressing the organ.

Finally, alcohol's impact on the gut and its relationship to the liver is important. Alcohol disrupts the gut barrier, allowing bacterial endotoxins to enter the bloodstream and travel to the liver, where they exacerbate inflammation. Known as "leaky gut," this condition allows more toxins into the liver, overwhelming its detoxification capacity and adding to liver strain and inflammation. This gut-liver interaction is a key contributor to the systemic impact of alcohol, affecting not only liver health but also immune function and inflammation levels throughout the body.

In summary, alcohol's biochemical effects on the body are widespread, with the liver bearing the brunt of its impact. Beyond merely processing alcohol, the liver experiences altered metabolism, fat accumulation, and inflammation. Over time, this metabolic disturbance contributes to conditions like fatty liver disease, hypertension, and impaired glucose regulation, making it crucial to understand these processes for managing or mitigating alcohol's health risks.

Advanced Glycation End Products (A.G.E.'s)

Understanding glycation and Advanced Glycation End Products (AGEs) is crucial in managing diabetes and preventing its complications. In diabetes, glucose levels in the bloodstream are frequently elevated, which leads to an increase in glycation, a process where sugars attach to proteins, lipids, or nucleic acids. When glycation becomes excessive, it forms AGEs—molecules that accumulate in tissues over time and are particularly damaging to cellular structures and functions. This section will explore why glycation and AGEs should not be overlooked, their role in diabetes, and how lifestyle interventions can help mitigate their harmful effects.

What is Glycation?

Glycation is a non-enzymatic reaction where sugars, particularly glucose, bond with proteins, lipids, and nucleic acids. Unlike enzymatic reactions, which are tightly regulated by the body, glycation happens spontaneously, depending on the availability of glucose. Glycation changes the structure and function of molecules, making them stiffer and less flexible, leading to cellular dysfunction and tissue damage. In diabetes, where blood sugar levels are consistently high, the rate of glycation increases, leading to accelerated formation of AGEs.

AGEs are molecules formed when glycated proteins, lipids, or nucleic acids undergo further modifications, a process accelerated in hyperglycemia. AGEs accumulate throughout the body, particularly in tissues with long-lived proteins such as collagen in the skin, lens proteins in the eye, and myelin in the nervous system. As these tissues accumulate AGEs, their functions decline, which is particularly concerning in diabetes where blood sugar levels are chronically elevated.

AGEs contribute to diabetes complications by:

Altering Protein Function: AGEs disrupt proteins' structural integrity, reducing their flexibility and functionality. For example, when AGEs modify collagen, it becomes stiff and resistant to repair, which can impact blood vessels and skin elasticity.

Inducing Inflammation: AGEs bind to specific receptors, known as RAGE (receptors for advanced glycation end products), triggering an inflammatory response. This inflammation leads to further tissue damage, a hallmark of diabetic complications like nephropathy and neuropathy.

Oxidative Stress: The interaction between AGEs and RAGE produces reactive oxygen species (ROS), molecules that damage cellular structures and contribute to oxidative stress. This stress damages cells in vital organs, particularly the eyes, kidneys, nerves, and heart, where diabetic complications are most severe.

Glycation and the Complications of Diabetes

In diabetes, elevated blood glucose levels expose the body to prolonged periods of glycation, amplifying the formation of AGEs and their harmful effects on various tissues. This glycation process plays a critical role in the development and progression of diabetic complications.

Cardiovascular Disease: AGEs accumulate in blood vessels, making them stiffer and less elastic, which is especially concerning given the prevalence of cardiovascular issues in diabetic individuals. This stiffness leads to higher blood pressure and vascular resistance, placing extra stress on the heart and increasing the risk of cardiovascular disease.

Retinopathy: Glycation affects the proteins in the retina, leading to structural damage and contributing to diabetic retinopathy, one of the leading causes of blindness in diabetes. AGEs disrupt the blood-retinal barrier, making blood vessels more susceptible to leaking, leading to vision impairment.

1. **Kidney Damage**: AGEs accumulate in the kidneys, particularly in the glomerular basement membrane, affecting the kidneys' filtering capacity. This contributes to diabetic nephropathy, a significant cause of kidney failure in diabetes. AGEs also lead to fibrosis, or scarring, of kidney tissues, further reducing kidney function over time.
2. **Nerve Damage**: Glycation disrupts nerve function by impairing myelin, a fatty sheath that insulates nerve fibers. The resulting nerve damage, known as neuropathy, can cause numbness, tingling, and pain in the extremities, significantly affecting quality of life for diabetics.
3. **Skin and Joint Damage**: AGEs accumulate in skin collagen, leading to decreased elasticity, wrinkles, and

impaired wound healing. In joints, AGEs stiffen collagen fibers, leading to limited flexibility and higher susceptibility to injury—a condition often referred to as "diabetic stiff hand syndrome."

Glycation as an Overlooked Factor in Diabetes Management

Most diabetes treatments focus on controlling blood sugar through medications and lifestyle changes, with less emphasis on preventing the formation of AGEs. However, because glycation has a significant impact on cellular function, targeting AGEs directly could be a crucial component of diabetes management. Despite the potential harm, the role of glycation is often underrepresented in standard diabetes care guidelines, which focus primarily on blood glucose, HbA1c levels, and insulin sensitivity.

To truly manage diabetes effectively, it is essential to understand and address glycation alongside blood glucose control. By targeting both, one can mitigate not only high blood sugar but also the long-term damage to tissues and organs that contribute to diabetic complications.

Lifestyle Interventions to Reduce Glycation and AGE Formation

Preventing or slowing the formation of AGEs in diabetes involves a multi-faceted approach, including dietary modifications, lifestyle changes, and targeted supplements. Here are several strategies that can help mitigate the harmful effects of glycation in diabetes.

1. Dietary Modifications

Certain dietary choices can reduce glycation and the formation of AGEs:

Low Glycemic Index Foods: Foods that release glucose slowly help to stabilize blood sugar levels, reducing spikes that accelerate glycation. Low-glycemic foods include vegetables, nuts, seeds, and lean proteins.

Limit Processed Foods: Processed foods often contain high levels of sugars and refined carbohydrates, which promote glycation. They also frequently contain high levels of AGEs formed during high-heat cooking processes.

Avoid Cooking at High Temperatures: AGEs form during cooking methods like grilling, frying, and roasting. Opting for steaming, boiling, or slow-cooking can help reduce dietary AGEs.

Choose Foods Rich in Antioxidants: Antioxidants like vitamins C and E, found in berries, leafy greens, and nuts, neutralize oxidative stress caused by AGEs. Polyphenols, such as those in green tea and turmeric, also help reduce AGE formation.

2. Exercise

Exercise has multiple benefits for diabetes management, and it also helps reduce glycation. Physical activity enhances insulin sensitivity, allowing the body to use glucose more effectively, which reduces blood sugar levels and glycation risk. Furthermore, exercise promotes antioxidant production, countering the oxidative stress associated with AGEs.

3. Fasting and Glycation

Intermittent fasting (IF) and other fasting strategies may be effective in reducing glycation by promoting lower blood sugar levels and encouraging autophagy, a cellular process that clears damaged proteins, including glycated ones. Fasting gives the body a break from glucose intake, which may slow the formation of new AGEs and help manage blood glucose levels in diabetes.

4. Supplements Targeting Glycation and AGEs

There are several supplements known to inhibit AGE formation or reduce their effects:

Alpha-Lipoic Acid (ALA): ALA has antioxidant properties that reduce oxidative stress from AGEs, and studies show it may reduce complications in diabetes.

Benfotiamine: A fat-soluble form of vitamin B1, benfotiamine reduces AGE formation and has shown promise in reducing symptoms of diabetic neuropathy.

Curcumin: The active compound in turmeric, curcumin is known for its anti-inflammatory and antioxidant properties and may inhibit AGE formation.

Vitamin C and E: These antioxidants reduce oxidative stress from AGEs and support overall metabolic health in diabetics.

Carnosine: An amino acid, carnosine can prevent glycation and reduce AGE formation, which has shown promise in animal studies.

The Importance of Monitoring Glycation Levels

Monitoring HbA1c levels is a common practice in diabetes management, as it provides a long-term view of blood glucose levels. However, HbA1c also reflects glycation levels in red blood cells, offering indirect insight into glycation in the body. High HbA1c levels indicate prolonged exposure to glucose and a greater likelihood of AGE formation, reinforcing the need for better glycation management.

However, more direct methods of measuring AGEs could be valuable in diabetes care, particularly for identifying patients at higher risk of complications. Non-invasive tests that measure AGEs in the skin are now being developed and could serve as useful diagnostic tools to predict diabetic complications, potentially helping to guide more individualized treatment approaches.

Why Glycation Should Not Be Overlooked

Glycation is a critical process in the development of diabetic complications, yet it often goes unaddressed in conventional diabetes treatment plans. By focusing only on blood sugar levels without considering glycation, healthcare providers miss an essential aspect of diabetes management that can impact long-term health outcomes.

Reducing Complications: Targeting glycation and AGE formation can help reduce the risk of complications like cardiovascular disease, retinopathy, and nephropathy, which are common in diabetes.

Improving Quality of Life: Managing glycation effectively can help maintain tissue health, flexibility, and functionality, enhancing overall quality of life for diabetic patients.

Preventing Cellular Aging: By mitigating AGE formation, we can slow down cellular aging and reduce oxidative stress, potentially extending healthy lifespan and reducing disability associated with diabetes.

The Future of Diabetes Management: Incorporating Glycation Awareness

Future diabetes management strategies would benefit from incorporating glycation awareness into standard care. While blood glucose and insulin levels are important markers of diabetic health, understanding glycation and AGEs offers a more comprehensive view of metabolic health. This expanded approach could lead to better preventive care, fewer complications, and more personalized treatment plans.

Incorporating routine glycation monitoring and interventions to prevent AGE formation could shift the paradigm in diabetes care. By understanding the impact of glycation, patients and healthcare providers can better address the root causes of diabetic complications, potentially improving health outcomes and reducing the burden of diabetes on the healthcare system.

Glycation and AGEs play a pivotal role in the progression of diabetes and its complications. Understanding the biochemical impact of glycation sheds light on why maintaining stable blood glucose levels alone is insufficient. By targeting glycation and AGE formation through lifestyle changes, dietary adjustments, exercise, and supplements, it is possible to reduce the damaging effects of diabetes and improve quality of life.

The importance of understanding glycation cannot be overstated. For individuals with diabetes, glycation awareness provides a pathway to proactive care—one that goes beyond blood sugar control to address the underlying cellular damage caused by prolonged hyperglycemia. As research progresses, a broader approach to diabetes management that includes glycation monitoring and intervention could lead to better health outcomes and a more sustainable way of reversing diabetes.

Foods For Insulin Resistant (Diabetic) People

While the proper human diet will be covered later, I wanted to include a section on foods for people with insulin resistance or diabetes. Managing carbohydrate intake is crucial for those dealing with insulin resistance or diabetes, as different types of carbohydrates can have varying impacts on blood sugar levels. To make informed dietary choices, it is essential to understand the concepts of the glycemic index (GI) and glycemic load (GL) and how they can guide better eating habits.

Understanding Glycemic Index (GI) and Glycemic Load (GL)

The glycemic index is a measure of how quickly a carbohydrate-containing food raises blood glucose levels after consumption. Foods are rated on a scale from 0 to 100, with higher numbers indicating a more rapid increase in blood sugar. For example, refined carbohydrates and sugary foods tend to have a high GI, while non-starchy vegetables and certain whole grains have a lower GI.

The glycemic load, on the other hand, takes into account both the GI of a food and the amount of carbohydrates it contains per serving. This provides a more comprehensive picture of a food's actual impact on blood sugar levels. For example, a food with a high GI but low carbohydrate content might have a moderate GL, making it less impactful on blood sugar than its GI alone would suggest.

Choosing the Right Carbohydrates for Better Health

While I will maintain that carbohydrates themselves are not optimal, I realize that to be realistic, many people will not go full carnivore, so I want to include this section. For individuals managing insulin resistance or diabetes, it is crucial to choose carbohydrates that have a low or moderate glycemic index and glycemic load to avoid rapid blood sugar spikes. Here are some guidelines for selecting healthier carbohydrate options:

1. **Avoid High-GI (Glycemic Index) Foods**:

Refined Sugars and Sweets: Foods such as candies, cakes, and pastries have a high GI and minimal nutritional value.

White Bread and Processed Grains: These foods are stripped of fiber and nutrients, leading to rapid spikes in blood glucose levels.

Sugary Beverages: Sodas, fruit juices, and other sweetened drinks contribute to quick rises in blood sugar and can exacerbate insulin resistance.

2. **Opt for Low- and Moderate-GI Foods**:

Non-Starchy Vegetables: Foods like leafy greens, broccoli, and peppers have a low GI and provide essential vitamins and minerals.

Whole Grains: When consumed in moderation, whole grains such as quinoa, barley, and oats can offer fiber and nutrients while maintaining a lower GI.

Legumes: Beans, lentils, and chickpeas have a low GI and are rich in fiber and protein, which can help regulate blood sugar levels.

Berries and Certain Fruits: While fruit intake should be moderated, berries and fruits with lower sugar content, such as strawberries and apples, can be better choices due to their lower GI and fiber content.

Why Glycemic Index Alone Isn't Enough

While the glycemic index can be a useful tool for gauging how a food might impact blood sugar, it has its limitations. The GI does not account for portion sizes, which is where *glycemic load* becomes particularly important. For example, watermelon has a high GI, but because it contains relatively few carbohydrates per serving, its GL is low. This means that eating a standard serving of watermelon is unlikely to cause a significant blood sugar spike, even though its GI number might suggest otherwise.

Practical Tips for Managing Carbohydrate Intake

Pair LOW Carbohydrate Food with Protein and Healthy Fats: Combining low-GI carbohydrates with protein and healthy fats can slow down digestion and reduce the overall impact on blood sugar levels.

Monitor Portion Sizes: Even low-GI foods can affect blood sugar when eaten in large amounts. Paying attention to portion sizes can help maintain better blood glucose control.

Limit Processed Foods: Processed foods often contain hidden sugars and refined carbohydrates that can elevate blood sugar more than expected.

Focus on Whole, Nutrient-Dense Foods: Prioritizing whole foods with minimal processing helps provide the body with essential nutrients and supports balanced blood sugar levels.

Understanding the difference between glycemic index and glycemic load can empower individuals to make more informed food choices, especially when managing insulin resistance or diabetes. By focusing on low- and moderate-GI foods and being mindful of glycemic load, it is possible to control blood sugar levels more effectively and support overall metabolic health. This knowledge, combined with an approach tailored to individual needs, can contribute to better long-term outcomes and improved quality of life.

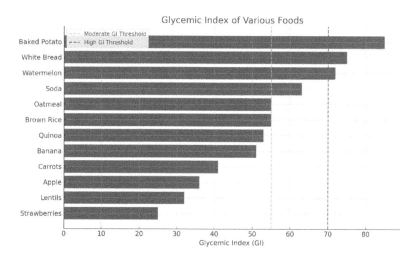

Glycemic Index vs Glycemic Load

The **Glycemic Index (GI)** and **Glycemic Load (GL)** are both tools used to measure the impact of carbohydrate-containing foods on blood sugar levels, but they serve different purposes and provide complementary information.

Glycemic Index (GI)

- **Definition**: The glycemic index is a measure of how quickly a carbohydrate-containing food raises blood glucose levels compared to pure glucose, which has a GI of 100. Foods are ranked on a scale from 0 to 100, with higher numbers indicating a faster and higher spike in blood sugar.
- **Classification**:
    - **Low GI**: 55 or less (e.g., lentils, apples, and oatmeal)
    - **Medium GI**: 56-69 (e.g., brown rice, bananas)

High GI: 70 or above (e.g., white bread, baked potatoes)

Limitations: GI only accounts for the quality of the carbohydrate and not the quantity consumed. A food may have a high GI but be eaten in a small portion that has minimal effect on blood sugar, or vice versa.

Glycemic Load (GL)

Definition: The glycemic load takes into account both the GI of a food and the amount of carbohydrates in a serving. It provides a more accurate picture of how a food will affect blood sugar levels when eaten in normal serving sizes.

Calculation: GL is calculated using the formula:

$$GL = \frac{GI \times \text{carbohydrates per serving (grams)}}{100}$$

- **Classification**:

Low GL: 10 or less (e.g., carrots, watermelon in small portions)

Medium GL: 11-19 (e.g., bananas, sweet potatoes)

High GL: 20 or more (e.g., white bread, large servings of high-GI foods)

Benefits: GL gives a better indication of the real impact of foods on blood sugar by incorporating both the type of carbohydrate (GI) and its quantity.

Key Differences Between GI and GL

GI: Measures the rate at which carbohydrates in a food raise blood glucose.

GL: Takes into account the GI and the portion size of the carbohydrate, providing a clearer understanding of how the food affects blood sugar levels in practical servings.

Practical Example:

Watermelon: Has a high GI (~72) but a low carbohydrate content per serving, resulting in a low GL. This means that while watermelon raises blood sugar quickly, the actual effect of a typical serving is minimal.

White Bread: Has a high GI and typically a higher GL, meaning it will both raise blood sugar quickly and in significant amounts when eaten in common serving sizes.

Why Both Matter

- **GI** helps individuals choose foods that have a slower impact on blood sugar, which is useful for general guidance.
- **GL** provides more actionable insights, particularly for those managing conditions like diabetes, as it reflects the real-world impact of eating specific portions of foods.

In summary, while the GI is helpful for understanding the potential impact of foods on blood sugar, the GL offers a more comprehensive perspective that accounts for portion size, making it a more practical tool for meal planning and blood sugar management.

Chapter Four Myths and Untruths:

This is an interesting chapter since it deals with so many misconceptions, myths, and flat out lies that people absolutely need to know and understand. I'll talk about several topics that need addressing.

Some of the topics covered will be:

1. Cholesterol and Fat
2. Statins and Medication
3. Seed Oils
4. "Calories In, Calories Out"
5. Whole Grains and Carbohydrates
6. Superfoods and Veganism
7. Meat and Religion
8. Fruits and Juice
9. Fiber

Cholesterol and Fat.

How many times have you heard someone say "You shouldn't eat that, it has too much cholesterol" or "The doctor says I have to take these pills because my cholesterol is too high"? well first and foremost, cholesterol does not cause heart attacks, cardiovascular disease, or anything of the sort. To villainize cholesterol for heart disease is like blaming the fire department for car accidents. "Well, every time I see an accident, the fire department seems to be there" is that logical?

To address the cholesterol myth, a key point is that cholesterol acts as an anti-inflammatory agent and a repair molecule, often responding to existing cardiovascular damage rather than causing it. When inflammation or damage occurs within blood vessels, the body deploys cholesterol to the area as part of its healing response, a process that sometimes forms arterial plaques as a protective measure. This natural repair mechanism is frequently misunderstood as causative, when in reality, cholesterol's presence at cardiovascular event sites highlights its role in countering inflammation, not initiating it.

A very good source of information on this is a book by Stephen Sinatra and Jonny Bowden. The book argues that cholesterol itself is not the main cause of heart disease but rather an indicator of underlying inflammation, insulin resistance, and oxidative stress. It challenges the idea that lowering cholesterol with medication directly reduces heart disease risk and instead suggests focusing on lifestyle changes that reduce inflammation, manage insulin levels, and decrease oxidative stress. If you want to dive deeper into cholesterol and its true function, go to a Dave Feldman lecture and you will learn everything you need to know.

LDL Cholesterol: The Carrier, Not the Culprit

LDL (Low-Density Lipoprotein) is a type of lipoprotein that carries cholesterol, triglycerides, and other lipids through the bloodstream to cells that need them. It's important to remember that LDL itself is not "bad"—it serves essential roles in delivering cholesterol, which is vital for cell membranes, hormone production, and other bodily functions.

The traditional focus on lowering total LDL cholesterol comes from studies showing that high LDL levels are correlated with an increased risk of heart disease. However, this is an **association**, not a direct cause. LDL is simply a carrier, not the underlying reason why plaque forms in the arteries.

The Real Risk: Small, Dense LDL Particles

What really matters in assessing cardiovascular risk is the **size and density of LDL particles**:

Small, Dense LDL Particles: These particles are more atherogenic (plaque-forming) because they can penetrate the arterial walls more easily, become oxidized, and trigger an inflammatory response. This process leads to the development of **atherosclerosis**, where plaque builds up in the artery walls, restricting blood flow and potentially leading to heart attacks or strokes.

Large, Fluffy LDL Particles: These are less likely to cause arterial damage because they are less dense and less prone to oxidation. Individuals with predominantly large, fluffy LDL particles may have a lower risk of cardiovascular disease, even if their total LDL cholesterol is high.

Lipoproteins: The Transport System

Lipoproteins like LDL and HDL are simply carriers that transport cholesterol and triglycerides through the bloodstream. They are essential for moving these hydrophobic substances, as cholesterol and triglycerides cannot dissolve in blood on their own. The focus on LDL being "bad" oversimplifies the role of lipoproteins:

LDL as a Carrier: LDL delivers cholesterol to cells where it's needed for cell repair, hormone synthesis, and other essential functions.

HDL as a Reverse Transporter: **HDL (High-Density Lipoprotein)** is often called "good" cholesterol because it helps remove excess cholesterol from the bloodstream, transporting it back to the liver for excretion or recycling.

Inflammation: The Underlying Factor

The presence of **small, dense LDL particles** becomes a problem when combined with **chronic inflammation**. Inflammatory processes make the arterial walls more susceptible to damage, allowing oxidized LDL particles to adhere and contribute to plaque formation. This is why simply focusing on LDL cholesterol levels without addressing inflammation can be misleading.

Root Causes and Addressing the Real Issue

The primary drivers of the production of small, dense LDL particles and chronic inflammation include:

Diet High in Refined Carbohydrates and Sugars: These promote insulin resistance and can increase the production of small, dense LDL particles.

Oxidative Stress: Leads to the oxidation of LDL particles, making them more likely to trigger an immune response and contribute to plaque buildup.

Lack of Physical Activity: Reduces HDL levels and promotes the formation of smaller LDL particles.

Chronic Stress and Poor Sleep: Elevates cortisol and other stress hormones, contributing to metabolic disruptions and inflammation.

The Misinterpretation of LDL Cholesterol

Focusing solely on total LDL cholesterol levels overlooks the complexity of cardiovascular risk. People with the same LDL levels can have very different risks depending on their **LDL particle size, HDL levels, triglycerides, and inflammatory markers**.

Comprehensive testing, including advanced lipid panels that measure LDL particle size and count, along with assessing inflammatory markers like **C-reactive protein (CRP)**, provides a clearer picture of cardiovascular risk.

LDL cholesterol is associated with heart disease due to its role as a carrier of cholesterol, but the real issue lies in the **type of LDL particles** and the presence of **chronic inflammation** and **oxidative stress**. Addressing these underlying causes through **diet, exercise, and lifestyle changes** can reduce the formation of small, dense LDL particles and lower overall cardiovascular risk more effectively than focusing solely on reducing total LDL cholesterol.

Incorporating this viewpoint into your chapter could involve breaking down:

Cholesterol as a Repair Molecule: Cholesterol plays a role in the body's healing response, arriving at inflamed or damaged arterial sites. However, it doesn't cause the damage—it's merely responding to it, suggesting that focusing solely on cholesterol misses the underlying inflammatory processes.

Role of Small Dense LDL Particles: It's not cholesterol in general but small, dense LDL particles (influenced by diet, stress, and lifestyle) that are most associated with atherosclerosis. These particles are more likely to oxidize and lead to plaque formation, whereas larger, fluffy LDL particles are less atherogenic.

Importance of Inflammation and Oxidative Stress: Reducing inflammation and oxidative stress is more effective in preventing heart disease than lowering cholesterol alone. The book promotes addressing root causes like high blood sugar, stress, smoking, and processed foods as primary drivers of cardiovascular risk.

Dietary Misconceptions: It debunks the low-fat, high-carb diet as counterproductive, advocating for a balanced approach rich in healthy fats, low-glycemic foods, and nutrient-dense options that support cardiovascular health without spiking insulin or promoting inflammation.

Another key researcher of cholesterol is Dave Feldman, who is the resident expert on cholesterol and its' purpose. Cholesterol is a waxy, fat-like substance found in every cell of the body. It's essential for building cell membranes, producing hormones (like estrogen, testosterone, and cortisol), making vitamin D, and forming bile acids that help digest fats. The body produces most of the cholesterol it needs, while the rest comes from dietary sources. Cholesterol travels in the blood carried by lipoproteins, mainly as low-density lipoprotein (LDL) and high-density lipoprotein (HDL), which play different roles in transporting and removing cholesterol. To understand cholesterol fully, especially in the context of cardiovascular health, it's crucial to see it as part of the body's healing response, rather than inherently harmful. Cholesterol is actually the body's way of responding to inflammation, oxidative stress, and vascular damage. In cases of injury or inflammation, cholesterol acts as a repair molecule, mobilized to areas where tissues need reinforcement or protection.

This concept is central to books like *The Great Cholesterol Myth*, which argues that inflammation and insulin resistance—rather than cholesterol itself—are primary drivers of cardiovascular disease. Cholesterol, often misunderstood as a causal factor, instead plays a supportive role in repairing damage to blood vessels.

Fats- The truth and the Worst Misconception

The topic of dietary fat has become one of the most controversial in modern nutrition, with endless myths clouding the true understanding of what's healthy and what's harmful. Many mainstream messages promote low-fat diets, associating fat with heart disease and weight gain. However, a more nuanced understanding shows that not all fats are created equal, and some are essential to health. Here, we'll explore the types of fats, their roles in the body, and reveal which ones actually support optimal health.

1. Types of Dietary Fats

Understanding fats starts with knowing the different types and their biological roles. Fats are broadly divided into four main categories:

Saturated Fats: Found primarily in animal products (meat, butter, and dairy) as well as tropical oils like coconut oil and palm oil. Saturated fats are solid at room temperature due to their stable chemical structure.

Monounsaturated Fats (MUFAs): Found in high amounts in olive oil, avocados, and some nuts (like macadamia nuts). MUFAs have one unsaturated (double) bond in their structure, making them liquid at room temperature but stable for cooking.

Polyunsaturated Fats (PUFAs): Present in many vegetable oils (like sunflower, soybean, and corn oils), nuts, seeds, and fatty fish. PUFAs are unstable due to their multiple double bonds, making them prone to oxidation, especially at high heat.

Trans Fats: These are artificially created through hydrogenation to make oils solid at room temperature, extending shelf life in processed foods. They're found in margarine, shortening, and many packaged foods. Trans fats are universally recognized as harmful.

Myth: "Saturated Fat is Harmful and Causes Heart Disease"

The demonization of saturated fats traces back to the 1950s and 60s when early research mistakenly linked saturated fats with heart disease. The famous "Seven Countries Study" by Ancel Keys, for instance, suggested a correlation between saturated fat intake and heart disease, though it overlooked key variables, including lifestyle and sugar intake.

What We Know Now: Current research reveals that not all saturated fats are equal and that, in fact, moderate consumption of natural sources of saturated fats may not harm cardiovascular health. Foods like butter, red meat, and dairy contain not only saturated fats but also essential nutrients, such as fat-soluble vitamins (A, D, E, K) and conjugated linoleic acid (CLA), which may have anti-inflammatory properties.

Metabolic Health: Studies now show that the harmful impact often attributed to saturated fats may be due to a diet high in refined sugars and processed foods rather than saturated fat itself. When consumed as part of a balanced diet low in processed carbs, saturated fats may not increase cardiovascular risk.

The Health Benefits of Monounsaturated Fats

Monounsaturated fats, especially from sources like olive oil, are widely praised for their health benefits. High in antioxidants and oleic acid, MUFAs are shown to have heart-protective effects, improve insulin sensitivity, and reduce inflammation.

Mediterranean Diet Evidence: Numerous studies, including large meta-analyses, highlight the benefits of MUFAs as part of the Mediterranean diet, which is associated with reduced cardiovascular disease and better longevity.

- **Cooking Stability**: Unlike PUFAs, MUFAs are more stable and less prone to oxidation, making them a healthier choice for moderate-temperature cooking.

Polyunsaturated Fats – A Double-Edged Sword

Polyunsaturated fats are essential as they include omega-3 and omega-6 fatty acids, both of which play roles in cellular function and inflammation regulation. However, the high consumption of omega-6 fats from processed seed oils (such as soybean and sunflower oils) is linked to inflammatory responses in the body.

The Omega-3 to Omega-6 Ratio: Historically, humans consumed a near-equal balance of omega-3 and omega-6 fats. Today's Western diets contain up to 20 times more omega-6 than omega-3, contributing to chronic inflammation.

Sources of Omega-3s: Fatty fish, flaxseed, and chia seeds are excellent sources of omega-3s, which support brain health, reduce inflammation, and improve cardiovascular markers.

Cooking Dangers: Omega-6 PUFAs are unstable and easily oxidize under heat, producing harmful free radicals. Frequent consumption of fried and high-heat-cooked PUFA oils can increase oxidative stress and inflammation in the body.

Trans Fats – The Real Culprit

The most universally acknowledged harmful fat, trans fats, have been linked to an array of health problems, from heart disease and insulin resistance to increased inflammation.

Health Risks: Trans fats are harmful because they interfere with healthy cellular function and lipid metabolism. They increase LDL (bad) cholesterol, lower HDL (good) cholesterol, and are associated with an elevated risk of heart disease, stroke, and type 2 diabetes.

The Shift Away from Trans Fats: Many countries have banned or limited trans fats due to overwhelming evidence of harm. Yet, small amounts may still exist in processed foods, making it essential to read labels.

Myth: "Eating Fat Makes You Fat"

A common misconception links fat consumption with weight gain. However, fats are essential to many bodily functions and can be metabolically neutral or even beneficial when consumed in moderation and from the right sources.

Satiety and Blood Sugar Stability: Unlike refined carbohydrates, fats digest slowly, promoting satiety and helping maintain steady blood sugar levels. Diets higher in healthy fats and lower in carbs can aid in weight management by reducing insulin spikes and enhancing fat utilization.

Insulin Sensitivity and Fat Storage: Studies suggest that diets higher in healthy fats (especially MUFAs and omega-3s) and lower in processed carbs improve insulin sensitivity, making the body less prone to fat storage, particularly in visceral fat.

The Role of Cholesterol and Fats in Heart Health

Cholesterol itself is not the enemy. Our body requires cholesterol to produce hormones, vitamin D, and bile acids. Dietary fats, particularly saturated fats, were once wrongly assumed to cause an increase in cholesterol and heart disease. Emerging evidence clarifies that it's more about the type of fat consumed.

HDL and LDL Cholesterol: Healthy fats, particularly omega-3s and monounsaturated fats, have been shown to increase HDL (good cholesterol) and improve the LDL particle profile, shifting it towards larger, buoyant particles that are less likely to clog arteries.

Inflammation as a Root Cause: Heart disease is increasingly recognized as an inflammatory condition. Processed carbohydrates, refined seed oils, and trans fats are the primary dietary drivers of inflammation, not naturally occurring fats from whole foods.

Revisiting Low-Fat Diet Recommendations

The "low-fat" craze of past decades contributed to an increase in carbohydrate-rich foods and added sugars, often used to replace fats for taste. This shift inadvertently worsened public health by increasing insulin resistance, obesity rates, and metabolic disorders.

Healthier Low-Carb, High-Fat Approaches: Studies on ketogenic and low-carb diets reveal that higher-fat diets (focusing on natural, unprocessed fats) are effective for managing weight, improving blood glucose, and reducing triglycerides.

Balanced Dietary Approach: Today's understanding of fats emphasizes balance, promoting natural fats from sources like fatty fish, avocado, eggs, nuts, and grass-fed meats as essential for overall health.

So you have "High Cholesterol" and your doctor prescribed statins:

Statins are among the most commonly prescribed medications for managing high cholesterol, especially LDL cholesterol, in an effort to reduce the risk of cardiovascular disease. While their effectiveness in lowering LDL cholesterol levels is well-documented, there is growing concern about the potential adverse effects of statins, particularly their impact on cellular health and mitochondrial function.

How Statins Work and Why They Are Prescribed

Statins function by inhibiting **HMG-CoA reductase**, an enzyme involved in cholesterol synthesis in the liver. This inhibition effectively lowers cholesterol production, which, in turn, reduces blood levels of LDL cholesterol. By decreasing LDL levels, statins aim to lower the risk of heart attacks, strokes, and other cardiovascular events, especially in individuals with a history of heart disease or multiple risk factors. However, the narrative that high cholesterol alone is a direct cause of heart disease has come under scrutiny, raising questions about the widespread use of statins as a primary preventive measure.

The Impact of Statins on Mitochondrial Function

One of the significant downsides of statins is their potential to impair mitochondrial function. Mitochondria, known as the **powerhouses of the cell**, are responsible for producing energy in the form of **adenosine triphosphate (ATP)**. Statins can interfere with mitochondrial health in several ways:

Coenzyme Q10 (CoQ10) Depletion: Statins inhibit the same pathway that produces cholesterol and also reduce the synthesis of **Coenzyme Q10**, a vital component for mitochondrial energy production. CoQ10 plays a crucial role in the electron transport chain, enabling efficient ATP production. A deficiency in CoQ10 can lead to decreased cellular energy and contribute to muscle pain, weakness, and fatigue, which are commonly reported side effects of statin therapy.

Oxidative Stress and Damage: Mitochondrial dysfunction can result in increased production of **reactive oxygen species (ROS)**, leading to oxidative damage. When statins deplete CoQ10 levels, the mitochondria are less equipped to neutralize ROS, resulting in oxidative stress that can harm cells and tissues. Chronic oxidative stress has been linked to accelerated aging and the development of various chronic diseases.

Muscle Health Implications: Statin-induced muscle symptoms, known as **statin-associated muscle symptoms (SAMS)**, range from mild myalgia to severe conditions like rhabdomyolysis, where muscle breakdown can lead to kidney damage. The link between statins and muscle issues is often attributed to mitochondrial dysfunction and the subsequent decline in cellular energy.

Broader Health Concerns and Risks

Beyond mitochondrial damage, statins may have other potential side effects and risks that should be carefully considered:

Diabetes Risk: Some research indicates that statin use can increase the risk of developing type 2 diabetes, particularly in individuals predisposed to insulin resistance. This effect may be related to how statins influence glucose metabolism and insulin sensitivity.

Cognitive Effects: Although the evidence is mixed, there have been reports of memory loss and cognitive decline associated with statin use. Mitochondrial dysfunction and reduced cholesterol levels—essential for brain function—may contribute to these cognitive issues.

Nutrient Depletion: Apart from CoQ10, statins may affect the levels of other essential nutrients and lipids, impacting overall cellular and systemic health.

Reevaluating the Use of Statins

While statins can be life-saving for certain high-risk patients, the broad prescription of these drugs for "high cholesterol" without considering the overall metabolic context has drawn criticism. The focus on lowering LDL cholesterol alone may overlook other critical factors in cardiovascular health, such as **inflammation, triglyceride levels, and LDL particle size**. For some patients, lifestyle interventions such as diet changes, regular physical activity, stress management, and targeted supplementation may offer an effective and safer alternative to statin therapy. Talk to your prescriber about alternative options.

A Balanced Perspective

It is essential for both doctors and patients to weigh the benefits and risks of statin use, particularly when prescribed for primary prevention (i.e., in patients without a history of heart disease). Understanding the potential mitochondrial implications and broader side effects of statins can lead to more informed decisions and alternative approaches for managing cholesterol and overall heart health.

Thoughts on Dietary Fats and Health

Understanding fats in their entirety—from saturated fats to trans fats—helps dismantle many of the myths that have led to widespread dietary confusion. The science is clear: not all fats are created equal. Embracing natural fats, particularly from whole, unprocessed foods, is a cornerstone of metabolic health, and the inclusion of such fats has shown benefits across various health markers, from cardiovascular health to weight management.

Incorporating a balanced perspective on fats—while avoiding processed foods, hydrogenated oils, and trans fats—leads to a diet that aligns more closely with our physiology and evolutionary needs. By focusing on whole-food sources of fat and understanding the science behind each type, individuals can make informed choices that prioritize long-term wellness.

Seed Oils: The Misleading "Heart-Healthy" Myth

In recent decades, seed oils such as soybean, corn, sunflower, and canola oil have become dietary staples. They're marketed as "heart-healthy" alternatives to saturated fats, endorsed by leading health organizations, and widely used in processed foods. Yet, despite their popularity, research is increasingly revealing the harmful effects of seed oils on health. Many of these oils carry a "heart-healthy" stamp, which consumers often take as a guarantee of their benefits, but this label is misleading. Seed oils are rich in omega-6 fatty acids, which can contribute to chronic inflammation, oxidative stress, and increased risk of metabolic diseases when consumed in excess. Understanding the reality behind seed oils and their impact on health can debunk the myths that continue to promote them as ideal cooking oils.

The Rise of Seed Oils and the "Heart-Healthy" Label

Seed oils emerged as dietary staples in the 20th century, largely due to the rise of industrialized agriculture and the push against saturated fats. As butter, lard, and coconut oil were demonized in favor of unsaturated fats, manufacturers sought affordable and scalable alternatives, which they found in seed oils. This shift was supported by studies like Ancel Keys' Seven Countries Study, which linked saturated fats to heart disease. The study, however, has been criticized for its selective data, which ignored countries with low rates of heart disease but high saturated fat intake.

To encourage the switch, health organizations like the American Heart Association (AHA) endorsed polyunsaturated fats—largely found in seed oils—as healthier for the heart. This endorsement gave rise to the "heart-healthy" label on seed oils, leading consumers to believe that these oils reduce heart disease risk. However, recent studies suggest that the health risks of seed oils may outweigh any supposed benefits, especially when they are a regular component of the diet.

The Omega-6 Problem: Inflammation and Imbalance

Seed oils are high in omega-6 fatty acids, a type of polyunsaturated fat. While omega-6 is an essential fatty acid, meaning the body requires it from food, consuming it in excessive amounts can lead to health problems. Omega-6 fats promote the production of pro-inflammatory compounds called eicosanoids. In contrast, omega-3 fatty acids, found in fatty fish, flaxseeds, and walnuts, produce anti-inflammatory eicosanoids. A balanced ratio of omega-6 to omega-3 is crucial for controlling inflammation, but the typical Western diet is heavily skewed toward omega-6, largely due to seed oils.

This imbalance contributes to chronic, low-grade inflammation, which is a precursor to numerous health issues, including heart disease, arthritis, obesity, and certain cancers. Studies have shown that populations consuming diets high in omega-6 and low in omega-3 have higher incidences of these conditions. Contrary to the "heart-healthy" claims, the inflammatory potential of omega-6 can actually increase the risk of heart disease rather than protect against it.

Oxidation and Toxicity: The Heat Sensitivity of Seed Oils

Seed oils are highly susceptible to oxidation due to their chemical structure. When oils oxidize, they produce harmful byproducts known as lipid peroxides and aldehydes, which can damage cells, DNA, and proteins in the body. This oxidative stress is linked to various chronic diseases, including cardiovascular disease and neurodegenerative conditions like Alzheimer's.

The problem with seed oils is that they are frequently used for cooking, often at high temperatures, which exacerbates their instability. High heat causes the omega-6 fats in seed oils to break down rapidly, producing toxic compounds that enter the bloodstream. Research has shown that these oxidized lipids can contribute to arterial plaque buildup, potentially increasing the risk of heart disease. Despite these risks, seed oils continue to be labeled as "heart-healthy" without clear guidelines on safe usage, misleading consumers into believing they're suitable for all cooking methods.

Misconceptions about Cholesterol and Saturated Fat

The "heart-healthy" claim for seed oils is largely based on outdated assumptions about cholesterol and saturated fat. Decades ago, cholesterol was blamed for clogging arteries and causing heart disease, leading to a widespread campaign against saturated fats. Seed oils, which contain no cholesterol and are low in saturated fat, were promoted as safe alternatives. However, recent research suggests that the relationship between cholesterol, saturated fat, and heart disease is far more complex than once believed.

Studies now indicate that saturated fats may not be the primary culprit in heart disease. Instead, factors like inflammation, oxidative stress, and the presence of small, dense LDL particles (rather than overall cholesterol levels) play a more significant role in cardiovascular risk. Unlike saturated fats, which are stable and resistant to oxidation, seed oils are prone to oxidize and create harmful compounds that can damage the arteries. The misconception that seed oils are inherently "heart-healthy" stems from outdated science that oversimplified the role of fats in heart disease.

Seed Oils and Metabolic Health: Links to Obesity and Insulin Resistance

The impact of seed oils extends beyond heart health to include metabolic conditions like obesity, insulin resistance, and diabetes. Omega-6 fatty acids, when consumed in excess, can disrupt metabolic processes and contribute to fat storage. Animal studies have shown that diets high in omega-6 fats can lead to weight gain, insulin resistance, and increased fat deposition, particularly around the liver. Although humans and animals metabolize fats differently, observational studies have linked high omega-6 intake to obesity and other metabolic diseases in humans as well.

One reason for this may be the role of linoleic acid, the primary omega-6 fatty acid in seed oils. Linoleic acid has been shown to promote the accumulation of fat cells and interfere with fat oxidation, making it harder for the body to burn stored fat. Additionally, excessive omega-6 intake can impair insulin sensitivity, which is a key factor in developing type 2 diabetes. By promoting seed oils as "heart-healthy," consumers may unknowingly be putting themselves at risk for metabolic conditions that go hand in hand with heart disease.

The Influence of Big Food and the Misleading "Heart-Healthy" Stamp

The widespread adoption of seed oils has been fueled by the influence of the food industry and its marketing strategies. Food manufacturers favor seed oils because they are cheap, abundant, and have a long shelf life. Organizations like the American Heart Association (AHA) have supported the use of seed oils, issuing guidelines that encourage replacing saturated fats with polyunsaturated fats. The "heart-healthy" label is frequently found on seed oil products, endorsed by reputable organizations, leading consumers to believe that these oils are beneficial.

However, these endorsements often fail to address the complexities of fat metabolism and ignore recent research highlighting the risks of excessive omega-6 intake. Critics argue that financial ties between health organizations and food manufacturers may play a role in these endorsements. For example, the AHA receives funding from food industry giants, raising questions about potential conflicts of interest in dietary recommendations. This relationship between industry and health organizations casts doubt on the validity of the "heart-healthy" label, as it may prioritize profit over public health.

Safer Alternatives to Seed Oils

Given the growing evidence against seed oils, many health experts advocate for the use of more stable fats in cooking and meal preparation. Oils that are less prone to oxidation include extra virgin olive oil, coconut oil, avocado oil, and animal-based fats like butter and ghee. These oils contain either monounsaturated fats (olive and avocado oil) or saturated fats (coconut oil, butter, and ghee), which are much more resistant to heat and less likely to produce harmful compounds when cooked.

Extra virgin olive oil, in particular, has been shown to have numerous health benefits, including anti-inflammatory properties, and is a staple of the Mediterranean diet, which is associated with lower rates of heart disease. Coconut oil and butter, although high in saturated fats, are more stable and less likely to oxidize at high temperatures. Switching to these alternatives can reduce exposure to the harmful byproducts of oxidized seed oils and provide healthier fats that support overall well-being.

Debunking the "Heart-Healthy" Myth of Seed Oils

The myth that seed oils are "heart-healthy" is a result of outdated science, aggressive marketing, and financial interests that have ignored the risks associated with high omega-6 intake and oil oxidation. Despite the claims made by health organizations and food manufacturers, seed oils may contribute more to chronic inflammation, metabolic issues, and oxidative stress than to cardiovascular health. The endorsement of seed oils as "heart-healthy" fails to consider the complex roles that different fats play in the body, misleading consumers into making choices that may be detrimental to their long-term health.

Understanding the true impact of seed oils and choosing healthier, more stable fats can help protect against the risks associated with a high omega-6 diet. By debunking the myth of the "heart-healthy" seed oil, we can promote more accurate, evidence-based dietary recommendations that support true cardiovascular health and overall well-being. For those looking to improve their health, reducing seed oils and incorporating more natural, stable fats is a crucial step toward a balanced, nourishing diet.

Calories in-Calories Out

This is something that has been said in gyms, dietitians' offices, doctor's offices, and anywhere you would have thought you can get reliable healthy information. Wrong. A calorie is not a calorie, and there's no way you can use this formula and be genuine about it. Calories come from different places, and act in different ways, depending on the origin.

Different types of calories—like those from refined carbs versus fats—have unique metabolic effects, impacting insulin, hunger hormones, and fat storage. For example, calories from sugars can promote insulin spikes and increase fat storage more than calories from protein or fats, leading to greater hunger and cravings. Furthermore, stress, sleep quality, gut health, and the body's adaptation to calorie intake can all alter how efficiently the body uses or stores energy. This is why focusing solely on calories disregards important hormonal and metabolic feedback mechanisms that influence body composition.

The CICO model posits that weight gain or loss depends solely on the difference between calories consumed and calories burned. At a basic level, if you consume more calories than you burn, you gain weight; if you burn more than you consume, you lose weight. However, this model doesn't account for the complexities of metabolism, hormone responses, or the quality and type of calories consumed.

Different macronutrients (carbs, fats, proteins) have distinct effects on the body's hormonal responses and metabolic processes:

Insulin Response: Carbohydrates, especially refined sugars, cause more significant insulin spikes than fats or proteins. Insulin promotes fat storage, so consuming high-carb, low-fat foods may lead to weight gain despite caloric balance due to frequent insulin responses and subsequent fat storage.

Thermic Effect of Food (TEF): The energy used to digest, absorb, and metabolize food varies by macronutrient. Protein, for example, has a higher thermic effect than fats and carbs, meaning it requires more energy to process and can slightly increase metabolic rate.

Hunger and Satiety: Caloric intake affects hunger hormones like ghrelin and leptin. High-calorie foods with low nutrient density can fail to satisfy hunger, leading to overeating, while nutrient-dense foods help regulate hunger more effectively.

The Role of Metabolism and Individual Factors

The body's metabolic rate adjusts to caloric intake over time—a process called metabolic adaptation. If calories are restricted for an extended period, the body can lower its energy expenditure to preserve fat stores, making sustained weight loss harder. Factors like genetics, sleep quality, stress, and even gut health can influence metabolic rate and how efficiently calories are utilized.

The Bigger Picture: Quality Over Quantity

A refined approach to weight management focuses on **nutrient quality and hormonal impact**, rather than just calorie counting. For example, whole foods, rich in fiber and protein, support satiety and stable blood sugar, which reduce cravings and overeating, whereas processed, sugary foods may increase fat storage and hunger. Don't let this mislead you into nutritional ignorance. Calories do matter, but not the way you might think.

Myth: Whole Grains are Healthy

So this is another myth that is absolutely ridiculous. "ancient gains"? "whole grains"? none of it is as good as you think. A box of your favorite breakfast cereal says "heart healthy" with an endorsement from the AHA (American Heart Association). I call BS.

Whole Grains: The Full Picture

Whole grains, such as oats, brown rice, and quinoa, are marketed as health-promoting foods due to their fiber and micronutrient content. However, it's essential to look deeper into their effects on metabolic health. Whole grains contain bran, germ, and endosperm—parts of the grain that offer vitamins, minerals, and fiber, which are stripped away in refined grains. Yet, not all whole grains are equal in health benefits, and their impact on blood sugar and insulin varies depending on the type and form consumed.

The Insulin Response

Although whole grains contain fiber, which can slow digestion, they still cause a significant insulin response due to their carbohydrate content. Regular consumption of high-carbohydrate grains can lead to frequent insulin spikes, similar to other carbohydrates, which over time may contribute to insulin resistance and metabolic syndrome.

Anti-Nutrients and Digestibility

Whole grains also contain anti-nutrients, like phytic acid, which can inhibit the absorption of essential minerals such as iron, zinc, and magnesium. Additionally, lectins in grains may irritate the gut lining in some individuals, leading to inflammation or digestive issues, especially if consumed in large amounts without proper preparation (like soaking or fermenting).

The Bioavailability of Nutrients

The nutrients in whole grains are not always fully bioavailable, meaning the body might not absorb them effectively due to these anti-nutrients. For individuals with specific metabolic goals or sensitivities, other nutrient-dense options may offer the same minerals and fiber without the associated insulin response or anti-nutrient concerns.

Whole Grains vs. Refined Grains

While whole grains are generally more nutritious than refined grains, they should still be consumed mindfully. Incorporating a variety of whole, lower-carbohydrate foods like certain low oxalate vegetables can often achieve the same fiber and nutrient benefits without the drawbacks of high insulin and blood sugar spikes that come with frequent grain consumption.

More on this in the section about the human diet.

Oatmeal has long been marketed as a "heart-healthy" breakfast staple, praised for its fiber content and cholesterol-lowering claims. However, the reality behind oatmeal's health profile is less favorable than many people realize. The idea that oatmeal is an ideal health food is often based on outdated or oversimplified nutrition science that doesn't account for the body's actual response to processed grains. Oatmeal, particularly the quick-cooking and instant varieties, is high in carbohydrates that rapidly break down into glucose, spiking blood sugar and insulin levels. This can lead to energy crashes and hunger shortly after eating, driving cravings and overconsumption. Over time, these blood sugar fluctuations may contribute to insulin resistance and weight gain, challenging the myth of oatmeal as a sustainable breakfast choice.

Moreover, oatmeal is high in anti-nutrients like phytic acid, which can inhibit the absorption of essential minerals such as iron, calcium, and zinc. This is particularly concerning for individuals who rely on grains like oats as a primary food source, as these anti-nutrients can lead to mineral deficiencies over time. Additionally, most commercial oatmeal products are heavily processed and often come with added sugars, artificial flavors, and preservatives, further reducing any potential health benefits. The "heart-healthy" label on oatmeal is largely a marketing tactic, ignoring these downsides and promoting oatmeal as an ideal food despite its potential to disrupt blood sugar, hinder nutrient absorption, and contribute to energy imbalances. For those seeking true health, more nutrient-dense, low-glycemic foods like eggs, avocados, and high-quality proteins can provide a more balanced and satiating start to the day.

Medication and the Reliance of Big Pharma

It's hard to discuss modern healthcare without examining the powerful role Big Pharma plays in shaping health outcomes. At the expense of sounding like a conspiracy theorist, the pharmaceutical industry, with its tremendous influence, has shaped the healthcare system in ways that arguably prioritize profit over genuine health solutions. Pharmaceutical companies wield significant control, shaping everything from medical education to the treatments doctors prescribe. Understanding how Big Pharma operates sheds light on why nearly **85% of medications prescribed today could potentially be replaced with lifestyle and dietary changes.**

Profit-Driven Motives

The pharmaceutical industry is one of the most profitable in the world, valued at nearly **$1.3 trillion globally**. Leading companies like Pfizer, Johnson & Johnson, and Roche earn billions in annual revenue—profits that hinge on a constant demand for medications. To maintain or increase profits, Big Pharma has a vested interest in promoting long-term medication use over sustainable health solutions. They benefit from patients managing symptoms rather than addressing the root causes of health issues. Medications for chronic conditions like hypertension, diabetes, and high cholesterol are often marketed as lifelong treatments, even when evidence suggests many cases could be managed or reversed through diet and lifestyle changes.

Influence on Medical Education and Research

Pharmaceutical companies also wield influence over medical education and research. Many medical schools rely on funding from Big Pharma, and studies have shown that the curricula often emphasize pharmacology over nutrition and lifestyle-based treatments. Doctors, therefore, are well-versed in prescribing medications but may lack a deep understanding of dietary and lifestyle approaches to managing health issues. Further, research funded by pharmaceutical companies often has a bias toward producing favorable results for drugs. An analysis of clinical trials found that **industry-sponsored trials were significantly more likely to report positive outcomes** compared to non-industry-sponsored studies, calling into question the objectivity of much of the data driving medication use.

The Decline of Health: Masking Symptoms Instead of Curing Diseases

The reliance on pharmaceutical treatments has contributed to the decline of overall health in modern society. Chronic diseases such as heart disease, diabetes, and obesity are at all-time highs, with many patients receiving medications that manage symptoms rather than resolve underlying health issues. For example, statins are commonly prescribed to lower cholesterol, but recent research suggests that cholesterol is not necessarily the root cause of heart disease—chronic inflammation and insulin resistance play significant roles. Instead of promoting dietary solutions to reduce inflammation, pharmaceutical companies push statins as the primary solution. This approach fails to address the true causes of the disease, leaving patients on lifelong medication without genuinely improving their health.

The Dietary Solution: 85% of Prescriptions Could Be Avoided

A growing body of evidence suggests that **85% of medications prescribed today could be replaced with dietary and lifestyle interventions**. For instance:

Diabetes: Type 2 diabetes is primarily driven by diet, specifically by excessive carbohydrate and sugar intake that causes chronic insulin spikes. Studies show that low-carb, high-fat diets can reverse Type 2 diabetes, yet metformin and insulin remain standard treatments.

Hypertension: High blood pressure is often treated with beta-blockers or ACE inhibitors, but a diet low in processed foods and rich in potassium can naturally lower blood pressure by reducing sodium retention and improving vascular health.

Cholesterol and Heart Disease: Statins are the standard for lowering cholesterol, but new research points to the benefits of anti-inflammatory diets that reduce arterial inflammation, a significant contributor to heart disease risk. Healthy fats, such as those found in fish and olive oil, saturated fat, along with reduced sugar intake, can naturally balance homeostasis without medication.

The Path Forward: Reclaiming Health Through Diet

The path to reclaiming public health starts with empowering people to make informed choices about diet and lifestyle. For too long, the healthcare system has treated symptoms with medications rather than addressing the core causes of health issues. A greater emphasis on whole foods, lower carbohydrate intake, and avoiding processed foods would lead to reduced inflammation, better insulin sensitivity, and overall improved metabolic health.

Educating the public and advocating for a shift away from medication dependency toward dietary and lifestyle solutions requires both transparency and systemic change. Organizations, policymakers, and medical professionals must prioritize patient health over pharmaceutical profits and recognize the power of food as medicine. By doing so, we could potentially reduce the prevalence of chronic diseases, minimize medication reliance, and improve quality of life across populations.

"Superfoods and Veganism"

The concept of "superfoods" has become a pervasive part of modern dietary culture, but its roots and reality are not as wholesome as many believe. The term was initially coined as a marketing strategy rather than a genuine health term, used to promote grains, fruits, and other plant-based foods under the guise of being nutrient-dense and essential for health. While grains, fruits, and vegetables can provide beneficial nutrients, most of these nutrients aren't fully bioavailable to the body. Bioavailability refers to how well a nutrient can be absorbed and utilized by the body, and many of the vitamins and minerals in plant-based "superfoods" are bound to anti-nutrients, such as oxalates and phytates, which hinder absorption. Thus, foods marketed as superfoods often fail to deliver on their nutritional promises, especially when compared to animal-based foods.

The Reality Behind "Superfoods"

The superfood label has been particularly effective in boosting sales of products like blueberries, chia seeds, quinoa, kale, and acai berries. While these foods do have beneficial properties, they lack essential nutrients in forms that are bioavailable. For instance, iron in spinach or other leafy greens is non-heme iron, which is much less efficiently absorbed by the body than heme iron found in meat. Moreover, plant sources of omega-3 fatty acids, like chia or flaxseeds, contain alpha-linolenic acid (ALA), which must be converted in the body to the active forms, EPA and DHA. This conversion process is inefficient in humans, making it challenging to get sufficient omega-3 from plant sources alone.

Animal-Based Superfoods: The Real Nutrient Powerhouses

In contrast, animal-based foods, particularly organ meats and egg yolks, provide a density and diversity of nutrients that are highly bioavailable, meaning the body can absorb and utilize them with much greater efficiency. Organ meats such as liver, kidney, and heart contain vast amounts of essential nutrients like vitamin A, B vitamins (especially B12), iron, zinc, and copper, in highly absorbable forms. Liver, for example, is one of the richest sources of vitamin A, an essential nutrient for vision, immunity, and reproduction, and it is present as retinol, which is the form our bodies can directly utilize.

Egg yolks are another example of an animal-based superfood. They contain essential fatty acids, choline (crucial for brain health), and high-quality proteins. Unlike plant proteins, animal proteins contain a full profile of essential amino acids, making them "complete" proteins. Additionally, egg yolks provide lutein and zeaxanthin, which support eye health, in forms that are immediately available for absorption.

Meat and the Myth of Plant-Based Superfoods

Animal products also come without the anti-nutritional factors present in many plant foods. For example, the oxalates in leafy greens can bind with calcium, potentially contributing to kidney stones. Phytates in grains and legumes inhibit the absorption of minerals like magnesium, calcium, and iron, limiting the body's access to these nutrients. While there are plant foods that can supplement a diet, animal products generally provide these nutrients in forms that do not come with such absorption blockers, making them more reliable sources for meeting human nutritional needs.

The Vegan Diet: Nutritional Gaps and Risks

Veganism has become increasingly popular, often promoted for health, ethical, and environmental reasons. However, the vegan diet can come with significant nutritional risks if not meticulously planned. For example, vitamin B12, which is vital for neurological health and blood formation, is virtually absent in plant foods. Deficiency in B12 can lead to irreversible nerve damage and cognitive decline, and this vitamin must typically be supplemented in vegan diets.

Additionally, essential fatty acids, as mentioned, are challenging to obtain in usable forms from plant foods alone. DHA, an omega-3 fatty acid crucial for brain function, is most readily available in fatty fish and other animal sources. Vegan diets, unless supplemented with algae-based DHA, may fail to provide adequate amounts of these fatty acids, potentially impacting brain health over time.

Iron is another concern for vegans, as plant-based iron is poorly absorbed compared to the iron in meat. Vegan diets are also generally lower in zinc, an essential mineral for immune health, and in choline, which supports brain and liver function. While these nutrients can be supplemented, the reliance on synthetic supplementation highlights a gap in the diet's natural completeness.

Ethical Considerations: The Order of Nature

The promotion of animal-based foods, however, does not disregard the importance of ethical and humane treatment of animals. Ethical omnivores advocate for responsible sourcing, sustainable practices, and respect for animal welfare. Recognizing the nutritional role of animal products does not mean endorsing cruelty but rather understanding the role of animals in the human food chain, as has been a natural order for millennia. Meat and animal products have always been essential in human diets, providing sustenance that plants alone cannot fully replicate.

In sum, the concept of "superfoods" is more a product of marketing than of science. While fruits and vegetables have their place in a balanced diet, their nutrients are not as accessible to the body as those found in animal-based foods, particularly organ meats and eggs. Furthermore, the vegan diet, while sustainable for some when properly supplemented, carries inherent risks due to its lack of naturally bioavailable essential nutrients. In future discussions, we'll explore how a balanced approach to eating can meet ethical and nutritional needs without compromising on health. The real "superfoods," from a bioavailability standpoint, are found in well-sourced animal products, not in the trendy foods that often carry the label today.

Meat and Religion

A common myth surrounding dietary practices is that many of the world's major religions discourage or outright forbid the consumption of meat. This idea is rooted in a misunderstanding of religious doctrines and an oversimplification of nuanced dietary laws. While certain religious beliefs encourage vegetarianism or place restrictions on the types and preparation of meat, most major religions do not fundamentally oppose meat consumption. Instead, they emphasize ethical guidelines, moderation, and respect for life, often framing meat consumption within a context of spiritual mindfulness. By exploring the actual stances of religions like Christianity, Judaism, Islam, Hinduism, and Buddhism, we can debunk the myth that meat is largely forbidden by religion and understand the broader role it plays in religious and cultural contexts.

Christianity and the Misconception of Meat Abstention

Christianity, in particular, is often mistakenly viewed as discouraging meat consumption. Some interpret Biblical teachings to imply that humans were meant to adopt a vegetarian diet, referencing passages like Genesis 1:29, where God gives Adam and Eve plants for food. However, this interpretation overlooks subsequent passages, such as Genesis 9:3, where God expands human diet to include meat, stating, "Every moving thing that lives shall be food for you." This permission came after the Flood, indicating a shift in dietary norms that permitted the consumption of animals alongside plant foods. This shift signifies that Christianity does not condemn meat consumption; rather, it frames dietary choices as permissible, provided they are accompanied by gratitude and respect.

Further evidence that Christianity does not discourage meat is found in the New Testament, where Jesus is depicted eating fish with his disciples (Luke 24:42-43), and lamb is traditionally part of the Passover meal, which Christians also observe. While some Christian sects and individuals choose to adopt vegetarianism or veganism as a means of compassion or personal choice, these practices are not doctrinally mandated. For many Christians, abstaining from certain meats during periods like Lent or practicing fasting on specific days is a form of discipline rather than a condemnation of meat. These practices reinforce a commitment to spiritual growth and self-control rather than suggesting that meat is intrinsically wrong or unhealthy.

The myth that Christianity opposes meat likely arises from individual interpretations rather than church teachings. Some modern Christians advocate vegetarianism based on compassion for animals or health concerns, but this is more of a personal or ethical choice than a religious requirement. Ultimately, Christianity leaves the choice of meat consumption open, underscoring the importance of moderation and thankfulness rather than restriction.

Judaism: Kosher Laws and the Principle of Ethical Eating

Judaism's dietary laws are often perceived as restrictive, leading some to believe that Jewish teachings discourage or disapprove of meat consumption. This misunderstanding stems from the complexity of kosher laws, which govern what kinds of meat can be eaten and how animals must be slaughtered. However, Judaism does not discourage eating meat; rather, it provides a framework that ensures meat consumption aligns with ethical and religious principles. Kosher laws, known as Kashrut, specify which animals are permitted (such as cattle, sheep, and poultry) and prohibit others (like pork and shellfish). This distinction is often misinterpreted as a ban on meat when, in reality, it is a guideline intended to elevate the act of eating to a mindful, respectful practice.

One of the critical aspects of Kashrut is **shechita**, the ritual slaughter process, which emphasizes humane treatment of animals. Shechita requires that animals be slaughtered quickly and with as little pain as possible, aligning with the Jewish value of Tza'ar Ba'alei Chayim, which discourages unnecessary suffering. Kosher laws do not prohibit meat but instead encourage ethical practices around its consumption, promoting the idea that life is sacred and should be respected, even in death. Rather than discouraging meat, these laws sanctify the act of eating, transforming it from a mundane activity to one of religious significance.

Judaism also contains various teachings that encourage thoughtful consumption of meat. For example, on Shabbat and during festivals, eating meat is traditionally seen as a way to celebrate God's blessings. However, meat is not to be eaten casually or wastefully; instead, it is viewed as a privilege and a gift, to be enjoyed with

93

gratitude and reverence. This distinction shows that Judaism's relationship with meat is about promoting awareness, ethical practices, and mindfulness rather than abstention or condemnation.

Islam: Halal and the Balance of Moderation

Islam, like Judaism, has dietary laws that specify the types of meat that are permissible and the methods by which they should be prepared. The concept of **halal** (permissible) encompasses not only the type of food but also the way in which it is sourced and prepared. Halal meat must come from animals that are slaughtered humanely, with a prayer invoked in God's name at the time of slaughter. This practice serves as a reminder of the sanctity of life and the interconnectedness between human beings, animals, and God. While some mistakenly view these laws as discouraging meat consumption, Islam permits and even encourages meat within the framework of respect and compassion.

Prophet Muhammad often advocated for moderation in all aspects of life, including diet. Islam encourages balance and advises against overindulgence in food, promoting health and spiritual well-being. Meat is regarded as a nutritious and beneficial part of the diet, but one that should not be consumed in excess or with disregard for the animal's life. By incorporating practices of humane slaughter and restraint, Islam aligns meat consumption with spiritual values, underscoring that food choices should respect creation and contribute to personal and community well-being.

The idea that Islam is opposed to meat is a misconception; rather, it values responsible consumption. Halal laws do not limit or discourage eating meat but ensure that it is done in a way that aligns with Islamic values. By fostering gratitude, respect, and compassion, these dietary laws uphold the importance of viewing food as a blessing, reminding Muslims to be mindful of the impact of their choices.

Hinduism: Ahimsa and the Nuanced Approach to Meat Consumption

In Hinduism, the principle of **Ahimsa** (non-violence) has led to the widespread adoption of vegetarianism among followers, with many Hindus choosing to avoid meat to prevent harm to living beings. This focus on non-violence is often mistaken as a religious prohibition against meat, but Hinduism's approach to diet is complex and regionally diverse. While vegetarianism is encouraged, it is not universally mandated, and some Hindus consume meat, particularly in regions where dietary customs include fish and other meats. Additionally, Hindu dietary practices can vary widely based on caste, sect, and personal choice, demonstrating that meat consumption is not wholly discouraged.

In Hindu tradition, cows are considered sacred and should not be harmed or eaten, contributing to the perception that Hinduism opposes all forms of meat. However, this prohibition specifically pertains to beef, reflecting the cow's symbolic role as a nurturing figure in Indian culture. Other meats are not necessarily forbidden, and individuals may choose their diet based on personal beliefs and regional customs. Hinduism's emphasis on self-discipline and respect for life extends to all food choices, whether vegetarian or not, encouraging followers to consider the ethical and spiritual implications of their diet.

While Hinduism highly values vegetarianism, it also respects personal choice and cultural variation. The myth that Hinduism entirely forbids meat fails to recognize the diversity of practices within the religion, where individuals and communities make dietary choices based on personal, spiritual, and cultural factors.

Buddhism: The Middle Path and Dietary Flexibility

Buddhism's stance on meat consumption is often associated with non-violence, leading many to assume that Buddhists are universally vegetarian. However, Buddhism, much like Hinduism, varies widely in its dietary practices. The **Middle Path** in Buddhism encourages moderation and discourages extremes, including rigid dietary restrictions. While the First Precept advises Buddhists to avoid harming living beings, interpretations of this precept differ among Buddhist traditions. For instance, Mahayana Buddhism often promotes vegetarianism as a way to avoid harming animals, but Theravada Buddhism is more flexible, allowing monks to eat meat offered to them, provided the animal was not killed specifically for them.

This diversity of practice highlights that vegetarianism in Buddhism is a personal choice rather than a universal rule. The Buddha himself did not explicitly forbid meat, and in many Buddhist cultures, meat consumption is common and accepted. The emphasis in Buddhism is on intention, mindfulness, and compassion in all actions, including eating, rather than an outright prohibition of meat.

The myth that Buddhism forbids meat is largely due to the prominence of vegetarianism in some sects, but Buddhism's approach to diet allows for flexibility based on personal choice and cultural norms. The focus remains on reducing suffering and practicing compassion, but how this is achieved can vary greatly among practitioners.

Debunking the Myth: Religion's Emphasis on Mindful and Ethical Eating

The myth that religion universally condemns meat is rooted in a misunderstanding of dietary laws and ethical practices. While many religions emphasize respect for life and encourage mindful eating, most do not outright forbid meat. Instead, they provide frameworks that ensure ethical treatment, moderation, and gratitude. Christianity, Judaism, Islam, Hinduism, and Buddhism each incorporate values of respect, compassion, and responsibility, offering followers the freedom to make dietary choices that align with their personal beliefs and cultural practices.

Ultimately, the idea that meat is forbidden across religions is a myth that oversimplifies complex doctrines. By understanding the true teachings of these religions, we can appreciate that they support a balanced approach to food, where meat consumption is often permitted and encouraged when done with mindfulness and respect. This view not only allows for personal freedom but also promotes health and spiritual well-being in a way that honors both cultural heritage and ethical principles.

Biblical Foundations for Meat Consumption

The Role of Animal Foods in the Bible:

Old Testament: The Bible contains numerous references to the consumption of animal products. In **Genesis 9:3**, after the Great Flood, God explicitly permits Noah and his descendants to eat meat: *"Every moving thing that lives shall be food for you. And as I gave you the green plants, I give you everything."* This passage underscores that meat consumption was seen as acceptable and even a provision from God.

Sacrificial Practices: In the Old Testament, animal sacrifices were part of worship, and certain parts of the animal were consumed by priests and the people, showing that meat was an integral part of religious and social practices.

New Testament Teachings:

Jesus and Meat: Jesus Himself consumed meat and fish, demonstrating that animal products were part of a righteous diet. **Luke 24:42-43** records Jesus eating fish with His disciples after His resurrection: *"They gave him a piece of broiled fish, and he took it and ate before them."* This illustrates that eating meat was consistent with Jesus' actions.

No Dietary Restrictions in the New Covenant: In **Mark 7:18-19**, Jesus declares all foods clean, emphasizing that dietary laws should not be a barrier to faith. This passage implies that Christians are not restricted from eating any type of food, including meat.

Christianity and the Value of Creation

Dominion and Stewardship:

The Bible teaches that humans were given **dominion over animals**. In **Genesis 1:28**, God commands Adam and Eve to "subdue" the earth and rule over the animals. This dominion suggests responsible stewardship, which can include the ethical use of animals for food. Christians can interpret this as a call to treat animals with respect while recognizing their role in human nourishment.

Animal Sacrifices as a Foreshadowing:

The use of animals in sacrificial rites, as seen in Leviticus and other Old Testament books, symbolizes that animals hold a significant place in God's creation and can be used to fulfill His purposes. While these sacrifices were primarily spiritual, they reinforce the idea that animals were viewed as an essential part of life and sustenance.

Spiritual Nourishment and Physical Health

The Body as a Temple:

1 Corinthians 6:19-20 states: *"Do you not know that your body is a temple of the Holy Spirit within you, whom you have from God? You are not your own, for you were bought with a price. So glorify God in your body."* This verse highlights the importance of caring for one's body as a gift from God. Proponents of the carnivore diet argue that animal-based foods are nutrient-dense and align with the goal of maintaining optimal health, thus honoring God through the care of one's body.

Spiritual and Physical Alignment:

Eating a diet that promotes health and well-being can be seen as fulfilling one's duty to maintain the body as a vessel for service to God. The carnivore diet, which emphasizes nutrient-dense foods such as meat, organs, and animal fats, can support this goal by providing essential vitamins, minerals, and proteins that are crucial for bodily function and vitality.

Misconceptions and Clarifications

Misinterpretation of Vegetarianism:

Some may argue that the Bible supports a plant-based diet based on **Genesis 1:29**, which refers to God giving plants for food. However, this verse pertains to the initial creation before the fall of man and subsequent changes in diet. After the flood in Genesis 9, the permission to consume animal flesh broadens the biblical dietary framework.

Dietary Choice and Christian Freedom:

Romans 14:2-3 states: *"One person believes he may eat anything, while the weak person eats only vegetables. Let not the one who eats despise the one who abstains, and let not the one who abstains pass judgment on the one who eats, for God has welcomed him."* This underscores that dietary choices should not be a point of contention among Christians, allowing for the freedom to choose a diet that aligns with individual beliefs and health needs.

The carnivore diet can be seen as aligning with Christian teachings by acknowledging the biblical acceptance of meat consumption, emphasizing the stewardship of God's creation, and supporting the goal of maintaining the body as a temple. While there is room for varied interpretations within Christianity, the allowance and respect for a diet that includes animal products are deeply rooted in Scripture and tradition. This understanding can foster a perspective that eating animal-based foods is not only permissible but can be a thoughtful way to honor the body and nourish the spirit.

Fruits: Overrated, Misunderstood, Modified, and Dangerous

Fruit has long been considered a staple of a healthy diet, touted for its vitamins, fiber, and antioxidants. However, the way fruit is consumed today has dramatically shifted from its original purpose, leading to potentially harmful effects on metabolic health. Understanding the evolutionary role of fruit, its modern modifications, and its impact on conditions such as non-alcoholic fatty liver disease (NAFLD) can help unravel the myths that surround its perceived health benefits.

The Original Role of Fruit in Human Diets

Historically, fruit was consumed seasonally, often during late summer and early fall when it was naturally available. This seasonal consumption provided bursts of energy and nutrition to prepare the body for the scarcity of food during winter months. Our ancestors relied on these short-term sources of fructose to signal the body to store energy as fat, a vital mechanism for surviving periods of food shortage. The occasional intake of fruit aligned with the natural cycles of harvest and hibernation.

Modern Modifications and Their Impact

Today, fruit has been bred and genetically modified to be larger, sweeter, and available year-round. These modifications, driven by agricultural advancements, have fundamentally altered the nutritional profile of fruit. The wild fruits our ancestors consumed were smaller, less sweet, and contained more fiber relative to their sugar content. Modern fruits, in contrast, are packed with higher amounts of fructose and glucose, which contribute to their sweet taste and larger size.

The implications of these changes are significant. Fructose, a type of sugar found abundantly in modern fruit, is metabolized exclusively by the liver. Unlike glucose, which is processed by nearly all body cells, fructose overloads the liver and can lead to fat accumulation, contributing to NAFLD. This condition, once rare, is now prevalent and closely linked to diets high in fructose, whether from processed sugars or excessive fruit consumption.

Fruit is not a "Superfood"

The widespread belief that fruit is a "superfood" has led many people to consume it in large quantities, under the impression that it can only benefit their health. We all know someone who proudly claims to "love fruit" and eats it throughout the day, believing it is the healthiest choice. This perception has been reinforced by decades of dietary advice that emphasizes fruits as a primary source of vitamins and natural sugars. While fruit does contain beneficial nutrients, its unchecked consumption poses risks that are often overlooked.

Fructose metabolism is unique in that it bypasses the normal regulatory pathways that control energy use. When consumed in high amounts, fructose tells the body to store energy as fat—a mechanism that would have been useful in ancient times to prepare for the winter. However, in the modern world, where food scarcity is no longer an issue, this storage leads to excess body fat and metabolic disorders.

The Hidden Dangers of Excessive Fruit Consumption

The metabolic pathway of fructose is particularly problematic because it contributes directly to fat synthesis in the liver. When consumed in large quantities, especially in combination with other macronutrients like fats, it can lead to advanced glycation end-products (AGEs), which are compounds that result from sugars binding to proteins and fats. This process, known as glycation, damages tissues and accelerates aging, contributing to chronic diseases such as diabetes and cardiovascular issues.

Furthermore, fruit is often consumed with high-fat foods—a combination that can exacerbate insulin resistance and amplify the storage of fat. This pattern of eating runs counter to the body's natural mechanisms for maintaining metabolic balance. The body's response to a sudden influx of fructose signals that it should store energy, creating an environment where fat accumulates without the subsequent winter-induced energy expenditure that would historically follow.

Rethinking the Role of Fruit in Diets

Modern society has been conditioned to view fruit as an unquestioned pillar of health. However, it is important to re-examine how fruit fits into a balanced diet. The evolutionary purpose of fruit was to aid in energy storage for times of scarcity—a scenario that no longer aligns with the year-round abundance most people experience. While occasional, moderate consumption of fruit can still be part of a healthy diet, eating it in excess under the guise of it being a "superfood" can contribute to metabolic imbalances, fat accumulation, and chronic diseases.

Dietary habits that prioritize constant fruit intake, particularly when combined with processed sugars and unhealthy fats, disrupt the natural metabolic processes. They send signals to the body to store energy as fat while creating conditions ripe for glycation and oxidative stress.

Understanding the true role of fruit in human health requires acknowledging its seasonal purpose, recognizing the effects of its modern modifications, and re-evaluating how it should be consumed in today's context. The idea that fruit is universally healthy has been ingrained in dietary culture, leading to excessive and potentially harmful consumption. The liver's exclusive role in fructose metabolism, coupled with the body's tendency to store fat in response, makes high fruit intake particularly risky. Reevaluating our approach to fruit consumption can promote better metabolic health and reduce the risk of conditions such as NAFLD, obesity, and insulin resistance. While fruit can still be enjoyed, it should be eaten mindfully and seasonally, with an awareness of its impact on overall health.

Fruit Juice is Absolute Garbage

Fruit juice has become a staple in many diets, marketed as a healthy and natural beverage packed with vitamins and nutrients. However, the reality of fruit juice consumption is far from its perceived benefits. While whole fruits have their drawbacks when consumed in excess, they still contain fiber that moderates the body's absorption

101

of sugars. In contrast, fruit juice strips away the only redeeming quality of whole fruit—fiber—and delivers a concentrated dose of sugar that can have detrimental effects on health. This section will explore the issues surrounding fruit juice consumption, its impact on metabolic health, and why it is one of the most misleading components of a so-called healthy diet.

The Problem with Fruit Juice: A Nutritional Perspective

Fruit juices, whether freshly squeezed or commercially processed, are essentially sugar-laden liquids devoid of the fiber that whole fruit contains. Fiber plays a crucial role in the body's metabolic response to sugar. It slows down the absorption of glucose and fructose in the digestive system, preventing sudden spikes in blood sugar and mitigating the strain on the liver. When the fiber is removed, as is the case with fruit juice, the body is left to deal with a flood of fructose, which must be processed by the liver.

The liver metabolizes fructose differently than glucose. While glucose can be utilized by almost every cell in the body for energy, fructose is primarily processed by the liver, where it is converted into triglycerides and stored as fat. This rapid influx of fructose taxes the liver and contributes to non-alcoholic fatty liver disease (NAFLD), a condition that has become increasingly common in both adults and children.

Juice as an Unhealthy Staple in Schools and Hospitals

One of the most troubling aspects of fruit juice consumption is its prevalence in settings that are meant to promote health, such as schools and hospitals. Juice is often served as part of a balanced meal or offered as a healthy alternative to soda. However, this practice perpetuates the misconception that juice is beneficial when, in reality, it contributes to a range of metabolic health issues. The routine consumption of fruit juice, especially among children, sets the stage for lifelong patterns of sugar overconsumption and metabolic imbalance.

Serving juice in schools is particularly problematic. Children's bodies are still developing, and establishing healthy dietary habits at a young age is crucial for long-term health. By serving juice in school cafeterias, educational institutions are effectively conditioning young palates to prefer sweet beverages, reinforcing the notion that juice is a healthy choice. This habit can extend into adulthood, where individuals continue to consume fruit juice, unaware of its potential harm. The high sugar content in juice can lead to weight gain, insulin resistance, and an increased risk of developing type 2 diabetes.

The Liver's Burden: Why Juice Taxes Your Body

The liver plays a central role in the metabolism of fructose. When fruit juice is consumed, the liver must work overtime to process the large amount of sugar it receives. Unlike whole fruits, where the fiber content slows down the absorption process, juice delivers an immediate load of fructose. This sudden influx can overwhelm the liver's ability to process the sugar efficiently, leading to the conversion of excess fructose into fat. Over time, this process contributes to the accumulation of fat in liver cells, which can progress to NAFLD.

NAFLD is a serious condition that affects millions of people worldwide. It is characterized by the buildup of fat in the liver without the presence of significant alcohol consumption. One of the main culprits behind the rise in NAFLD is the overconsumption of fructose, particularly from sources like fruit juice. The condition can lead to liver inflammation, fibrosis, and, in severe cases, cirrhosis or liver failure. The fact that fruit juice, a product often marketed as a health drink, can contribute to such serious health issues highlights the need for a reevaluation of its role in our diets.

Juice Consumption and Weight Gain

Another critical issue with fruit juice is its contribution to weight gain. Fruit juice is often consumed in large quantities because it is perceived as "healthy." Unlike whole fruit, which contains fiber and requires more time and effort to eat, juice can be consumed quickly and in large amounts. A single glass of orange juice, for example, may contain the sugar equivalent of four to five whole oranges. Most people would not eat that many oranges in one sitting, but they can easily drink that amount of juice without feeling full.

This ease of consumption leads to a higher intake of calories without the feeling of satiety that comes from eating whole fruit. The rapid absorption of sugar from juice also triggers a quick release of insulin, the hormone responsible for managing blood sugar levels. Frequent spikes in insulin can lead to insulin resistance over time, a condition that is closely associated with weight gain, obesity, and type 2 diabetes.

The Glycation Process and Chronic Disease

The high sugar content in fruit juice contributes not only to liver fat storage but also to the formation of advanced glycation end-products (AGEs). Glycation occurs when sugars bind to proteins or lipids in the body, leading to the formation of harmful compounds that accelerate aging and contribute to chronic diseases such as diabetes, cardiovascular disease, and even neurodegenerative conditions. The combination of high sugar and the absence of fiber in fruit juice exacerbates this process, making it particularly damaging when consumed regularly.

The glycation process is one of the lesser-discussed consequences of excessive sugar consumption, but it has significant implications for health. AGEs can damage tissues and organs, promote inflammation, and interfere with normal cellular function. The chronic intake of fruit juice, therefore, not only stresses the liver but also sets the stage for systemic inflammation and long-term damage throughout the body.

Mixing Juice with High-Fat Foods: A Recipe for Disaster

One dietary pattern that compounds the negative effects of fruit juice is the tendency to consume it alongside high-fat foods. This combination can worsen insulin resistance and amplify fat storage. The body's metabolic response to a meal that includes both high sugar and fat is more pronounced, leading to increased triglyceride levels and greater fat accumulation. When fruit juice is consumed with foods that are already high in unhealthy fats, such as pastries or fried snacks, the risk of developing metabolic syndrome and related conditions is heightened.

Why Fruit Juice Should Not Be Considered Healthy

Despite the pervasive belief that fruit juice is a healthy alternative to sugary drinks, its nutritional profile tells a different story. The absence of fiber, the high concentration of fructose, and its rapid absorption make juice a poor choice for maintaining metabolic health. The fact that juice is served in schools and hospitals further complicates public perception, as these institutions are seen as authorities on health. Promoting fruit juice as a healthy option undermines efforts to improve public health and combat obesity and metabolic diseases.

Fruit juice is often viewed as a natural source of vitamins, particularly vitamin C, which is essential for immune function and skin health. However, the vitamin content does not offset the detrimental effects of the high sugar load. If vitamin C is the primary concern, it can be obtained from other sources that do not carry the same metabolic risks, such as leafy greens, bell peppers, and berries.

Re-evaluating the Place of Juice in Diets

For those seeking to improve their health, it is crucial to rethink the role of fruit juice in their diets. While whole fruits, when eaten in moderation, can provide beneficial nutrients and fiber, fruit juice should be viewed more critically. The practice of serving juice in schools, hospitals, and even at home needs to be reconsidered, as it reinforces unhealthy consumption patterns that contribute to metabolic dysfunction.

Replacing juice with water, herbal teas, or even whole fruits that contain fiber can help mitigate the risks associated with excessive sugar intake. Public health policies should focus on educating people about the true nature of fruit juice and promoting healthier alternatives. Addressing these misconceptions is an essential step toward reducing the prevalence of obesity, NAFLD, and related metabolic conditions. Juice is NO BETTER than soda or anything else with sugar.

Dietary Fiber

Fiber has been long regarded as an indispensable part of a healthy diet, often cited as essential for digestive health, regular bowel movements, and preventing various diseases. The narrative that "you need fiber" is so ingrained in modern nutritional advice that it is rarely questioned. However, the necessity of fiber warrants a closer examination, especially in the context of diets that align more closely with human evolutionary patterns. This section will dissect the myths surrounding fiber and explain why it may not be as essential as commonly believed, particularly for those following an ancestrally appropriate diet such as carnivore.

Why Fiber Is Recommended

The common reasons for recommending fiber include its role in promoting bowel regularity and preventing constipation. Fiber is found in plant-based foods and comes in two main forms: soluble and insoluble. Soluble fiber dissolves in water and forms a gel-like substance that can help moderate digestion, while insoluble fiber adds bulk to the stool and is believed to aid in facilitating the movement of material through the digestive system.

These perceived benefits have led to a strong push for high-fiber diets in public health guidelines. Fiber supplements and high-fiber processed foods are marketed as solutions for digestive issues and as components of a balanced diet. But is fiber truly essential, or is it just compensating for the standard modern diet?

The Carnivore Diet and the Fiber Debate

Proponents of the carnivore diet—a diet consisting entirely of animal-based foods—argue that fiber is not necessary for optimal health. This diet excludes all plant-based foods, which means it contains zero dietary fiber. Despite this, many who follow a strict carnivore diet report thriving digestive health and do not experience the constipation or digestive issues often attributed to low fiber intake. How is this possible?

The answer lies in how the body processes and utilizes the nutrients it receives. In a carnivore diet, the foods consumed are highly bioavailable and nutrient-dense, meaning the body can efficiently absorb and utilize the majority of what is ingested. As a result, less waste is produced, leading to smaller, more infrequent bowel movements. This can be misinterpreted as constipation by those accustomed to larger and more frequent stools resulting from high-fiber diets. However, this is not true constipation; it is simply the body efficiently using what it consumes, with minimal waste.

Fiber as a Response to a Suboptimal Diet

The modern, carbohydrate-heavy diet often contains processed foods full of additives and low-quality ingredients. These foods can create digestive disturbances and other health issues that fiber is then used to mitigate. Fiber acts as a bulking agent and can help push indigestible substances through the digestive tract, but it does not address the root cause of the problem—the intake of foods that are not optimal for the body.

In a diet based on nutrient-dense, easily digestible foods such as animal proteins and fats, the body does not require fiber to maintain regular digestion. The absence of fiber in such a diet does not result in a build-up of waste or digestive issues because the body is better equipped to handle and absorb these foods. Claims that fiber is essential for preventing constipation and promoting bowel health fail to account for this perspective.

The Myths About Fiber and Gut Health

A prevalent myth is that fiber is essential for gut health and that a lack of fiber leads to severe digestive issues. While it is true that some people on fiber-rich diets experience benefits such as regular bowel movements, it is equally true that others report improvements in digestive health after reducing or eliminating fiber from their diets. For individuals with conditions such as irritable bowel syndrome (IBS), diverticulitis, or other digestive disorders, reducing fiber intake can sometimes lead to reduced symptoms and greater comfort.

The belief that fiber is universally beneficial fails to consider the varying responses different people have to it. The idea that all people need high levels of fiber comes from generalized dietary guidelines that do not take individual variation into account.

Why "Less Waste" Does Not Mean Constipation

One common concern with low- or no-fiber diets is that they result in fewer bowel movements, which some interpret as constipation. However, true constipation involves hard, dry stools and difficulty passing them. In contrast, those on carnivore or low-fiber diets often produce smaller, well-formed stools that are easy to pass. This is because their bodies are efficiently utilizing the majority of the food consumed, leaving little to expel as waste.

The modern emphasis on frequent, bulky stools as a sign of health is rooted in the high-fiber diet model. When most of the diet consists of plant-based foods that are not fully digestible, the body produces more waste. This increased volume can create the illusion of a healthy digestive system when, in reality, it may simply be a sign of excess, indigestible material passing through the body.

Rethinking Fiber's Role in an Ancestrally Appropriate Diet

An ancestrally appropriate diet—one that closely resembles what our ancestors ate—often does not include the high levels of fiber found in modern diets. Historically, human diets varied greatly depending on the region and available food sources, but many were centered around animal-based nutrition. These diets were rich in proteins and fats and contained minimal to no fiber, yet ancient humans thrived.

The idea that fiber is essential comes from a modern context where diets are filled with processed and unnatural foods. In contrast, when people eat diets composed of whole, nutrient-dense foods, such as those found in carnivore or paleo approaches, the body manages digestion efficiently without the need for added fiber.

The notion that fiber is an essential component of a healthy diet is worth reevaluating. While it may play a role in helping to manage the effects of a modern, processed diet, it is not a requirement for those following an ancestrally appropriate diet that consists of nutrient-dense, bioavailable foods. In such cases, the body can utilize most of what it consumes, leading to efficient digestion and reduced waste. For those who experience better health and digestion on low- or no-fiber diets, the idea that "you need fiber" is not only misleading but also unnecessary. Fiber should be seen as a tool that may be beneficial for some dietary contexts but is not universally essential for everyone, especially those thriving on a carnivore or low-fiber diet.

Chapter 5 History of Human Diets

There are fad diets, trends, and different theories about what the proper human diet is and what works best for everyone. The truth is different people from different geographical locations (with different environments) have different DNA. Not to mention different genetics. Many things come into play when determining what the optimal diet is for human beings. That said, let's talk about what we were eating as humans long before there were convenience stores, fast food restaurants, and Mom's spaghetti. You may have heard that processed foods are bad, and they are something you should avoid. This is 100% true but let's talk about the word *processed*. Generally, we view processed foods as anything that doesn't come naturally from nature, or that is made in a factory. Also keep in mind that even "Natural" foods may not be what you think they are (more on that later) but for this section, let's define processed foods. If you put fruit in a blender, that is processing food. As you know, that's why they call it a food processor. Once you blend fruits, or juice them, they immediately become processed and lose 90% of the desirability of that food. It is extremely important to consider ancestral habits to determine what is proper for humans. Think about the things we have heard. Saturated fat is bad. Red meat is bad. We evolved on these things and thrived. We MUST focus on the truth, and we must shift our perspectives.

Let's go back a few thousand years.

The Evolutionary Human Diet: A Meat-Centric Approach to Survival and Metabolic Health

1. The Foundation of Early Human Diets: High Meat Consumption

Anthropological evidence reveals that early humans predominantly relied on meat and animal products as their primary food source. Hunting large game was a high-reward activity, providing essential nutrients not easily found in plants, such as complete proteins, B vitamins, and omega-3 fatty acids. Meat and animal fats offered a concentrated source of calories critical for survival, especially in harsh environments where plant availability fluctuated.

Organ meats, in particular, provided essential vitamins (A, D, and K2), minerals like iron and zinc, and bioavailable forms of other nutrients, supporting everything from brain development to immune function. This focus on animal-based foods contributed significantly to the growth of the human brain and likely influenced our species' evolutionary success.

2. Minimal Reliance on Plants: Seasonal and Secondary in Diet

While early humans did consume plant foods, these were typically seasonal and represented a smaller fraction of the diet compared to meat. Fruits, for example, were available only in certain regions and seasons, and they were less sweet, fibrous, and far less calorie-dense than modern fruit varieties. Early plants also contained high levels of natural toxins and antinutrients, which often required processing (like cooking or fermentation) to reduce their potential harm.

In regions where plant foods were more accessible, they supplemented an already nutrient-rich diet but did not provide the bulk of energy or nutrients. Edible wild plants provided fiber and some carbohydrates but were generally limited by seasonal availability and lower caloric density compared to animal-based foods.

3. The Advent of Agriculture and the Rise of Grain Consumption

About 10,000 years ago, agriculture began transforming human diets by introducing a reliance on grains and legumes. While agriculture allowed for stable food supplies and population growth, it also shifted the human diet away from nutrient-dense animal foods to calorie-dense, carbohydrate-rich plant foods like wheat, barley, and rice. This shift led to an increase in antinutrients such as phytates, which hinder the absorption of minerals, and lectins, which can cause digestive issues and immune responses.

Anthropological data reveal that early agricultural societies experienced more malnutrition, shorter lifespans, and higher rates of diseases related to nutrient deficiencies, such as anemia and bone disorders. These health declines highlight the challenges of relying on plant-based foods as dietary staples without the nutritional diversity offered by a meat-based diet.

4. The Role of Antinutrients: Phytates and Lectins in Grains and Legumes

Many plant foods contain natural compounds known as antinutrients, which can reduce nutrient absorption and even cause digestive distress. Phytates, for example, are found in grains, seeds, and legumes and bind to minerals like calcium, magnesium, iron, and zinc, preventing the body from absorbing them efficiently. This effect can lead to deficiencies in individuals relying heavily on plant-based diets, particularly if they do not consume adequate animal-based nutrients.

Lectins, another group of antinutrients, are proteins present in legumes, seeds, and some vegetables. In their raw form, lectins can disrupt cell membranes, causing inflammation and irritation in the gut lining. While cooking can reduce lectin content, the presence of these compounds often requires more energy for digestion and can compromise gut health over time. Early humans likely avoided many of these issues by consuming minimal amounts of lectin-rich foods and focusing on animal sources of protein and nutrients.

5. The Physiological Adaptations for Meat Consumption and Fat Metabolism

Human physiology reflects an adaptation to a high-fat, high-protein diet, with digestive and metabolic mechanisms optimized for processing animal products. Our stomach acidity is one of the highest among mammals, aiding in the breakdown of dense protein and minimizing bacterial load from animal foods. Additionally, humans possess limited ability to ferment plant cellulose in the gut, a capability seen in herbivores, underscoring our evolutionary preference for meat over plants.

Ketogenesis, a metabolic pathway in which the liver converts fat into ketone bodies for energy, is another evolutionary adaptation that aligns with a meat-centric diet. Early humans likely spent extended periods in ketosis, particularly during times when food was scarce or during fasting periods between hunts. This ability to switch between glucose and ketone metabolism provided flexibility, allowing humans to thrive even when carbohydrate sources were unavailable.

6. Genetically Modified Fruits and Vegetables: A Modern Phenomenon

The fruits and vegetables found in supermarkets today differ significantly from their wild ancestors. Through selective breeding and genetic modification, modern agricultural practices have enhanced traits such as sweetness, size, and shelf-life, often at the expense of nutrient density. For example, wild apples were smaller, fibrous, and sour compared to today's large, sugar-laden varieties, which contribute to higher insulin spikes when consumed.

Modern fruits are now available year-round, an unnatural phenomenon that encourages overconsumption and higher sugar intake. This availability contrasts sharply with the seasonal, sporadic access to fruit that characterized the diets of early humans, who consumed fruit primarily in autumn to build fat stores for winter. The increased sugar content in modern fruits, combined with constant availability, has had unintended metabolic consequences, including promoting insulin resistance and fat storage.

7. The Impact of a Meat-Based Diet on Modern Metabolic Health

Ancestral populations consuming primarily meat experienced low rates of metabolic diseases such as diabetes, cardiovascular disease, and obesity. Hunter-gatherer groups, like the Inuit and Maasai, consumed diets high in animal fats and proteins without experiencing the metabolic disorders common today. This absence of disease suggests that human physiology may be better suited to a diet that minimizes carbohydrates and emphasizes high-quality fats and proteins.

Modern diets, rich in refined carbohydrates, sugars, and processed foods, have drastically altered insulin and blood glucose regulation, leading to widespread insulin resistance. In contrast, diets high in animal products do not stimulate insulin production as intensely, helping to maintain stable blood sugar levels and reducing the risk of metabolic syndrome.

8. Reintroducing the Ancestral Diet for Health Restoration

Given the health implications of a carbohydrate-heavy diet, many experts advocate a return to an ancestral-inspired diet focusing on nutrient-dense animal foods. This dietary shift involves prioritizing meats, fish, eggs, and other animal-based foods while limiting processed carbohydrates and sugars. By following a low-carbohydrate, high-fat diet, individuals can lower insulin levels, improve metabolic flexibility, and support overall health.

This approach also involves being selective with plant foods, choosing those with minimal antinutrient content or employing preparation methods, like soaking and fermenting, to reduce phytates and lectins. Adopting these practices can help minimize digestive distress and nutrient interference, enabling a diet more aligned with our evolutionary biology.

9. The Long-Term Impact of Ancestral Eating on Health and Longevity

Studies indicate that populations adhering to diets similar to those of our ancestors, such as the Mediterranean or ketogenic diets, experience lower rates of chronic diseases and increased longevity. By consuming foods in their whole, unprocessed forms, these diets naturally reduce the glycemic load and insulin demands placed on the body. This dietary approach helps prevent obesity, type 2 diabetes, and heart disease—conditions that are nearly absent among hunter-gatherers but prevalent in modern societies.

Returning to a diet focused on nutrient-dense, animal-based foods offers a pathway to better health, reducing the metabolic stress associated with processed foods. By understanding the evolutionary underpinnings of our dietary needs, individuals can make informed choices that support long-term wellness and metabolic resilience.

Looking at modern diets compared to those of early human history indeed shows the sharp contrast between natural food sources and the highly processed, convenience-oriented diet common today. In ancient times, especially before the agricultural revolution, humans relied heavily on whole foods available in their environment, primarily meat from hunting and gathering with occasional seasonal fruits and fibrous vegetables.

For the majority of our evolutionary history, our ancestors consumed a diet that was naturally low in carbohydrates and rich in animal fats and proteins, which played a crucial role in human development. The belief that frequent meals are necessary to "keep the metabolism up," or that natural sugars from fruit are essential every day, overlooks this history. Early humans thrived on fewer, nutrient-dense meals, often fasting between hunting cycles. This pattern is supported by our body's response to fasting, which triggers metabolic pathways that optimize energy use, conserve glucose for the brain, and increase ketone production for sustained energy – adaptations that likely evolved from periods of food scarcity.

The agricultural revolution, which began around 10,000 years ago, shifted human diets significantly. With the domestication of grains and an increase in carbohydrate-rich crops, the intake of refined carbohydrates and sugars spiked, leading to changes in metabolic health over generations. This shift intensified with the introduction of processed foods in the 20th century, along with genetically modified crops that altered the nutritional profile of many plants to emphasize yield, sweetness, and shelf stability over nutrient density.

For instance, today's fruit is much sweeter than ancient varieties due to selective breeding and genetic modification, emphasizing high fructose levels that are now linked to increased insulin resistance and metabolic syndrome. These modifications make it difficult to compare "natural" foods from our past to their modern counterparts. The focus on "superfoods" and sugars as essential parts of the diet disregards how human biology adapted to a low-carb, high-fat regimen over millennia, not a diet centered around refined carbs, sugars, or frequent eating.

These dietary changes coincide with the rise in chronic health conditions, such as obesity, diabetes, and cardiovascular disease, which are now linked to the overconsumption of refined carbs, sugars, and processed foods. It's increasingly evident that returning to a diet closer to our ancestral eating patterns—prioritizing whole foods, healthy fats, and natural proteins—can help mitigate these issues and support long-term health.

Today, we live in a society where convenience is prioritized over quality, and where cravings for sweet, sugary foods have become the norm rather than the exception. From a young age, we're conditioned to believe that frequent snacking, sugary treats, and ultra-processed foods are normal parts of daily life. Advertisements for fast food and sugary drinks surround us, reinforcing the message that these foods are both harmless and desirable. But as we're now starting to understand, these "normal" eating habits come with severe, often unseen consequences for our physical and mental health.

This is the time to take a step back, reflect, and reevaluate the decisions we make about food. We have to become not only more self-aware but also more aware of our environment, the cues that shape our eating habits and the effects they have on us. When we begin to question the current norms around food, we start to see that our modern cravings for sugar and convenience are far from harmless. Instead, they are driving an epidemic of metabolic and mental health issues.

The history of human diet is deeply intertwined with survival, evolution, and environmental adaptation. For the majority of our existence as a species, humans have relied on natural resources available in their surroundings. Our ancestors did not have the convenience of supermarkets or restaurants but survived and thrived through hunting, gathering, and adapting to what the land could provide. This section delves deeper into how our diet has evolved in response to environmental challenges and opportunities and how it shaped our biology.

The Role of Hunting and the Development of Tools

Early humans were initially scavengers before developing the skills to hunt animals. Scavenging and hunting required ingenuity and resourcefulness, leading to the creation of stone tools and weapons. These advancements allowed humans to obtain high-quality animal meat more consistently, making it a staple of their diet. Unlike plant foods, meat provided a rich source of essential nutrients that were easily accessible and bioavailable. Hunting also required teamwork, complex planning, and communication skills, fostering social structures that were integral to early human communities.

The emphasis on hunting likely drove evolutionary changes in humans, such as the development of larger brains. Meat is calorie-dense and nutrient-rich, supplying fats and amino acids that are critical for brain growth and cognitive function. This focus on animal foods supported the development of advanced cognitive abilities and laid the foundation for the sophisticated societies that would eventually emerge.

The Importance of Fat in Human Evolution

Fats from animal sources provided early humans with a reliable energy source that sustained them through long periods without food. Unlike carbohydrates, which are burned quickly, fats provide a more sustained release of energy, making them essential during times of scarcity. Human metabolism adapted to efficiently use fat for energy, particularly through ketogenesis—a process where fats are converted into ketones that can fuel the brain and muscles during fasting or low carbohydrate intake.

This metabolic flexibility, the ability to switch between using glucose and fat as fuel, is an evolutionary advantage. It allowed early humans to survive in diverse environments, from cold, barren landscapes where plant foods were scarce to tropical regions where food was more abundant. This adaptability highlights the importance of a diet rich in animal fats in early human survival, which contrasts sharply with today's carbohydrate-heavy diets.

Seasonal Diet Variability and Nutrient Cycling

While meat was a primary component of the diet, early humans also consumed plant foods when available. However, plant foods were seasonal and highly variable in nutrient content. Wild fruits, for instance, were smaller, more fibrous, and less sweet than today's cultivated varieties. These natural variations in the diet contributed to what scientists call "nutrient cycling," where different nutrients were consumed in varying amounts depending on the season.

This cycling likely provided a range of vitamins, minerals, and phytochemicals, though not in the consistent quantities seen in modern diets. For instance, in colder months, early humans might have relied solely on animal sources, which provided essential nutrients, while in warmer months, they could gather berries, tubers, and other wild plants. This periodic shift in nutrient intake reflects how human physiology evolved to handle dietary fluctuations rather than continuous, abundant access to food.

The Agricultural Revolution and Dietary Transition

Around 10,000 years ago, the advent of agriculture marked a significant dietary shift. The domestication of grains and legumes allowed for settled communities and a stable food supply, supporting larger populations. However, this stability came with a cost. Agriculture introduced a dependence on carbohydrate-rich crops like wheat, barley, and rice, which lack many of the essential nutrients found in animal products.

This reliance on grains led to increased intake of phytates and lectins—antinutrients that impair the absorption of minerals such as calcium, magnesium, and iron. This shift had profound health consequences. Skeletal remains from early agricultural societies show evidence of malnutrition, such as bone deformities, tooth decay, and shorter stature, suggesting that the transition from a meat-centric diet to a grain-based one came at the expense of nutritional health. Populations became more susceptible to nutrient deficiencies, infectious diseases, and other health issues that had been rare among hunter-gatherers.

How Early Agricultural Societies Adapted

Despite these challenges, early agricultural societies developed methods to mitigate the effects of antinutrients in plant-based diets. Fermentation, for example, was widely practiced to reduce the antinutritional factors in grains and legumes, making them more digestible and enhancing their nutrient availability. Soaking, sprouting, and cooking were other techniques used to minimize the impact of phytates and lectins.

While these methods helped, they did not entirely compensate for the loss of nutrients that had been plentiful in the hunter-gatherer diet. The human body, which evolved on nutrient-dense animal foods, had to adapt to a less diverse and often nutrient-limited diet. Over generations, this adaptation resulted in genetic and epigenetic changes that may have made certain populations more tolerant to grains, though not without health costs.

The Modern Diet and Its Disconnect from Evolutionary Needs

The evolution of the human diet reached a new turning point in the 20th century with the introduction of processed foods and industrial agriculture. Food production focused on convenience and profitability rather than nutritional value, leading to an abundance of calorie-dense, nutrient-poor foods. Refined sugars, seed oils, and processed grains became dietary staples, contributing to the rise of metabolic diseases that were virtually unknown among early humans.

Modern agriculture also led to genetic modifications and selective breeding of plants to enhance traits like sweetness, size, and shelf stability. These modifications created fruits and vegetables vastly different from their wild counterparts, often with higher sugar content and lower fiber levels. This continuous access to high-sugar fruits and refined carbohydrates has altered human metabolism, contributing to conditions like insulin resistance, obesity, and type 2 diabetes.

The Rise of Food-Related Chronic Illnesses

Today, chronic illnesses related to diet—such as obesity, heart disease, diabetes, and certain cancers—are among the leading causes of death worldwide. These conditions are largely attributed to the consumption of processed foods, excessive sugar, and refined carbohydrates. Unlike the intermittent fasting and nutrient cycling of early human diets, modern diets expose the body to a constant influx of calories and sugars, disrupting metabolic homeostasis.

In addition to metabolic diseases, autoimmune disorders have also increased, potentially due to overconsumption of processed foods and a lack of nutrient diversity. The immune system, which evolved to handle occasional dietary antigens from natural foods, is now exposed to artificial additives, preservatives, and novel proteins that may trigger inflammatory responses.

Revisiting Ancestral Diets in the Modern World

Given the negative impact of modern diets on health, there is growing interest in returning to ancestral eating patterns. Diets that mimic the nutrient composition of early human diets—such as paleo, ketogenic, and carnivore diets—focus on whole, unprocessed foods, emphasizing meats, healthy fats, and low-glycemic vegetables. These dietary approaches aim to restore metabolic health by reducing insulin levels, improving nutrient absorption, and supporting the body's natural energy regulation mechanisms.

Studies on low-carbohydrate, high-fat diets show promising results for reversing metabolic syndrome, reducing inflammation, and promoting weight loss. These findings align with the eating patterns of early humans, who thrived on diets that minimized carbohydrates and emphasized fats and proteins.

The Evolutionary Advantage of Intermittent Fasting

Intermittent fasting has also gained popularity as a dietary practice that aligns with ancestral eating patterns. Early humans did not have continuous access to food, so their bodies adapted to periods of fasting between successful hunts or foraging cycles. Fasting triggers metabolic processes like autophagy, where cells clear out damaged components and regenerate, supporting longevity and reducing disease risk.

Modern research supports the benefits of intermittent fasting, showing improvements in insulin sensitivity, reduced inflammation, and enhanced fat oxidation. By incorporating intermittent fasting, people can better align their eating habits with evolutionary adaptations, potentially improving their health and reducing dependency on constant food intake.

Understanding Ancestral Nutrition as a Guideline for Health

The study of ancestral nutrition reveals that humans are not biologically adapted to the high-carb, high-sugar, processed foods prevalent in the modern diet. Rather, our physiology favors nutrient-dense, whole foods that provide a balanced mix of fats, proteins, and essential vitamins and minerals. While it may not be feasible to replicate early human diets entirely, understanding these principles offers a valuable framework for improving health.

Adopting a diet that emphasizes whole foods and minimizes processed ingredients can reduce the risk of chronic illnesses and support overall wellness. Recognizing our evolutionary dietary needs empowers individuals to make informed food choices that align with the biological processes honed over thousands of years of adaptation.

Concluding Thoughts on the Historical Evolution of the Human Diet

In sum, the human diet has undergone dramatic changes from the nutrient-dense, meat-centered diets of early humans to today's processed and carbohydrate-heavy diets. These shifts have contributed to the rise in metabolic diseases and highlight the need to re-evaluate our food choices in light of evolutionary principles. By adopting elements of ancestral diets—such as consuming whole foods, practicing intermittent fasting, and prioritizing quality fats and proteins—modern individuals can work toward restoring metabolic health and fostering resilience against chronic disease. The path forward may lie in embracing the wisdom of the past, respecting our evolutionary heritage, and choosing a dietary approach that aligns with our natural biology.

The Science of Sugar and Dopamine

Sugar, like drugs, acts on the brain's reward centers by triggering the release of dopamine—a neurotransmitter linked to pleasure and reward. When you eat something sweet, your brain releases dopamine, giving you a quick sensation of pleasure and satisfaction. This dopamine "hit" feels good, and it makes you want more. Over time, as with any addictive substance, the brain becomes accustomed to these dopamine bursts. The more you consume, the more your body craves the same feeling, and soon, a vicious cycle of sugar dependency is established.

Much like nicotine in cigarettes, sugar doesn't just give you pleasure in the moment; it changes your brain chemistry over time. With each sugary snack or drink, you reinforce the dopamine pathway, strengthening your brain's association between sugar and pleasure. This cycle of craving and consumption can be extremely difficult to break, especially because we're exposed to sugar at nearly every turn, from the office break room to advertisements on social media. WE MUST RECOGNIZE THIS.

Killing Me Softly: Sugar's Long-Term Effects on Health

While a sugary snack or a sweet drink might seem harmless, repeated exposure over time can lead to devastating health outcomes. Similar to how smoking one cigarette won't kill you, but years of smoking certainly could, consuming sugar-laden foods on a regular basis contributes to a host of health issues that accumulate and worsen over time. These include obesity, type 2 diabetes, cardiovascular disease, and even mental health issues like depression and anxiety.

One of the major problems with sugar is that it contributes to chronic inflammation in the body. When you consume large amounts of sugar, your body goes into overdrive to metabolize it, producing byproducts that can be toxic to cells. This cellular damage leads to inflammation, which has been linked to nearly every chronic illness, including heart disease, cancer, and neurological disorders. In this sense, sugar acts as a slow-acting poison—its effects are not immediate, but they build up over years, eroding health and contributing to early mortality.

Eating Frequency and Its Impact on Health

Along with our sugar dependence, modern society has conditioned us to believe that eating every couple of hours is healthy and necessary. The idea that we need three large meals a day, with snacks in between, has become deeply ingrained in our culture. But from a physiological perspective, this constant eating disrupts our body's natural metabolic processes.

When we eat frequently, our bodies are constantly producing insulin, a hormone that helps manage blood sugar levels. Frequent insulin spikes can eventually lead to insulin resistance, a condition where the body becomes less responsive to insulin and blood sugar levels remain elevated. Insulin resistance is a hallmark of metabolic syndrome and is closely linked to conditions like type 2 diabetes, obesity, and heart disease. Additionally, constant eating prevents our bodies from entering a state of fasting, which is essential for cellular repair and the elimination of damaged cells.

The belief that eating every few hours is normal is largely a product of marketing by the food industry. Snacks, convenience foods, and sugary beverages are constantly promoted as necessary for energy and health. However, if we step back and examine human history, we find that our ancestors thrived without constant access to food. They ate intermittently, allowing their bodies to fully digest and utilize nutrients, and they maintained strong health without the modern epidemic of metabolic diseases.

Cultivating <u>Self-Awareness</u> and Environmental Awareness

To break free from the conditioning around sugar and frequent eating, we need to cultivate self-awareness and environmental awareness. Self-awareness involves paying attention to our physical and emotional responses to food, understanding our cravings, and recognizing when we're eating out of habit rather than hunger. This can be as simple as asking yourself why you're reaching for a snack. Are you truly hungry, or is it a momentary craving influenced by stress, boredom, or convenience?

Environmental awareness means recognizing the cues around you that encourage unhealthy eating. Our environment is filled with triggers that push us toward sugar and convenience. Grocery stores are stocked with processed foods at eye level, advertisements glamorize sugary treats, and social gatherings often revolve around food. By becoming aware of these influences, we can start to make conscious choices rather than reacting to environmental cues. This might mean choosing not to keep sugary snacks in the house, packing whole foods for work, or setting boundaries around social eating.

Building Resilience Against the Modern Food Environment

To counteract the conditioning around sugar and convenience, we need to build resilience. Resilience involves creating habits that support healthy choices and protect against the constant temptation of processed, sugary foods. This might mean cooking more meals at home, planning meals ahead of time, or finding substitutes for sugary snacks. It also involves surrounding yourself with a supportive community—friends, family, or online groups who share your commitment to healthier choices.

One powerful way to build resilience is through intermittent fasting, a practice that aligns more closely with our evolutionary biology. Fasting helps reset the body's hunger signals, improves insulin sensitivity, and allows for cellular repair. Over time, fasting can help break the cycle of sugar cravings and reduce dependency on constant eating, allowing your body to function optimally.

Redefining What's Normal

Finally, we need to redefine what we consider normal when it comes to food and eating habits. The current norms around sugar and convenience are not only unhealthy, but they're also unsustainable for long-term health. By challenging these norms and making conscious choices, we can create a new normal—one where whole foods, balanced meals, and mindful eating are the standards.

This shift begins with individuals taking ownership of their health and rejecting the belief that cravings for sugar and constant eating are normal. It's time to look beyond the conditioning of the modern food industry and make choices that support our well-being, not just in the present, but for years to come. With each conscious choice, we reclaim our health and build a stronger foundation for future generations.

Chapter 6 : Fasting – Understanding Intermittent and Prolonged Fasting

Fasting has become an increasingly popular practice in recent years, not only for weight management but for its significant benefits to metabolic health. Yet, fasting is not a new concept; humans have practiced it for millennia, whether by necessity or through cultural and religious traditions. Today, scientific research supports the benefits of fasting, including its role in managing insulin resistance, reducing inflammation, and supporting cellular repair processes like autophagy. In this chapter, we'll explore two primary types of fasting—Intermittent Fasting (IF) and Prolonged Fasting (PF)—and examine the science behind how each can help optimize health.

When I first began my research and self-experimentation, I adopted prolonged fasting and was met with reactions like, "That can't be healthy," or "Aren't you tired?" The truth is that fasting, when combined with the proper diet for each individual's unique circumstances, is more powerful than most people realize. Humans have evolved to thrive in a fasting state, yet we've lost touch with this natural way of eating. By moving away from eating purely for pleasure or social reasons, we can truly understand the transformative benefits fasting has to offer. Once a month, I do a 72 hour fast and it does wonders for me. More energy, more clarity, revitalization.

The primary goal of fasting is to optimize your fuel source. Most of us are locked into running on glucose, and for generations, this has been the default. But the human body is, in fact, a hybrid fuel-burning machine, capable of switching between glucose and fat as energy sources, with fat being the optimal fuel for sustained energy and mental clarity. This shift from glucose to fat-burning involves entering a state of ketosis, an ancient metabolic state far older than the glucose-burning metabolism we're used to today.

Thousands of years ago, our ancestors weren't eating every two hours, let alone consuming cereal and oatmeal for breakfast. Eating constantly was simply not possible or necessary. Instead, they relied on stored fat as a consistent energy source. While a fasting and fat-fueled lifestyle may not be feasible for every person today, raising awareness about fasting and the benefits of a balanced diet closer to what humans historically thrived on can move the needle in improving the nation's health.

Fasting: Unlearning the Myths of Food and Energy

For decades, we've been told that regular meals and constant snacking are essential for maintaining energy levels, preventing hunger, and even managing weight. The food industry and mainstream media have built an entire narrative around the idea that eating every few hours is necessary to keep our metabolism running and prevent lethargy. But this view is misleading and deeply flawed. When we step back and think ancestrally, we see that fasting, rather than constant eating, is how our bodies are truly designed to function. Our hunter-gatherer ancestors went days without food, relying on their bodies' stored energy to fuel them. In fact, fasting doesn't make us weak and lethargic; rather, it optimizes our body's ability to create and utilize energy, keeping us sharp and resilient in times of scarcity. By unlearning the myths about constant eating, we can tap into the body's innate energy systems, which have evolved over thousands of years.

The Myth of Constant Eating for Energy

One of the biggest misconceptions we've absorbed is that we need a steady stream of calories throughout the day to sustain energy. We're told to eat three meals plus snacks, fearing that skipping even one could cause our energy levels to plummet. But this approach ignores how our bodies were designed to function. Our ancestors didn't have pantries full of food or a fast-food drive-thru at every corner. They endured cycles of feast and famine, relying on stored body fat for energy during times of scarcity. Human physiology evolved with this pattern, where fasting was not only common but essential for survival.

When food was scarce, the body adapted by switching to stored fat as a primary fuel source. This process, called **ketosis**, allows the body to break down fat into ketones, which fuel the brain and muscles efficiently. The ability to function well in a fasted state was crucial for survival; a hunter weakened by hunger would be at a disadvantage, unable to chase prey or find food. Therefore, humans evolved to maintain focus, strength, and stamina even after days without food. Far from being a cause of weakness, fasting triggers adaptations that enhance mental clarity, energy levels, and physical endurance.

Ketosis: Unlocking the Body's Natural Energy Reserves

Ketosis is a metabolic state that becomes essential during fasting, when the body transitions from relying on glucose (sugar) to using stored fat as a primary fuel source. This shift is a powerful adaptation developed over millennia, allowing humans to survive and even thrive in periods of food scarcity. In ketosis, the liver converts fatty acids into **ketones**—small molecules that provide a steady, efficient source of energy for the brain, muscles, and other organs. Ketones offer a unique fuel alternative to glucose, which becomes limited when we're fasting. The process of ketosis is not just a survival mechanism but also an optimized metabolic state that allows for improved mental clarity, endurance, and resilience—qualities that were essential for our ancestors.

In the first 24 hours of fasting, the body typically uses up its glycogen stores—its stored form of glucose located in the liver and muscles. Once glycogen is depleted, the body shifts to breaking down stored fat for energy. This metabolic state marks the beginning of ketosis, where fatty acids are transformed into ketones. These ketones then circulate in the bloodstream and are used to fuel vital organs, especially the brain, which requires a constant energy supply. Unlike glucose, which spikes insulin levels and can lead to energy fluctuations, ketones offer a more stable energy source, allowing the body to function at a high level without the need for continuous food intake.

Ketosis and Evolutionary Survival: Why the Body Uses Ketones During Fasting

For our ancestors, food was not readily available in abundance, and fasting wasn't a choice but a natural part of life. They would often go days between successful hunts or gathering expeditions, relying on stored energy reserves to carry them through periods without food. If humans couldn't perform without constant eating, they would have been at a severe disadvantage in the wild. Instead, ketosis equipped them with a way to function optimally during these fasted periods. Ketones provided the brain with an alternative energy source, fueling their physical and mental tasks with stable energy that didn't depend on meal frequency.

In ketosis, rather than becoming weak and lethargic, the body actually enters a state of heightened focus and alertness. This is partly due to increased production of **adrenaline** and **noradrenaline** during fasting, which help the body remain alert and capable, even without food. This counteracts the myth that not eating leads to weakness or lack of focus; instead, fasting prompts the body to maximize its resources, tapping into fat stores and preserving muscle tissue while maintaining energy. This metabolic adaptability underscores the incredible resilience of the human body, allowing us to survive and perform at a high level even in the absence of food.

How Ketosis Works: The Role of Ketones in Energy Production

When glucose stores are low, the liver begins producing ketones by breaking down fatty acids, which are released from stored fat. The primary ketones produced are **beta-hydroxybutyrate (BHB)**, **acetoacetate**, and **acetone**. These ketones circulate in the bloodstream and serve as alternative fuel, especially for the brain, which cannot directly utilize fatty acids for energy. The brain relies heavily on glucose in a fed state, but during ketosis, it switches to using ketones, which provide a more stable and efficient fuel source.

Ketones are particularly advantageous for the brain because they can cross the blood-brain barrier and provide a clean, efficient source of energy without the oxidative stress that can result from constant glucose metabolism. This shift to ketones as a primary fuel source supports cognitive function and can even have neuroprotective benefits. Many people who enter ketosis through fasting report experiencing greater mental clarity and focus, which is likely due to ketones' stable, long-lasting energy compared to the short-lived spikes and crashes associated with glucose. Ketones support the brain in a way that aligns with how our ancestors needed to stay sharp while navigating challenges in a fasted state.

The Hormonal Benefits of Ketosis and Muscle Preservation

One concern people often have about fasting is the potential for muscle loss, but ketosis helps preserve muscle tissue by increasing levels of **human growth hormone (HGH)**. HGH is known to play a key role in muscle maintenance and fat metabolism. During fasting, as the body enters ketosis, HGH levels rise significantly, especially during prolonged fasting periods. This hormonal response prevents the body from breaking down muscle tissue for fuel, instead encouraging it to use fat stores for energy. The result is that fasting and ketosis allow for fat-burning without sacrificing muscle mass, a key benefit for anyone concerned about maintaining strength and physical performance while fasting.

Ketosis also lowers insulin levels, creating a state of **insulin sensitivity** that enhances the body's ability to utilize fat as fuel. Low insulin levels signal the body to access stored fat, promoting fat oxidation while maintaining lean muscle. This is why, contrary to the fear of muscle wasting, ketosis supports a balanced approach to weight management, energy production, and muscle preservation. The steady energy derived from ketones allows the body to function smoothly without the constant need for external food sources, empowering individuals to rely on their own stored energy and achieve metabolic efficiency.

Brain Health and Ketones: Enhancing Mental Clarity and Focus

One of the most powerful aspects of ketosis is its impact on brain health. Ketones, particularly BHB, are a highly efficient source of energy for the brain, and studies show that they may even support neurogenesis—the growth and repair of neurons. The brain typically relies on glucose, but in a fasted state, ketones serve as its primary energy source, leading to increased mental clarity, focus, and cognitive resilience. The brain's adaptation to ketones likely provided our ancestors with a cognitive edge, helping them stay alert and focused during hunts and survival activities.

Research suggests that ketones can help reduce **oxidative stress** in the brain, as they produce fewer free radicals than glucose during metabolism. This reduction in oxidative stress is linked to improved cognitive function and may even help protect against neurodegenerative diseases like Alzheimer's and Parkinson's. Some researchers are exploring the use of ketogenic diets and fasting as potential therapeutic approaches for these conditions due to their neuroprotective effects. Ketosis, therefore, is not only about surviving without food but also about tapping into an energy source that can potentially improve brain health and longevity.

The Metabolic Efficiency of Ketosis: Fueling the Body from Within

One of the primary benefits of ketosis is metabolic flexibility—the body's ability to switch between glucose and fat as energy sources. In today's carbohydrate-heavy diet culture, metabolic flexibility is often compromised, leading people to depend on constant carbohydrate intake for energy. This dependency on glucose can lead to frequent energy crashes, sugar cravings, and insulin resistance over time. Ketosis offers a solution by promoting the body's ability to use fat as a sustainable, long-term energy source, even in the absence of dietary intake.

In ketosis, the body can tap into stored fat reserves, which contain thousands of calories that can fuel activities for days, if not weeks. This adaptation was crucial for early humans, who needed reliable energy between meals. Ketosis allowed them to go extended periods without eating, relying on their own body fat as a reservoir of energy. This is a stark contrast to the misconception that going without food depletes energy. Instead, ketosis enables the body to fuel itself efficiently and avoid the highs and lows that come with a glucose-dependent metabolism.

Ketosis vs. Glucose: Debunking the Energy Crash Myth

A key misconception surrounding fasting and ketosis is that the body will become weak or lethargic without regular glucose intake. However, people often feel energized, not depleted, once they enter ketosis. This energy boost occurs because ketones provide a consistent fuel source that doesn't cause the blood sugar spikes and crashes associated with high-carb diets. The steady energy from ketones allows for prolonged mental and physical endurance without the constant need to refuel.

This energy stability in ketosis challenges the myth that fasting leads to lethargy. Rather than depending on external food sources, ketosis allows the body to tap into its own fat reserves, which offer sustained energy throughout the day. Many people report feeling more alert and focused while in ketosis, as ketones prevent the roller-coaster effect that glucose dependency can create. Ketosis essentially frees people from the need for constant snacking, supporting energy and focus in a way that aligns with how the human body is designed to operate.

Ketosis and Health Benefits Beyond Energy: Supporting Longevity and Cellular Repair

Beyond energy production, ketosis activates processes like **autophagy**—a cellular "cleanup" mechanism that clears out damaged cells and promotes cellular repair. Autophagy, which is triggered in a fasted state, has been linked to longevity and reduced risk of diseases. This process helps the body rejuvenate at a cellular level, supporting functions that are compromised by constant eating. By cycling through periods of fasting and ketosis, the body optimizes cellular repair and resilience, underscoring the benefits of this ancient energy system.

Furthermore, ketosis has been associated with lower levels of inflammation, as ketones like BHB possess anti-inflammatory properties. This reduction in inflammation can benefit everything from cardiovascular health to metabolic function, suggesting that ketosis isn't just a tool for surviving without food but a pathway to supporting holistic health.

Embracing Ketosis as a Natural State

Ultimately, ketosis is not a "hack" or a recent health trend; it's a natural metabolic state that aligns with how our ancestors functioned for thousands of years. By relying on stored fat and ketones for energy, the body accesses a sustainable energy reserve, allowing us to maintain physical endurance and mental clarity in the absence of food. Ketosis supports a balanced, flexible metabolism, which can protect against modern health issues associated with constant eating and carb dependency.

As we continue to challenge the myths about fasting and constant eating, understanding ketosis empowers us to reconnect with our bodies' natural mechanisms for energy production. Far from being a starvation mode, ketosis allows us to thrive, adapt, and remain resilient. It's a reminder that our bodies are designed to withstand periods of food scarcity and perform at a high level, making ketosis an essential part of the fasting process and a testament to human adaptability.

The Body's True Energy System: Fasting and Metabolic Flexibility

Modern diets high in refined carbs and sugars encourage our bodies to rely on glucose as a primary fuel source, conditioning us to crave food every few hours. But this constant intake disrupts **metabolic flexibility**—the body's natural ability to switch between burning glucose and stored fat. When we fast, however, the body begins to shift to fat stores for energy, a process that's far more sustainable and energy-dense. One pound of body fat contains roughly 3,500 calories, a vast energy reserve that the body can tap into during fasting.

In contrast, glucose is a short-term fuel, quickly used up, which is why people experience energy crashes after carb-heavy meals. With fasting, the body becomes efficient at using stored fat for fuel, resulting in sustained energy. This is why people who practice intermittent fasting or prolonged fasting often report feeling more focused, energized, and mentally clear. It's a stark contrast to the narrative that going without food leaves you tired and weak.

Additionally, when we fast, the body initiates a process called **autophagy**—a cellular "clean-up" mechanism that removes damaged cells and regenerates new ones. Autophagy is crucial for longevity and disease prevention, and it is triggered in a fasted state, not when we're constantly eating. Essentially, fasting allows the body to perform vital maintenance that is neglected when we're in a fed state all the time. This is another reason fasting aligns with our evolutionary biology; our bodies are designed to cycle between eating and fasting, benefiting from both.

Ancestral Insight: Thriving in a Fasted State

Imagine an early human going days without food while on the hunt. Would evolution have favored lethargy and weakness in this state? Absolutely not. If early humans became lethargic or unable to function after a few hours of hunger, they simply wouldn't have survived. Instead, fasting would have primed their bodies to be sharp, energized, and capable. Fasting activates hormones like **adrenaline** and **noradrenaline**, which boost energy and focus, essentially putting the body on high alert. These hormones ensure that a fasted individual can perform tasks with high intensity, whether that's hunting for food or engaging in physical activity.

There's also the **human growth hormone (HGH)** factor. During fasting, the body increases HGH production, which preserves muscle mass and enhances fat-burning. This is a survival mechanism to prevent muscle breakdown and optimize fat stores for energy. Rather than causing us to waste away, fasting helps maintain muscle mass and even improve physical performance. Ancient humans, far from being sluggish, were likely at their physical peak when fasting, as their bodies were primed to find food.

Modern Misinformation: The Food Industry's Role

The modern emphasis on constant eating is not only scientifically unsound but also heavily influenced by the food industry. Processed food companies benefit from a culture that encourages eating multiple times a day, and they capitalize on the fear that skipping meals will harm us. The snack industry, for example, is worth billions, with products marketed as "healthy" snacks to keep us going between meals. However, these foods are often high in sugars, refined carbs, and unhealthy fats, causing blood sugar spikes and crashes, which create dependency on frequent eating.

The "breakfast is the most important meal of the day" mantra originated from marketing campaigns rather than nutritional science. Research now shows that breakfast is not universally essential and that many people experience better focus and energy levels by fasting through the morning. Despite this, the idea that we must eat breakfast persists, largely due to media and marketing influences that have ingrained these habits in our culture.

Health Benefits of Fasting: Reclaiming Our Metabolic Health

When we stop eating constantly, our bodies begin to return to their natural, optimized state. Fasting has been shown to improve **insulin sensitivity**, which is crucial for preventing type 2 diabetes and managing weight. In a constantly fed state, the body is exposed to frequent insulin spikes, which over time can lead to insulin resistance—a precursor to metabolic disorders. Fasting reduces these spikes, giving the body a break from insulin production and allowing cells to reset their sensitivity.

Furthermore, fasting supports **brain health** by increasing the production of **brain-derived neurotrophic factor (BDNF)**, a protein that supports neuron growth and cognitive function. This means that fasting can improve focus, mental clarity, and even protect against neurodegenerative diseases. Ancient humans needed this mental edge to survive, and fasting triggers cognitive benefits that align with our ancestral needs.

Debunking the Myth of Constant Hunger

One reason people fear fasting is the assumption that they'll be constantly hungry or unable to concentrate. However, the sensation of hunger is largely influenced by eating patterns and hormones like **ghrelin**, the "hunger hormone." Ghrelin levels rise in response to habitual eating times, which is why many people feel hungry around noon if they're used to eating lunch at that time. But with fasting, ghrelin adapts, and the sensation of hunger becomes manageable, often fading after the first few days of adjusting to a fasting routine.

In fact, many people report that fasting reduces cravings and helps them feel more in control of their eating habits. Without constant food intake triggering blood sugar fluctuations, they experience fewer cravings and a steadier appetite. This is a significant departure from the snack-driven culture we've been led to believe is necessary for stable energy.

Undoing the Damage: Embracing Fasting in a Modern World

For many, embracing fasting means unlearning the fear of hunger and challenging the deeply rooted misconceptions about food and energy. The modern food industry, with its vested interest in continuous consumption, has perpetuated myths that disconnect us from our natural metabolic processes. By reintroducing fasting into our lives, we tap into a system designed to optimize energy, focus, and resilience.

Fasting doesn't mean deprivation or starving; it means giving our bodies the space to operate as they're meant to. Intermittent fasting, for instance, can involve eating within an 8-hour window and fasting for 16 hours, a cycle that fits comfortably into many people's schedules while providing the benefits of an extended fast. This approach allows people to experience improved energy, focus, and metabolic health without drastic lifestyle changes.

Fasting as a Return to Our Natural State

Fasting aligns with human evolution and biological needs in a way that constant eating does not. It allows the body to burn fat, trigger autophagy, and maintain muscle—all essential adaptations that helped our ancestors survive. While the food industry promotes myths around the need for frequent eating, fasting challenges these misconceptions, proving that our bodies are resilient and capable without constant food intake.

In a world of abundant food and relentless marketing, fasting offers a counterbalance, reconnecting us to our body's true energy system. By embracing fasting, we reclaim a natural rhythm that supports optimal health and vitality, dispelling the myth that we need to be constantly fed to thrive.

1. What is Fasting, and Why Does it Matter?

Definition of Fasting: Fasting is the voluntary abstinence from food and, in some cases, from caloric beverages for a set period. During fasting, the body switches from an anabolic (building and storing) to a catabolic (breaking down) state, which can initiate numerous health benefits.

The Evolutionary Perspective: Fasting isn't just a trend but a part of human history. Our ancestors faced periods without food and adapted to function optimally in fasting states. This biological adaptation forms the basis for why fasting has such profound effects on modern health.

The Science Behind Fasting: The body uses glucose as its primary energy source when food is readily available. During fasting, however, the body shifts to burning stored fat as fuel, increasing metabolic flexibility and potentially aiding in weight management.

2. Intermittent Fasting (IF): Variations and Benefits

Intermittent Fasting involves cycling between periods of eating and fasting within the same day or week. Here's an overview of popular IF methods and their associated health benefits:

- **Popular IF Protocols**:

16:8 Method: Fasting for 16 hours, eating within an 8-hour window.

5:2 Diet: Eating normally for five days and consuming minimal calories (around 500-600) on two non-consecutive days.

Alternate-Day Fasting: Alternating between regular eating days and fasting days, where calories are restricted to a small percentage of usual intake.

OMAD (One Meal a Day): Eating only one meal per day, typically within a one-hour window.

- **Benefits of Intermittent Fasting**:

Insulin Sensitivity: IF has been shown to improve insulin sensitivity, helping to regulate blood sugar levels and reduce the risk of type 2 diabetes.

Weight Loss and Body Composition: By limiting the eating window, IF can reduce overall caloric intake, aiding in weight management. Fasting also shifts the body towards fat burning, which can help in losing body fat while preserving lean mass.

Cellular Autophagy: IF promotes autophagy, a process where cells remove damaged components, recycling them for energy and reducing oxidative stress. Autophagy is essential for longevity and preventing chronic diseases.

Inflammation Reduction: Short-term fasting has been shown to lower inflammatory markers, which can reduce the risk of heart disease, certain cancers, and other chronic conditions.

Intermittent Fasting (IF) offers several benefits for metabolic health, weight management, and cellular repair, largely influenced by hormonal responses and alignment with our natural circadian rhythm. One of the primary ways IF supports these benefits is through the hormone ghrelin, commonly referred to as the "hunger hormone." Ghrelin levels naturally rise when it's time to eat and fall after eating, playing a crucial role in regulating hunger and signaling the body's need for energy intake. With regular intermittent fasting, ghrelin can begin to follow a more stable rhythm, decreasing hunger spikes and making fasting periods easier over time. This adjustment can contribute to better appetite control, helping individuals maintain a healthier weight.

IF also interacts positively with our circadian rhythm, the body's internal 24-hour clock that governs various physiological processes, including metabolism, hormone release, and sleep-wake cycles. Research suggests that aligning eating patterns with natural daylight hours—avoiding late-night eating and focusing on daylight hours—can optimize metabolic efficiency. Our bodies are more insulin-sensitive during the day and tend to burn energy more efficiently, meaning that eating during this time and fasting at night can help improve blood sugar regulation and fat oxidation.

Additionally, intermittent fasting supports cellular repair mechanisms, such as autophagy, where cells remove damaged components and regenerate. This process is promoted during fasting and has implications for aging and disease prevention. Together, ghrelin regulation and circadian alignment not only make fasting easier over time but also work synergistically to optimize energy metabolism, support weight loss, and promote overall health.

3. Prolonged Fasting (PF): Taking Fasting to the Next Level

Prolonged Fasting extends beyond 24 hours, often lasting 48 to 72 hours or more. While longer fasting periods can be challenging, they provide unique physiological benefits that are not achieved through shorter fasting windows.

- **How Prolonged Fasting Works**:

After 24 hours of fasting, glycogen stores are depleted, prompting the body to burn fat for fuel.

By the 48-hour mark, autophagy increases significantly, supporting cellular repair and rejuvenation.

Around 72 hours, studies show the body initiates stem cell regeneration, particularly in the immune system, enhancing long-term health.

- **Benefits of Prolonged Fasting**:

Deeper Cellular Repair: The body enters an intensified state of autophagy and cellular cleanup, helping eliminate dysfunctional cells and potentially reducing cancer risks.

Improved Immune System: Prolonged fasting stimulates stem cell production, aiding in the regeneration of immune cells. This process can enhance immune function, especially after illness.

Increased Ketosis: After around two days, the body produces more ketones, which provide a steady energy source for the brain and may enhance mental clarity and focus.

Insulin and Blood Sugar Control: Longer fasting periods allow insulin levels to stay low for extended periods, reducing insulin resistance and improving glucose metabolism.

Breaking a prolonged fast and entering a prolonged fast are two essential phases that significantly impact the experience and benefits of fasting. Entering a fast with intention and understanding prepares the body for optimal adaptation, while breaking a fast with care prevents digestive distress and helps maintain the metabolic benefits achieved during the fasting period. This section will delve into both stages, providing guidance on approaching prolonged fasting with safety, efficiency, and mindfulness.

Entering a Prolonged Fast

Entering a prolonged fast involves preparing the body and mind for an extended period without food. While many people focus solely on the fasting period itself, the hours leading up to a fast can make a significant difference in how the body handles the transition. A thoughtful entry into fasting can set the stage for reduced hunger, stable energy levels, and a more comfortable experience overall.

1. Gradual Reduction in Carbohydrate Intake

One of the best ways to prepare for a prolonged fast is by gradually reducing carbohydrate intake a few days before fasting. High-carb diets cause the body to rely heavily on glucose for energy, meaning a sudden shift to fasting can lead to energy crashes and intense cravings. By tapering off carbohydrates beforehand, you encourage the body to start tapping into fat stores and increase ketone production. This process, called ketosis, enables the body to use fat as its primary energy source, making the transition into fasting smoother and reducing the likelihood of experiencing a "keto flu," characterized by fatigue, headaches, and irritability.

2. Eating Nutrient-Dense Foods

As you approach the fasting period, focus on consuming nutrient-dense meals rich in healthy fats and proteins. These macronutrients provide a slow, steady release of energy, helping you feel satisfied and energized longer into your fast. Omega-3-rich fats from sources like fatty fish, avocados, and olive oil are particularly beneficial, as they help reduce inflammation and support brain health during fasting. Additionally, nutrient-dense foods loaded with vitamins, minerals, and electrolytes provide the body with the essential building blocks it needs during a prolonged period without food intake.

3. Hydration and Electrolytes

Hydration is crucial for any fast, but it's especially important when entering a prolonged one. Dehydration is one of the most common issues people face during fasting, often exacerbating symptoms like fatigue and headaches. In the days leading up to the fast, increase your water intake to ensure your body is fully hydrated. Including electrolytes—such as sodium, potassium, and magnesium—also helps prevent imbalances that can occur when you're not consuming food. Consider drinking an electrolyte solution or incorporating foods like leafy greens, nuts, and seeds to boost electrolyte levels. Proper hydration and electrolytes will help you avoid common pitfalls of fasting, such as dizziness and muscle cramps.

4. Mental Preparation and Setting Intentions

Fasting can be a challenging mental endeavor, especially for those new to the practice. Taking time to mentally prepare can help you stay committed and focus on the benefits of fasting rather than any temporary discomfort. Setting clear intentions—such as promoting metabolic health, mental clarity, or spiritual growth—can keep you motivated. Remind yourself of these goals when challenges arise during the fasting period.

The Prolonged Fasting Period

Once you've entered the fasting state, your body gradually shifts into a mode that prioritizes energy conservation, cellular repair, and ketone production. During prolonged fasting, it's essential to pay attention to your body's signals and understand what's happening physiologically.

1. Embracing Ketosis and Fat Adaptation

As glucose levels decrease, the body begins producing ketones from stored fat to provide an alternative energy source, particularly for the brain. By around 24 to 48 hours, ketone production increases, leading to a state of ketosis. This metabolic shift not only supports energy needs but also offers cognitive benefits such as improved mental clarity and focus. Many people report experiencing a "fasting high" due to increased ketone levels, which is a period of heightened energy and mental clarity.

2. Autophagy and Cellular Repair

Around 24 hours into a fast, autophagy—a cellular process that removes damaged components—becomes active. Autophagy plays a key role in removing toxins, misfolded proteins, and damaged cells, which can contribute to aging and disease. Prolonged fasting enhances autophagy, promoting cellular repair and regeneration. The body enters a "clean-up" phase, where it breaks down dysfunctional proteins and recycles them. This has profound implications for aging, as it can reduce the buildup of cellular waste products linked to age-related diseases.

3. Monitoring and Managing Symptoms

During a prolonged fast, it's common to experience symptoms such as fatigue, mild headaches, or nausea, particularly during the initial transition. While these symptoms usually subside as the body adjusts, it's essential to monitor them. If symptoms become severe or unmanageable, it may indicate that the body is not ready for a prolonged fast, and it's best to break the fast gradually. Staying hydrated, consuming electrolyte-infused water, and practicing deep breathing or light stretching can alleviate mild symptoms and help the body stay balanced during the fasting period.

Breaking a Prolonged Fast

Breaking a fast is as important as entering it, especially after a prolonged period without food. A thoughtful approach to breaking a fast can maximize the benefits, prevent digestive discomfort, and support a smooth transition back to regular eating.

1. Start with Small, Gentle Foods

After an extended fast, the digestive system needs time to reactivate and prepare for regular food intake. Start with small portions of easily digestible foods. Bone broth, for instance, is an excellent choice because it's rich in collagen and amino acids, which help support the gut lining and aid digestion. Smoothies with low-sugar fruits and greens or lightly steamed vegetables are also gentle options that provide nutrients without overwhelming the digestive system. Avoid rich, fatty, or high-carb foods initially, as these can be difficult to digest and may lead to stomach upset or even a blood sugar spike.

2. Reintroduce Nutrients Gradually

Following an extended fast, the body's insulin sensitivity is heightened, so it's important to be mindful of carbohydrate intake when reintroducing foods. Starting with protein and healthy fats, such as eggs, avocados, or a small portion of lean meat, allows the body to ease back into digestion without causing large insulin spikes. Over the course of a day or two, gradually reintroduce a broader range of foods, focusing on nutrient-dense, whole foods that support your goals, whether they're related to fat loss, metabolic health, or general wellness.

3. Hydration and Electrolytes Post-Fast

The hydration requirements post-fast are similar to those pre-fast, as rehydrating the body and balancing electrolytes is essential for a smooth transition. Drinking water with added electrolytes or consuming natural sources of electrolytes, like coconut water or bone broth, can prevent dehydration and support overall recovery. Electrolytes play a significant role in maintaining muscle function, nerve signaling, and energy levels, especially as the body readjusts to regular nutrient intake.

4. Avoiding Overeating and Digestive Distress

It's natural to feel a strong urge to eat a large meal after a prolonged fast, but overeating can overwhelm the digestive system and negate some of the benefits gained during fasting. Start with small meals and allow your body to signal when it's ready for more. Eating mindfully and taking time to chew food thoroughly can prevent digestive discomfort and allow you to appreciate each flavor and texture. Gradually working up to larger meals over a day or two will support a comfortable transition back to regular eating patterns.

The Psychological Aspects of Breaking a Fast

Just as entering a fast requires mental preparation, breaking a prolonged fast also involves a psychological adjustment. It's common for people to feel heightened awareness around food and hunger cues post-fast. Embracing this awareness and practicing mindful eating can reinforce the sense of accomplishment from the fast, helping to build a healthier, more intentional relationship with food.

1. Reinforcing Healthy Eating Patterns

One of the major benefits of fasting is the opportunity to reset habits and develop a mindful approach to eating. Use the transition back to regular eating to focus on nutrient-dense, whole foods that align with your health goals. Reinforcing healthy choices after fasting can help you avoid the temptation to indulge in processed or high-sugar foods, which may diminish the metabolic benefits gained from fasting.

2. Maintaining an Adaptive Mindset

Prolonged fasting can be both physically and mentally challenging, and breaking the fast can often evoke mixed emotions. Some people may feel anxious about reintroducing food, while others may feel a sense of loss after ending the fasting period. Recognize that these feelings are normal and that adopting a balanced mindset can help you transition smoothly. Embrace the progress made during the fast and see the post-fast period as a chance to continue building resilience and self-awareness.

Incorporating Prolonged Fasting into a Health Routine

Once you've experienced a prolonged fast, you may want to consider how it fits into your broader health routine. Prolonged fasting can offer profound benefits when practiced periodically, but it's essential to approach it with balance and respect for your body's needs. Establishing a consistent pattern, such as incorporating intermittent fasting between prolonged fasts, can help maintain the metabolic and cellular benefits while avoiding overextending your body's resources.

1. Listen to Your Body

Each individual's capacity for fasting varies, and what works well for one person may not be suitable for another. Pay attention to your body's signals and respect them. Over time, you'll develop a better understanding of your ideal fasting schedule and the appropriate length for each fasting period. This individualized approach ensures that fasting remains a beneficial tool rather than a source of stress or strain.

2. Combining Fasting with Other Health Practices

Fasting pairs well with other health practices such as exercise, meditation, and nutrient-rich eating. Physical activities, like light exercise or walking, can enhance the benefits of fasting by promoting circulation and reducing stress. Meditation and mindfulness practices can also help maintain focus and resilience throughout the fasting period, making the experience more fulfilling.

Both entering and breaking a prolonged fast are essential components of the fasting process, influencing the body's response and overall experience. Approaching a fast mindfully, preparing the body in advance, and gradually reintroducing foods afterward are all integral to harnessing the full benefits of fasting. By listening to your body, respecting its signals, and fostering a balanced approach, you can turn fasting into a powerful tool for health, resilience, and self-awareness. Through thoughtful practice, fasting can become an effective and sustainable part of your health journey.

3. How Fasting Affects Metabolic Health and Metabolic Syndrome

Insulin and Fat Storage: High insulin levels prevent fat burning and contribute to metabolic dysfunction. Both IF and PF keep insulin levels low, which is beneficial for those with metabolic syndrome.

Benefits for Heart Health: Fasting has been linked to improved cholesterol and triglyceride levels, key factors in cardiovascular health.

Effect on Blood Pressure: IF and PF can reduce blood pressure by allowing the body time to restore balance, free from the constant insulin spikes that come with frequent eating.

Impact on Inflammation and Oxidative Stress: By reducing inflammation and promoting cellular repair through autophagy, fasting addresses two major factors in metabolic syndrome and related diseases.

4. Debunking Common Fasting Myths

Myth: Fasting Slows Down Metabolism: Contrary to popular belief, fasting does not decrease metabolism. In fact, short-term fasting can increase metabolic rate by promoting the release of norepinephrine, a hormone that stimulates metabolism.

Myth: Fasting Causes Muscle Loss: When done correctly, fasting preserves muscle mass. The body adapts by increasing growth hormone, which supports lean muscle and minimizes muscle breakdown.

Myth: Fasting is Dangerous: While fasting isn't suitable for everyone, especially those with specific medical conditions, studies confirm that both IF and PF are safe for healthy individuals when done under proper guidance.

Fasting is often misunderstood, with many myths surrounding its safety and effectiveness. A common misconception is that fasting slows down metabolism, leading to long-term weight gain. In reality, short-term fasting can actually boost metabolism. During fasting, levels of norepinephrine increase, which helps release stored fat and provides a surge in energy. Studies show that intermittent fasting or periodic fasting for a few days doesn't significantly lower metabolism, especially when followed by a nutrient-dense diet. Prolonged, extreme calorie restriction for weeks on end can lower metabolism, but intermittent fasting, combined with proper eating, has been shown to maintain metabolic health without leading to long-term metabolic slowdowns.

People often assume that without a constant intake of protein, the body will start breaking down muscle for fuel. However, the body first uses glycogen stores for energy before shifting to fat reserves, a process called ketosis, which spares muscle tissue. In fact, fasting can actually boost human growth hormone (HGH) levels, which helps preserve muscle and encourages fat burning. For those who exercise during fasting periods, studies show that strength training while fasting can maintain, or even increase, muscle mass.

There's also a widespread belief that fasting is unhealthy for the brain, leading to mental fog and fatigue. While some people may experience initial hunger pangs or lightheadedness as they adjust, research shows that fasting can enhance cognitive function. Fasting has been linked to the production of brain-derived neurotrophic factor (BDNF), a protein that supports neuron growth and cognitive resilience. Rather than causing brain fog, fasting has been found to support clearer thinking, improved memory, and even protection against neurodegenerative diseases.

These myths often arise from misunderstandings of how the body adapts to fasting. When paired with balanced refeeding and nutrient-rich foods, fasting offers a safe and effective approach to improving metabolic health without compromising muscle, metabolism, or mental function.

5. How to Approach Fasting Safely and Effectively

Start Small: If you're new to fasting, begin with the 16:8 method before moving to longer fasting periods. This approach allows your body to adjust gradually.

Listen to Your Body: Fasting is meant to benefit health, not hinder it. If you feel overly fatigued or lightheaded, break the fast and consult a healthcare provider if necessary.

Stay Hydrated: Hydration is crucial during fasting. Drinking water, herbal teas, and electrolyte solutions (if needed) can prevent dehydration and support energy levels.

Mind Your Electrolytes: Longer fasts, especially PF, can lead to electrolyte imbalances. If fasting for more than 24 hours, consider supplementing with sodium, potassium, and magnesium.

It's crucial for pregnant individuals to approach fasting with caution and consult their healthcare provider before making any changes to their eating patterns. Pregnancy is a time of increased nutritional needs to support both the mother and the developing baby. Fasting, especially prolonged fasting, can affect blood sugar levels, nutrient intake, and energy reserves, all of which are essential for a healthy pregnancy.

While intermittent fasting may have potential health benefits for some individuals, the needs of pregnant people differ. Nutrients like folate, iron, calcium, and protein are especially important during pregnancy for fetal development and maternal health. Skipping meals or reducing intake might limit the ability to meet these needs, potentially affecting both the mother and the baby. Consulting with a healthcare provider will help ensure that any dietary changes are safe and appropriately adapted to support a healthy pregnancy.

6. Combining Fasting with a Healthy Diet

While fasting alone offers numerous benefits, pairing it with a nutrient-dense diet amplifies the positive effects on health. Prioritize whole foods, avoid processed foods, and focus on low-carb, high-protein meals during eating windows to keep insulin levels in check.

Healthy Fats: Avocado, olive oil, and nuts provide steady energy and support mental focus without causing insulin spikes.

Lean Proteins: Foods like fish, poultry, and eggs maintain muscle mass, particularly beneficial after prolonged fasting.

Low-Carb Vegetables: Leafy greens, cruciferous vegetables, and other non-starchy vegetables provide fiber, vitamins, and minerals, supporting digestion and nutrient absorption.

Combining fasting with a nutrient-dense diet is a powerful approach to optimizing health and preventing chronic disease. Fasting allows the body time to rest from constant digestion, promoting cellular repair, reducing inflammation, and enhancing insulin sensitivity. When you pair this with nutrient-dense foods—those rich in essential vitamins, minerals, healthy fats, and lean proteins—you amplify these effects, helping the body stabilize blood sugar, reduce cravings, and build resilience against metabolic imbalances.

One of the key benefits of fasting with a nutrient-dense diet is its effect on insulin regulation. Constant eating, particularly of carbohydrate-heavy foods, keeps insulin levels elevated, leading to insulin resistance over time—a precursor to numerous chronic conditions, including type 2 diabetes and heart disease. By incorporating intermittent fasting, you allow insulin levels to drop and facilitate the body's shift from glucose to fat as the primary energy source. Foods that are high in protein, fiber, and healthy fats, like leafy greens, fish, eggs, and avocados, support this process by providing sustained energy and keeping blood sugar stable without unnecessary insulin spikes.

A balanced, whole-food approach also complements fasting by reducing inflammation, which is central to many health issues. Nutrient-rich foods supply antioxidants and omega-3 fatty acids that counterbalance inflammatory foods and promote healing. Meanwhile, fasting gives the body a break from inflammatory triggers and supports processes like autophagy, where the body cleans up damaged cells. Together, these approaches encourage a healthy metabolic environment, fostering weight control, mental clarity, and overall well-being, making fasting and a nutrient-dense diet a sustainable and effective combination for long-term health.

7. Final Thoughts on Fasting for Health

Fasting can be a powerful tool for achieving metabolic health, reducing inflammation, and potentially extending lifespan. By helping to regulate insulin levels, support cellular repair, and promote autophagy, both intermittent fasting (IF) and prolonged fasting (PF) offer unique advantages that help counter the damaging effects of today's processed, high-carb diets. In a world where constant eating and refined foods are commonplace, fasting stands out as a natural way to reset the body's metabolic balance.

However, fasting isn't a one-size-fits-all solution, and it's crucial to approach it thoughtfully. Factors like individual health conditions, nutritional needs, and lifestyle all play into finding the right balance of fasting and nutrient-dense eating. Done correctly, fasting can be a transformative practice for modern health challenges, providing our bodies with the metabolic "break" they need to thrive.

Fasting is one of the most natural practices for the human body, yet in our modern world, it's viewed as something unusual, even extreme. To understand why fasting is not only natural but beneficial, we need to shift our perspective back to ancestral times and see how it aligns with our biological design.

For thousands of years, humans lived in environments where food wasn't available on demand. Our ancestors would go days, or sometimes even longer, between successful hunts. Between kills, they naturally entered periods of fasting. This was not a choice; it was simply the reality of life. Our bodies evolved to adapt to these cycles of feast and famine, developing systems that allow us to store energy when food is available and to efficiently use stored energy during times when food is scarce. This natural cycle of fasting and eating is part of our genetic blueprint, a survival mechanism that has shaped human physiology for millennia.

Our bodies are resilient and incredibly intuitive when it comes to managing hunger and energy. When we're sick, for instance, we often lose our appetite. Think about the last time you had the flu—you probably weren't craving food every few hours. This is a natural response, as our body's energy shifts toward healing rather than digesting. When we listen to these signals, we allow our bodies to perform optimally. However, in today's world, we often ignore these natural cues, frequently eating because it's "time to eat" or because food is constantly accessible, rather than because we're truly hungry.

One reason we feel hungry more often now than our ancestors did is because we've disrupted the natural balance of our hormones. Modern diets, high in processed foods and carbohydrates, have led to hormonal imbalances that impact hunger and satiety. Foods loaded with sugars and refined carbs spike insulin levels and lead to fluctuating blood sugar, which drives constant hunger. In contrast, fasting allows our hormones, especially insulin, to recalibrate, bringing our natural hunger cues back into alignment. As insulin levels stabilize, our body becomes better at utilizing stored fat for energy, reducing the frequency and intensity of hunger pangs.

Fasting, therefore, is not just a trend or a fad but a practice deeply rooted in our evolution. It's a natural, ancestral way of living that aligns with how our bodies were designed to function. Rather than questioning nature, we should embrace this powerful tool as a means to restore metabolic balance, improve resilience, and reconnect with our body's innate wisdom.

For those interested in diving deeper into the science and applications of fasting, *The Complete Guide to Fasting* by Dr. Jason Fung, a nephrologist based in Canada, offers an inspiring and comprehensive look into how fasting can positively impact health. His book is a highly recommended resource for anyone considering fasting as part of their wellness journey.

Chapter 7 Inflammation

Inflammation is a natural, essential process for healing, but when it becomes chronic, it turns from a protective mechanism into a contributor to disease. Our dietary and lifestyle choices play a crucial role in either promoting or reducing this persistent inflammation. Chronic inflammation is now understood to be a root factor in many modern diseases, including heart disease, diabetes, autoimmune disorders, mental health conditions, and certain cancers. Addressing inflammation through diet and lifestyle changes offers a proactive approach to health—targeting the underlying causes rather than just managing symptoms. By adopting an anti-inflammatory lifestyle, we can harness the healing power of inflammation while preventing it from becoming a driver of disease. This dual understanding empowers us to use inflammation for recovery and resilience while safeguarding long-term health.

To fully grasp the effects of chronic inflammation, it's important to understand how the inflammatory response functions at a biological level and why certain factors in our modern lifestyle and diet are driving it to dangerous, prolonged levels. This chapter delves into the biochemistry of inflammation, how it manifests in the body, and practical methods for reducing chronic inflammation for long-term health.

Understanding Inflammation as a Homeostatic Response:

Inflammation is the body's complex biological response to harmful stimuli such as pathogens, damaged cells, or toxic compounds. This process is essential for initiating healing and restoring homeostasis. While **acute inflammation** is beneficial and necessary for fighting infections and repairing tissue damage, chronic inflammation is where problems arise. It becomes detrimental when the inflammatory response persists over time and contributes to various chronic diseases, including metabolic syndrome, diabetes, cardiovascular disease, and autoimmune disorders.

Fever: The Body's Natural Defense Mechanism:

Fever is an example of how the body's inflammatory response functions to restore balance. When an infection occurs, the body raises its temperature to create an environment less hospitable to pathogens and enhance the activity of immune cells. This natural response promotes recovery and helps the body fight off the infection more effectively. However, common medical practice often involves the use of **antipyretics** (fever reducers) to lower fever, which may sometimes hinder the body's natural healing processes. While there are situations where reducing a high fever is necessary to prevent potential complications (e.g., febrile seizures in children), routine suppression of moderate fevers might not always be the best approach.

A Call for Reevaluation in Medical Practice:

Medical practitioners should weigh the benefits and risks of suppressing inflammation in each case. Chronic use of anti-inflammatory drugs, such as NSAIDs, for minor or moderate conditions could interfere with the body's natural healing mechanisms and potentially contribute to long-term issues. Furthermore, this practice can mask underlying problems rather than addressing the root causes of inflammation.

Encouraging doctors and patients to understand the dual nature of inflammation—both as a protector and, when unchecked, a contributor to disease—can lead to a more **holistic approach** to treatment. This would include promoting lifestyle interventions that support the body's natural inflammatory responses while preventing chronic inflammation, such as diet modifications, stress management, and physical activity.

Reframing Inflammation as a Positive Force:

By framing **inflammation as the body's attempt to regain homeostasis**, you highlight the importance of viewing acute inflammatory responses, including fever, as beneficial under many circumstances. This perspective can promote better patient education, where people understand that not every fever or sign of inflammation needs to be suppressed immediately. Instead, the focus can be on **supporting the body through the process**, ensuring hydration, rest, and nutrient-rich foods to enhance recovery, reserving medication for when it is truly necessary.

Revisiting how inflammation and fever are managed in medical practice can lead to better health outcomes. Understanding the body's natural defense mechanisms and respecting their role in maintaining homeostasis will help shift the paradigm from quick symptomatic relief to long-term health maintenance and resilience. Emphasizing this concept in your book will help readers appreciate the fine balance between beneficial and harmful inflammation and support a more **informed and balanced approach** to health interventions.

Biochemistry of Inflammation At its core, inflammation is a complex biological response involving various cells and signaling molecules. When the body detects an injury or infection, white blood cells are activated and begin releasing cytokines, which are small proteins that signal other cells to initiate a response. Key players in inflammation include:

1. **Cytokines and Chemokines**: These signaling molecules (such as IL-6 and TNF-alpha) are produced by immune cells and help recruit other cells to the site of infection or injury.
2. **Macrophages**: These large immune cells digest cellular debris and pathogens and are pivotal in both initiating and resolving inflammation.
3. **Histamines**: Released by immune cells, histamines dilate blood vessels, allowing more immune cells to reach the affected area.

While acute inflammation, like that from a cut or infection, is temporary and beneficial, chronic inflammation involves sustained levels of cytokines and other inflammatory markers, which damage healthy cells over time. This ongoing immune response is particularly dangerous because it creates an environment of oxidative stress and tissue damage, which disrupts cellular functions and increases disease risk.

Types of Inflammation and Triggers

- **Acute Inflammation**: Acute inflammation is the body's rapid response to injury or infection. For example, if you get a cut, blood flow increases to the area to bring white blood cells and platelets to help fight infection and clot the blood. Redness, heat, swelling, and pain are typical symptoms, and once the infection is cleared or the tissue is repaired, the inflammation subsides.

- **Chronic Inflammation**: Unlike acute inflammation, chronic inflammation lingers, often with no clear injury or infection to resolve. Chronic inflammation occurs when the body's immune system is continually activated. Over time, this damages tissues and organs, increasing the risk of various disease

Pathways of Acute vs Chronic Inflammation

Acute Inflammation	←	Immune Response	←	Healing & Recovery
Chronic Inflammation	←	Sustained Immune Activation	←	Tissue Damage & Disease Risk

Triggers of chronic inflammation include:

Dietary Factors: Diets high in sugar, refined carbs, and processed foods contribute to inflammation. Inflammatory oils such as soybean, canola, and corn oil contain omega-6 fatty acids, which can imbalance the body's omega-6 to omega-3 ratio, exacerbating inflammation.

Lifestyle: Sedentary behavior, lack of sleep, and chronic stress are significant contributors to inflammation. Stress hormones like cortisol, when elevated long-term, promote an inflammatory state.

Environmental Toxins: Exposure to pollutants, chemicals, and toxins found in air, water, and consumer products can trigger chronic inflammation.

Gut Microbiome Imbalances: A poor diet and high levels of stress can lead to an imbalance in gut bacteria (dysbiosis), promoting inflammation through the gut-brain and gut-immune system connections.

The Role of Inflammation in Disease Chronic inflammation is a key driver in the development of many modern diseases:

Metabolic Syndrome and Insulin Resistance: Inflammation plays a role in obesity and insulin resistance, two primary components of metabolic syndrome. Inflammatory markers like TNF-alpha interfere with insulin signaling, causing cells to become insulin-resistant. As insulin resistance progresses, it disrupts glucose metabolism and fuels a vicious cycle of inflammation and metabolic dysfunction.

Cardiovascular Disease: Inflammation contributes to the development of atherosclerosis, where plaques form in artery walls. Inflammatory cytokines damage the endothelium (the inner lining of blood vessels), which leads to plaque buildup and restricts blood flow, significantly increasing the risk of heart attacks and strokes.

Autoimmune Disorders: Conditions such as rheumatoid arthritis, lupus, and multiple sclerosis occur when the immune system mistakenly attacks the body's own tissues. Chronic inflammation is both a cause and a symptom of these autoimmune disorders.

Cognitive Health: Chronic inflammation is linked to neurodegenerative diseases like Alzheimer's. Inflammatory cytokines can cross the blood-brain barrier, leading to brain inflammation, which contributes to the formation of amyloid plaques and tau tangles, key markers of Alzheimer's.

Cancer: Prolonged inflammation can lead to DNA damage, increasing the likelihood of mutations and cancer development. Inflammatory cells produce reactive oxygen species **Lifestyle Factors and Their Influence on Inflammation** Chronic inflammation isn't solely caused by diet. Various lifestyle factors also impact inflammatory processes:

1. **Physical Activity**: Exercise has been shown to reduce inflammatory markers like CRP (C-reactive protein) and IL-6. Physical activity promotes anti-inflammatory responses and can lower the risk of conditions such as cardiovascular disease and diabetes.
2. **Stress**: Chronic stress elevates cortisol levels, a hormone that, when sustained, leads to inflammation. Mindfulness, meditation, and relaxation techniques can help mitigate this effect by lowering cortisol and promoting an anti-inflammatory state.
3. **Sleep**: Poor sleep quality or insufficient sleep increases inflammatory markers and weakens the immune system.

Quality sleep is essential for tissue repair and for the immune system to reset.

4. **Gut Health**: The gut microbiome plays a crucial role in inflammation. Beneficial bacteria help to regulate the immune system, while an imbalance of harmful bacteria (dysbiosis) promotes inflammation. Probiotics, prebiotics, and a diverse diet rich in fiber support a healthy gut microbiome.

Practical Strategies to Combat Inflammation To address chronic inflammation effectively, a holistic approach that includes diet, lifestyle changes, and stress management is essential:

Dietary Adjustments: Minimize sugar, refined carbs, and seed oils while focusing on anti-inflammatory foods like leafy greens, berries, and omega-3 sources such as salmon and walnuts.

Lifestyle Changes: Engage in regular physical activity, practice stress management techniques, and prioritize sleep. These factors reduce cortisol levels and help the body maintain a balanced immune response.

Reducing Toxin Exposure: Choose natural, non-toxic household products, reduce processed foods, and try to minimize exposure to pollutants when possible.

Inflammation Relating to Diet and Health

Inflammation, a natural and necessary biological response, is crucial for healing and protecting the body from harm. Yet, when inflammation becomes chronic, it can set the stage for numerous diseases, from cardiovascular conditions to autoimmune disorders. A significant factor in controlling inflammation is the balance of omega-3 and omega-6 fatty acids in our diet. The optimal ratio of omega-3 to omega-6 fatty acids is around 1:1, meaning an equal intake of both types. Unfortunately, in the modern American diet, this ratio has been severely disrupted, with intakes often reaching 1:20 or even 1:30, heavily skewed in favor of omega-6. This imbalance has drastic implications for inflammation and health, as omega-6 fats are known to promote inflammatory pathways while omega-3s play a counterbalancing, anti-inflammatory role.

Omega-6 and Omega-3 Fatty Acids: The Balance Dilemma

Omega-3 and omega-6 fatty acids are essential polyunsaturated fats that the body cannot produce independently. Thus, they must be obtained from our diet. Omega-3 fats, found in fatty fish (like salmon and mackerel), flaxseeds, walnuts, and chia seeds, are critical for reducing inflammation, supporting heart health, and maintaining brain function. Omega-6 fats, on the other hand, are abundant in vegetable oils (like corn, soy, and sunflower oils) as well as processed foods and grains, and while necessary in small amounts, they become problematic when consumed in excess. The ratio of Omega-3 to Omega-6 in our body should be 1:1. The average American has a ratio closer to 1:25 and declining as we speak, which is extremely bad news.

The excessive consumption of omega-6 fats is largely a byproduct of modern dietary habits. Many processed foods are laden with omega-6-rich oils due to their affordability, long shelf life, and presence in almost every packaged snack or meal. Additionally, animals raised on grain-based diets (as opposed to grass-fed diets) also have higher levels of omega-6 fatty acids in their meat, which further contributes to the imbalance in our diets. This cumulative effect creates a skewed ratio in favor of omega-6, leading to an inflammatory environment in the body. Inflammation itself is an immune response, but when constantly triggered, it creates conditions that stress the body, disrupt cellular health, and contribute to chronic diseases.

How Chronic Inflammation Harms the Body

When the body senses a "foreign" substance—be it a pathogen, toxin, or injury—it triggers inflammation to protect and heal the affected area. This reaction is typically localized, with white blood cells rushing to the site of injury or infection, releasing chemicals to repair tissue and neutralize invaders. This form of inflammation, called acute inflammation, is beneficial as it aids in healing.

However, chronic inflammation differs significantly. Instead of being a temporary response, chronic inflammation is a prolonged, low-grade response that continues even without an immediate threat. Instead of helping the body, this prolonged state of inflammation causes cellular damage, disrupts normal tissue function, and increases the risk of several diseases. The body's immune system remains in a heightened state, continually producing inflammatory markers and cytokines that can damage healthy cells, weaken immune responses, and contribute to tissue degeneration.

Modern Diets and the Inflammatory Cascade

Today's typical diet, which is high in refined carbohydrates, sugars, and processed foods, is a recipe for chronic inflammation. Refined carbs, found in foods like white bread, pastries, and sugary drinks, rapidly spike blood sugar levels, prompting the body to release insulin to bring these levels down. Frequent blood sugar spikes and insulin surges can lead to insulin resistance, a condition closely linked to metabolic syndrome, obesity, and Type 2 diabetes—all of which are associated with chronic inflammation.

In addition, sugar itself can be an inflammatory agent. High sugar intake triggers an immune response, leading to the release of inflammatory markers. It also promotes the formation of advanced glycation end-products (AGEs), which are compounds created when proteins or fats combine with sugars in the bloodstream. AGEs accumulate in tissues and blood vessels, causing oxidative stress, damaging cells, and contributing to inflammation.

The problem compounds with the widespread consumption of trans fats and omega-6-rich oils. Trans fats, found in fried foods, baked goods, and margarine, increase "bad" LDL cholesterol levels and reduce "good" HDL cholesterol levels, a combination that promotes inflammation and the buildup of plaque in arteries. Similarly, excess omega-6 fatty acids, as previously mentioned, stimulate inflammatory pathways, perpetuating chronic inflammation when they far outnumber omega-3s in the diet.

The Role of Omega-3 Fatty Acids in Reducing Inflammation

Omega-3 fatty acids serve as potent anti-inflammatory agents, and their presence in the body helps counterbalance the inflammatory actions of omega-6 fats. There are three main types of omega-3s: EPA, DHA, and ALA. EPA (eicosapentaenoic acid) and DHA (docosahexaenoic acid) are primarily found in marine sources like fish, while ALA (alpha-linolenic acid) is found in plant sources, such as flaxseeds and walnuts.

EPA and DHA, in particular, are instrumental in reducing inflammation at a cellular level. They get incorporated into cell membranes and influence the production of signaling molecules known as eicosanoids, which play a direct role in the inflammatory response. When cells contain higher levels of EPA and DHA, they produce fewer inflammatory eicosanoids, thereby reducing inflammation. Research has shown that diets high in omega-3 fatty acids are associated with lower levels of C-reactive protein (CRP), an inflammatory marker, and reduced risk of chronic diseases, including heart disease, arthritis, and certain cancers.

To reduce inflammation effectively, it is essential to adjust the omega-6 to omega-3 ratio. Striving for a 1:1 or 2:1 ratio, as seen in ancestral diets, can significantly reduce inflammatory markers in the body. This adjustment involves not only increasing omega-3 intake through dietary sources like fatty fish, flaxseeds, and chia seeds but also reducing omega-6 intake by limiting processed foods, vegetable oils, and grain-fed meats.

The Body's Natural Response to Foreign Substances

The human body is highly attuned to maintaining balance, known as homeostasis. When something foreign enters the body, whether it's a toxin, chemical, or pathogen, the body's immune system initiates a response to eliminate it and restore balance. Inflammation is a part of this protective process, helping the body rid itself of harmful invaders and repair damaged tissues. This mechanism has served humans well in an evolutionary context, as acute inflammation is critical for survival.

However, chronic exposure to modern dietary toxins, artificial ingredients, and an imbalance of fatty acids puts the body in a constant state of vigilance. In a sense, the body interprets the presence of these unnatural substances as a threat, leading to chronic low-grade inflammation. Over time, this state of persistent inflammation can damage healthy cells, weaken immune defenses, and impair organ function. For instance, inflammation in blood vessels can lead to endothelial damage, contributing to atherosclerosis (plaque buildup in the arteries), while inflammation in the digestive tract can increase the risk of inflammatory bowel diseases.

The Damaging Impact of Chronic Inflammation

The effects of chronic inflammation extend to nearly every system in the body. In the cardiovascular system, inflammation contributes to atherosclerosis and increases the risk of heart attacks and strokes. In the brain, chronic inflammation is linked to cognitive decline, dementia, and depression. In the joints, it exacerbates conditions like arthritis, and in the endocrine system, it can disrupt hormone function, contributing to conditions such as polycystic ovarian syndrome (PCOS) and hypothyroidism.

Moreover, inflammation is a primary driver of insulin resistance, a condition where cells no longer respond effectively to insulin. As insulin resistance develops, blood sugar levels remain elevated, leading to a cascade of metabolic disturbances, including increased fat storage, weight gain, and heightened inflammation. This vicious cycle perpetuates metabolic syndrome and heightens the risk of Type 2 diabetes.

Moving Toward an Anti-Inflammatory Diet

To combat chronic inflammation, dietary changes are essential. An anti-inflammatory diet focuses on whole, unprocessed foods that are low in sugar and refined carbohydrates while being rich in antioxidants, fiber, and essential nutrients. Key dietary practices include:

Increasing Omega-3 Intake: Incorporate fatty fish like salmon, sardines, and mackerel into your diet to boost EPA and DHA levels. For plant-based sources, add chia seeds, flaxseeds, and walnuts.

Reducing Omega-6 Fatty Acids: Limit vegetable oils like corn, soy, and sunflower oil, which are high in omega-6 fats. Instead, opt for olive oil, avocado oil, or coconut oil, which have healthier fat profiles.

Eliminating Trans Fats: Avoid foods with trans fats, commonly found in baked goods, fried foods, and processed snacks, as these fats contribute significantly to inflammation.

Reducing Sugar and Refined Carbohydrates: Minimizing sugar intake helps prevent blood sugar spikes and reduces the risk of insulin resistance. Replace refined carbs with whole grains like quinoa and oats.

Incorporating Antioxidant-Rich Foods: Foods like berries, dark leafy greens, and nuts are rich in antioxidants, which combat oxidative stress and reduce inflammation at the cellular level.

Choosing Grass-Fed or Pasture-Raised Animal Products: These options generally contain higher levels of omega-3s and fewer inflammatory compounds than grain-fed products.

Staying Hydrated: Proper hydration supports cellular function and helps the body flush out toxins that could otherwise contribute to inflammation.

Chronic inflammation is a central factor in numerous diseases and a symptom of modern lifestyle imbalances. By focusing on dietary adjustments, improving sleep, managing stress, and engaging in regular physical activity, we can reduce inflammation and improve overall health. Tackling inflammation at its root provides a pathway not only to preventing diseases but also to enhancing the quality of life for long-term wellness. Understanding and addressing the underlying causes of inflammation empowers us to live healthier, more resilient lives.

Gut Health "Protect the Liver...Feed the Gut"

Gut health has emerged as one of the most critical areas of focus for understanding overall health. Far more than just the site of digestion, the gut plays a fundamental role in numerous bodily systems and has profound implications for long-term wellness. The human gut, often referred to as the "second brain," houses trillions of microorganisms that impact not only digestion but also immune function, mental health, and metabolic balance. As Dr. Robert Lustig aptly states, "Protect the liver, feed the gut," a guiding principle that underscores the intricate relationship between gut health and overall bodily health.

Understanding the Gut Microbiome

The gut microbiome consists of a diverse community of bacteria, viruses, fungi, and other microorganisms that live primarily in the intestines. These microorganisms help break down food, synthesize vitamins, regulate metabolism, and support immune function. The balance of these microorganisms is crucial for maintaining health; when disrupted, it can lead to a state known as dysbiosis. Dysbiosis has been linked to numerous health conditions, including

157

inflammatory bowel disease (IBD), irritable bowel syndrome (IBS), obesity, type 2 diabetes, and autoimmune disorders.

The gut is also home to the majority of the body's immune cells. Approximately 70% of the immune system resides in the gut-associated lymphoid tissue (GALT), highlighting the direct connection between gut health and immune function. A well-balanced gut microbiome contributes to a robust immune response, while an imbalanced microbiome can lead to chronic inflammation and a weakened ability to fight off pathogens.

Gut Health and Inflammation

Chronic inflammation is a major contributor to many of today's most prevalent diseases, including heart disease, metabolic syndrome, and autoimmune disorders. The gut plays a significant role in modulating the body's inflammatory response. When the gut barrier is compromised—a condition often called "leaky gut syndrome"—harmful substances such as toxins and partially digested food particles can pass through the intestinal wall and into the bloodstream. This triggers the immune system to respond, resulting in systemic inflammation.

A healthy gut lining acts as a barrier, preventing these harmful substances from escaping into the bloodstream. Supporting the gut's integrity and maintaining a balanced microbiome are thus essential for minimizing chronic inflammation. A diet that prioritizes gut health—rich in nutrient-dense, whole foods—helps support the gut lining, bolster immune function, and reduce systemic inflammation.

The Gut-Brain Connection

The gut-brain axis is a two-way communication system between the gut and the brain, involving the central nervous system, the enteric nervous system, and biochemical signaling through the bloodstream. This connection means that the gut not only affects physical health but also has a significant impact on mental health and cognitive function. The gut produces neurotransmitters such as serotonin, a chemical that contributes to feelings of well-being and happiness. In fact, around 90% of the body's serotonin is produced in the gut.

Dysbiosis or poor gut health can disrupt the production of these neurotransmitters, leading to mood imbalances and mental health disorders such as depression and anxiety. This further emphasizes that taking care of gut health is not just about physical wellness but also about mental and emotional well-being.

Metabolic Health and the Role of the Gut

Dr. Robert Lustig's principle, "Protect the liver, feed the gut," encapsulates the importance of gut health in metabolic processes. The liver and the gut work in tandem to manage the body's metabolism and energy balance. A well-functioning gut aids in the efficient digestion and absorption of nutrients, which are essential for proper liver function. When gut health is compromised, it can lead to increased stress on the liver as it processes toxins and manages nutrient imbalances.

Moreover, the gut microbiome helps regulate blood sugar levels and insulin sensitivity. Beneficial gut bacteria produce short-chain fatty acids (SCFAs) such as butyrate, acetate, and propionate, which help modulate glucose metabolism and reduce inflammation. SCFAs play a critical role in maintaining the gut lining, promoting healthy lipid profiles, and preventing the development of insulin resistance. Conversely, a lack of SCFAs due to poor gut health can exacerbate metabolic dysfunction and contribute to the onset of metabolic syndrome and type 2 diabetes.

Diet and Lifestyle Factors for Optimal Gut Health

Supporting gut health involves a holistic approach that incorporates dietary choices, lifestyle habits, and stress management. Here are key strategies for promoting a healthy gut:

Nutrient-Dense Diet: Prioritize whole foods rich in vitamins, minerals, and fiber (if applicable to the diet). Foods such as fermented vegetables, bone broth, and grass-fed meats provide the building blocks for a healthy gut lining and diverse microbiome.

Fermented Foods and Probiotics: Including fermented foods like kefir, sauerkraut, kimchi, and yogurt can introduce beneficial bacteria that support the gut microbiome. Probiotics, whether from food or supplements, can help replenish and maintain gut flora.

Avoiding Processed Foods and Excess Sugars: Processed foods and refined sugars can promote the growth of harmful bacteria and lead to dysbiosis. Reducing or eliminating these foods can help restore balance to the gut microbiome.

Stress Management: Chronic stress negatively impacts gut health by altering the composition of gut bacteria and increasing gut permeability. Practices such as mindfulness, meditation, and regular physical activity can mitigate stress and support gut health.

Hydration: Adequate water intake is essential for maintaining the mucosal lining of the intestines and facilitating the smooth movement of food through the digestive tract.

The Long-Term Importance of Gut Health

The implications of maintaining gut health extend far beyond digestion. A well-balanced gut microbiome contributes to a strong immune system, reduced risk of chronic disease, better mental health, and improved metabolic function. Conversely, neglecting gut health can lead to a cascade of health issues, starting with digestive discomfort and escalating to systemic inflammation and chronic disease.

Given the interconnected nature of the gut with various bodily systems, it becomes clear why Dr. Lustig's adage, "Protect the liver, feed the gut," is a vital mantra for holistic health. By prioritizing gut health through appropriate dietary choices and lifestyle changes, we can support not just the gut but the body as a whole. This approach paves the way for sustained energy, better mental clarity, and a resilient immune system—key components of long-term health and well-being.

Foods To Improve Gut Microbiome

Foods that improve gut microbiome health are typically those rich in beneficial bacteria, prebiotics, and fiber (for those who include it in their diet). These foods help maintain a diverse and balanced gut microbiota, which supports digestion, immunity, and overall well-being. Here are key food categories that promote gut health:

1. Fermented Foods

Yogurt: Contains live cultures such as *Lactobacillus* and *Bifidobacterium* that can improve gut flora.

Kefir: A fermented milk drink with a high probiotic content and diverse strains of bacteria.

Sauerkraut: Fermented cabbage rich in probiotics and fiber.

Kimchi: A traditional Korean dish made from fermented vegetables, often cabbage and radishes, which contains *Lactobacillus* and other beneficial strains.

Miso: A fermented soybean paste used in Japanese cuisine, packed with probiotics.

Tempeh: Fermented soybeans that provide probiotics and protein.

2. Prebiotic-Rich Foods

- **Garlic**: Contains inulin, a prebiotic fiber that feeds beneficial gut bacteria.
- **Onions**: Rich in inulin and fructooligosaccharides that promote the growth of healthy gut bacteria.
- **Bananas**: Particularly green bananas, which contain resistant starch, a type of prebiotic.
- **Asparagus**: Contains inulin, supporting the growth of good bacteria in the gut.
- **Leeks**: High in prebiotics that support digestive health.
- **Chicory Root**: One of the richest sources of inulin.

3. High-Fiber Foods (For Non-Carnivore Diets)

- **Whole Grains**: Oats, barley, and other whole grains provide soluble fiber and beta-glucans that feed beneficial bacteria.
- **Legumes**: Lentils, chickpeas, and beans offer both fiber and resistant starch.
- **Berries**: Blueberries, raspberries, and strawberries are high in antioxidants and fiber that support gut health.

4. Polyphenol-Rich Foods

- **Green Tea**: Contains polyphenols that are metabolized by gut bacteria and have anti-inflammatory effects.
- **Dark Chocolate**: In moderation, provides polyphenols that feed beneficial gut microbes.
- **Red Wine**: Rich in polyphenols that can help improve gut microbiome diversity when consumed in small amounts.
- **Olive Oil**: Contains polyphenols that promote a healthy gut environment.

5. Bone Broth

- Contains gelatin and amino acids like glycine and glutamine, which support the gut lining and overall digestive health.

6. Healthy Fats

- **Saturated Fats:** Yes folks, you read right. Saturated fats are vital for health, despite what you may have heard from the 1950's, eating saturated fat WILL NOT make you fat.
- **Omega-3 Fatty Acids**: Found in fatty fish like salmon, mackerel, and sardines, these fats have anti-inflammatory properties that benefit the gut.
- **Avocado**: Provides healthy monounsaturated fats and fiber for gut health.

7. Probiotic Supplements

- While not technically a food, high-quality probiotic supplements can be helpful, particularly for those who may not get enough fermented foods in their diet.

Incorporating a variety of these foods can help support a balanced gut microbiome, reduce inflammation, and improve digestion and overall health. For those on specialized diets like the carnivore diet, fermented foods and nutrient-dense bone broths may provide similar benefits without the fiber component.

Chapter 8 The Proper Diet for *You*

In today's world, diet trends come and go, and everyone seems to have an opinion on what constitutes the "best" diet. From the Zone Diet, popularized in fitness circles with its 40/30/30 ratio of carbohydrates to proteins to fats, to an antiquated regimen like the South Beach Diet, there is no shortage of opinions on what we should be eating. But here's the thing: these popular diets often fail to address the individual needs of the human body, nor do they consider our evolutionary history, a key mistake. The concept of "balanced" macros might sound scientifically sound, but I believe it's missing the mark entirely.

As a nutrition and scientific analyst, I'm convinced that carbohydrates, at least in the forms and quantities widely consumed today, have no essential place in the human diet. While this view may seem radical, it's based on both an evolutionary perspective and the adverse metabolic effects I've seen in clients and in research. In this chapter, we'll break down what people are currently eating, how human diets have changed drastically over millennia, and the dietary patterns I believe best support human health. By looking at our nutritional past and the impact of modern foods on metabolism, my goal is to help clarify what we really should be eating as human beings for optimal health.

From evolutionary insights to practical applications, I hope to guide you toward a dietary pattern that nourishes your body according to its design—not according to food industry trends or outdated nutritional myths. Let's get into why and how carbohydrates could be working against your body, and what an ideal diet looks like for long-term wellness.

It should be noted that while I will tell you that fats and proteins are what the majority, if not totality of what you consume should be, but I will mention other foods that I believe are NOT optimal but are the lesser of other evils. For example, whole grains. Do I eat whole grains? I do not, nor do I think they are healthy, but they're LESS harmful than other foods. I will cover the hierarchy of foods in another chapter.

For hundreds of thousands of years, humans evolved as hunter-gatherers, surviving on the foods they could hunt or forage. This diet was predominantly made up of animal-based sources, including nutrient-dense organ meats, fatty tissues, and occasionally, fibrous plants or seasonal fruits. Carbohydrate intake was scarce and inconsistent; fruits and tubers were only available seasonally and varied significantly in nutrient and sugar composition compared to today's varieties. Unlike our modern high-carb diet, early humans didn't consume grains, processed sugars, or refined carbohydrates in any significant amount. Instead, they relied on fats and proteins to sustain energy, and their bodies adapted to use these macronutrients efficiently.

Our ancestors' reliance on animal-based foods and the minimal role of carbohydrates is crucial in understanding the human body's metabolic preferences and adaptability. The infrequent intake of carbohydrates also meant that early humans were not frequently experiencing the spikes and falls in blood sugar levels that are common today. This dietary pattern, low in carbs and high in fats and proteins, shaped our metabolism in ways that are still fundamental to our health today.

The Randle Cycle: Why Carbohydrates Aren't Necessary

The **Randle Cycle**, or the **glucose-fatty acid cycle**, provides a foundational understanding of how the body prioritizes fuel sources and highlights why a high-carbohydrate diet may not be ideal for metabolic health. According to the Randle Cycle, cells can only prioritize one primary fuel—either glucose or fat—at a time. When fat is available for energy, the body inhibits glucose utilization, and when glucose is abundant, the body limits fat burning. This metabolic mechanism illustrates that high dietary carbohydrate intake interferes with the body's ability to efficiently burn fat, promoting fat storage and, over time, contributing to insulin resistance.

In a high-carbohydrate diet, glucose levels in the bloodstream are consistently elevated, leading the body to prioritize glucose as a primary fuel source. This frequent reliance on glucose decreases the body's natural capacity to burn fat, ultimately leading to the accumulation of fat stores. As insulin is released to manage blood glucose, high levels over time may contribute to **insulin resistance**, a central characteristic of metabolic syndrome. In essence, the Randle Cycle indicates that an excess of dietary carbohydrates

164

disrupts fat metabolism, keeping the body dependent on glucose and diminishing its fat-burning efficiency.

From an evolutionary perspective, our ancestors likely existed in a metabolic state that prioritized fat as a primary fuel source, given the scarcity of high-carbohydrate foods and the reliance on animal fats and proteins. In this state, the body was naturally geared toward burning fat, a more efficient fuel for extended energy. Reducing carbohydrate intake and shifting to a fat-based fuel source can help modern individuals replicate this ancestral metabolic state, minimizing the risk of insulin resistance and metabolic dysfunction. By allowing fats to become the primary fuel, the body becomes metabolically flexible, leading to more stable energy levels, improved fat metabolism, and a reduced risk of metabolic syndrome and its associated conditions.

Gluconeogenesis: The Body's Ability to Produce Its Own Glucose

A common argument in favor of carbohydrates is that the body "needs" them for essential functions, especially for fueling the brain. While glucose is indeed necessary for some bodily functions, the body has a built-in mechanism to ensure it always has a sufficient supply, regardless of dietary carbohydrate intake. This process is known as gluconeogenesis, in which the liver and kidneys convert non-carbohydrate substrates—such as amino acids from proteins and glycerol from fats—into glucose.

Gluconeogenesis is an adaptive process that enables humans to survive without direct carbohydrate intake. In a low-carbohydrate or ketogenic state, the body relies primarily on fats and ketones for energy, with gluconeogenesis providing the minimal glucose needed to maintain homeostasis. The body's capacity to generate glucose internally eliminates the necessity of carbohydrates in the diet, reinforcing that they are not an essential macronutrient. This ability has allowed humans to thrive on varied diets, from the fatty, animal-based diets of Arctic populations to the meat-and-milk-based diets of pastoralist societies.

Protein and Fat

A diet consisting solely of protein and fat would align closely with what many consider to be the diet of early humans, as well as that of modern carnivorous populations. Without carbohydrates, the body enters a metabolic state where it relies predominantly on fats and proteins to fuel itself. This dietary model is often referred to as a ketogenic or carnivore diet, where fat becomes the primary energy source, and protein provides the building blocks for muscle, hormones, and immune function.

In this state, fats are converted into ketones, a highly efficient energy source, especially for the brain. The body also undergoes gluconeogenesis, where small amounts of protein are converted into glucose, supplying energy for cells that require it, such as red blood cells. This approach reduces insulin spikes and supports a more stable energy profile throughout the day, avoiding the blood sugar fluctuations associated with carbohydrate-heavy diets. High-fat, moderate-protein diets can also reduce inflammation, as they minimize insulin production, lower oxidative stress, and decrease fat storage, which is closely linked to inflammation.

From a nutritional standpoint, a diet with only protein and fat can provide all essential nutrients. Organ meats, eggs, fish, and fatty cuts of meat offer ample vitamins and minerals, including B vitamins, iron, zinc, and fat-soluble vitamins A, D, E, and K, which are vital for immune and hormone function, bone health, and cellular repair. Additionally, essential fatty acids like omega-3s, found in fatty fish and animal products, support brain health, cardiovascular health, and help regulate inflammation. A diet rich in these foods can also optimize cholesterol and lipid profiles, with fats encouraging HDL (the "good" cholesterol) production and supporting healthy hormonal balance.

This high-protein, high-fat model promotes satiety and sustained energy, as fats are more energy-dense than carbs and take longer to metabolize. This naturally reduces cravings and may lead to weight management benefits without the need for calorie counting. While the absence of carbohydrates may seem unconventional by modern dietary standards, the body adapts efficiently, prioritizing nutrient-dense foods and metabolic stability. A protein-and-fat-only diet aligns with both evolutionary eating patterns and many individuals' modern health goals, potentially supporting metabolic health, reducing inflammation, and improving overall well-being.

Dairy in the Human Diet

Dairy products have long been promoted as a primary source of calcium and other essential nutrients, yet from an evolutionary and biological standpoint, dairy consumption in adulthood is unusual. By nature, humans are designed to consume Mother's milk during infancy, at which point our bodies are well-equipped with the enzyme lactase to digest lactose, the primary sugar in milk. However, as we age, most people experience a decline in lactase production, which can lead to lactose intolerance, resulting in digestive discomfort, bloating, and other gastrointestinal symptoms when dairy is consumed. This is because cow's milk, like human milk, is designed specifically for the growth and development of the young within that species—baby cows, in this case—not for the continued consumption by adult humans. Listen to your body.

Nutrient Dense Foods

Per 100gram Serving	Salmon Roe	Beef Liver	Ribeye Steak	Oysters	Lamb Chops	Eggs	Wild Salmon	Pork	Anchovies	Cheese
Vitamin A	10%	870%	–	1%	–	18%	1%	–	1%	22%
Vitamin E	66%	3%	–	15%	1%	7%	132%	2%	22%	2%
Vitamin D	58%	8%	–	–	–	10%	–	13%	9%	3%
Vitamin K2	1%	88%	1%	–	7%	80%	–	61%	–	30%
Thiamin (B1)	9%	15%	8%	9%	8%	3%	19%	34%	7%	2%
Riboflavin (B2)	21%	263%	34%	5%	16%	35%	29%	29%	28%	29%
Niacin (B3)	11%	109%	29%	8%	42%	–	49%	34%	124%	6%
Pantothenic Acid (B5)	35%	–	–	3%	13%	31%	33%	15%	18%	35%
Pyridoxine (B6)	12%	79%	28%	4%	16%	10%	48%	21%	12%	10%
Folic Acid (B9)	23%	73%	2%	5%	4%	12%	6%	1%	3%	9%
Cobalamin (B12)	333%	3464%	142%	675%	93%	37%	133%	45%	37%	51%
Choline	45%	76%	8%	25%	23%	53%	40%	18%	15%	3%
Selenium	93.6%	60%	66%	116%	40%	56%	66%	68%	124%	26%
Iron	3%	62%	20%	32%	9%	11%	4%	10%	26%	2%
Zinc	9%	37%	100%	345%	32%	12%	6%	42%	22%	24%
Potassium	6%	9%	8%	3%	6%	3%	10%	7%	12%	5%
Calcium	3%	–	–	3%	2%	4%	1%	4%	18%	41%
Copper	11%	1621%	16%	82%	13%	8%	28%	16%	38%	4%
Magnesium	5%	5%	6%	8%	5%	3%	7%	6%	16%	5%
Phosphorus	40%	49%	19%	7%	13%	16%	16%	21%	20%	31%
Manganese	–	15%	–	17%	1%	1%	1%	1%	4%	–
Omega-3 Fatty Acids	200%	1%	1%	24%	29%	3%	108%	7%	131%	17%

The Lactose Issue and Enzyme Deficiency

While some populations have evolved a genetic adaptation that allows for lactose persistence into adulthood, a significant percentage of the global population lacks this ability. This is why lactose intolerance is common worldwide, particularly in regions where dairy was not a traditional dietary staple. The absence of lactase leads to undigested lactose in the digestive system, fermenting and causing discomfort. Even for those who can digest lactose, the question remains whether dairy is an optimal or necessary part of an adult diet. From a physiological perspective, humans have no nutritional requirement for dairy, as all essential nutrients can be obtained from other foods.

Calcium, Vitamin K2, and the Risks of Misplaced Calcium

A major reason for the popularity of dairy is its high calcium content, essential for bone health. However, the way calcium is utilized in the body is far more complex than simple intake; without proper guidance, calcium may end up in places it doesn't belong, like soft tissues, arteries, and organs, rather than being deposited in the bones. This misplaced calcium can lead to calcification in the arteries, increasing the risk of cardiovascular disease.

This is where vitamin K2 comes into play. Vitamin K2 acts as a regulatory nutrient, directing calcium to the bones and teeth where it's needed and away from soft tissues where it can cause harm. Osteoblasts are the bone-building cells that help deposit calcium into bone tissue, while osteoclasts break down bone tissue to release calcium when it's needed elsewhere. Vitamin K2 activates osteocalcin, a protein that binds calcium to the bone matrix, and matrix GLA protein (MGP), which prevents calcium from depositing in the blood vessels and soft tissues.

Many dairy products, especially those from grain-fed cows, contain minimal vitamin K2, meaning that even if they're rich in calcium, they lack the tools to ensure it ends up in the right place. K2 is found in greater quantities in animal products such as grass-fed dairy, organ meats, egg yolks, and certain fermented foods like natto (fermented soybeans).

The Takeaway on Dairy and Bone Health

While dairy is rich in calcium, it doesn't necessarily translate to improved bone health if calcium isn't properly regulated within the body. In fact, excessive dairy consumption without sufficient K2 intake may lead to arterial calcification rather than stronger bones. Focusing on a diet that includes natural sources of K2, along with other sources of calcium like leafy greens, sardines, and almonds, can support bone health without the potential risks associated with dairy. For those who are lactose intolerant or prefer to avoid dairy, these alternatives offer safe and effective ways to maintain a strong bone structure, guided by a nutrient profile that aligns with the body's natural needs.

To Each His Own

We all have different DNA, needs, genetics, and tolerance levels, and that's crucial when determining what works best for us individually. The needs of a competitive athlete won't look the same as someone with sensitivities or someone managing health conditions. Recognizing these individual differences is essential if we want to optimize our health based on our unique makeup.

Let's be clear: food should first serve its purpose for sustenance, over pleasure or social expectations. It doesn't mean we need to eliminate enjoyment or social gatherings from eating entirely, but being aware of ourselves allows us to make choices aligned with our health goals. If we continue as we are, with convenience and pleasure dominating, health and longevity will continue to decline sharply. The worst part? This decline will impact future generations even more heavily. It's heartbreaking to think that our children will carry this burden, but it's within our power to turn things around.

Starting **now**, we owe it to ourselves and to future generations to recognize what's at stake.

Veganism

Veganism has gained significant traction in recent years, largely due to its perceived benefits for the environment and animal welfare. While these motives are commendable, the nutritional reality of a vegan diet often diverges from its idealized image. Nutritional challenges arise when individuals switch to a vegan diet without considering the implications of eliminating animal products from their nutrition entirely. Prominent figures, like Mikhaila Peterson, have shared stories of health decline associated with vegan diets, or just simply consuming vegetables, and highlighted the potential risks for those who may be sensitive to plant-based compounds or require nutrient density typically found in animal-based foods.

Processed Foods in the Vegan Diet

One significant concern with modern veganism is the reliance on processed foods. In order to replace meat, many people turn to heavily processed "fake meats" and other plant-based substitutes that are often loaded with additives, preservatives, and high levels of sodium. These items are far from the wholesome, plant-based staples that veganism initially promoted. Processed vegan products are crafted to mimic meat in texture and flavor but frequently lack essential nutrients, and the body often has difficulty digesting and absorbing nutrients from these products. This can lead to nutrient deficiencies over time, including protein, B12, iron, and zinc.

Lectins, Oxalates, and the Dangers of Plant Compounds

A key factor that often goes unaddressed is the presence of lectins and oxalates in many plant foods, which can have negative health effects, particularly for individuals with sensitivities. Lectins, for example, are found in legumes and grains, staples in a vegan diet, and can be hard on the digestive system, contributing to inflammation or digestive discomfort in some people. Oxalates, found in foods like spinach, nuts, and some grains, can bind to minerals like calcium, potentially leading to kidney stones or hindering mineral absorption.

For those who choose veganism as a lifelong approach, these issues may accumulate over time. Oxalates and lectins may not harm everyone, but for people with underlying sensitivities or autoimmune conditions, they can worsen symptoms and complicate nutrient absorption. This is why some prominent former vegans, like Peterson, experienced health improvements after reintroducing animal-based foods and focusing on nutrient density from bioavailable sources.

The Environmental Perspective vs. Nutritional Realities

Much of the modern vegan movement is driven by environmental concerns, with advocates suggesting that plant-based diets are more sustainable for the planet. While reducing the environmental impact of food production is important, it's crucial to balance environmental goals with the need for nutrient-dense, health-supportive diets. Veganism is far from optimal nutritionally, as it lacks certain key nutrients primarily found in animal products—nutrients like vitamin B12, DHA, heme iron, and highly bioavailable proteins. Without these, vegans often need supplements or highly fortified foods, which introduces a level of artificiality into the diet that might seem contradictory to its natural ethos.

The reality is that animal foods provide a level of nutrition and bioavailability that plants struggle to match. While it's possible to structure a well-planned vegan diet, it often requires extensive knowledge and supplementation to meet all nutrient requirements adequately. Unfortunately, many people do not approach it with this level of planning, which leads to common nutrient deficiencies.

The Health Risks Associated with Long-Term Veganism

Over time, people who follow a vegan diet without proper planning or supplementation may experience deficiencies that affect their overall health, particularly if they are in stages of life that demand higher nutritional density, such as childhood, pregnancy, or advanced age. Deficiencies in vitamin B12, iron, and protein can impact brain function, muscle health, and energy levels. Additionally, some people may develop sensitivities to soy or gluten, which are often over-relied upon in vegan diets, potentially leading to autoimmune issues or digestive discomfort.

Dangers of Vegetable and Seed Oils

A significant, yet often overlooked, concern in vegan and plant-based diets is the reliance on vegetable and seed oils, such as soybean, canola, sunflower, and corn oil. These oils are frequently promoted as healthier, plant-based alternatives to animal fats and are a staple in many vegan recipes and processed foods. However, the high use of vegetable and seed oils in vegan diets can lead to several health issues due to their biochemical composition and the way they're processed. Let's break down why these oils pose risks.

High Omega-6 Fatty Acid Content

One of the primary concerns with vegetable and seed oils is their high content of omega-6 fatty acids. While both omega-6 and omega-3 fatty acids are essential for health, they need to be consumed in balance. The ideal omega-6 to omega-3 ratio is around 1:1, as this ratio promotes an anti-inflammatory environment in the body. However, the modern Western diet—especially one rich in processed vegan foods—pushes the ratio closer to 20:1 or even higher, tipping the body toward chronic inflammation.

Excessive omega-6 fatty acids are metabolized into inflammatory compounds in the body. Chronic inflammation is linked to numerous health issues, including heart disease, autoimmune disorders, and metabolic syndrome. By contrast, omega-3 fatty acids (primarily found in fatty fish and grass-fed animal products) promote anti-inflammatory pathways, supporting cardiovascular, brain, and joint health. Vegan diets heavy in seed oils can lack sufficient omega-3s and may lead to an inflammatory imbalance that has detrimental long-term health effects.

Oxidative Stress from High Heat Processing

Vegetable and seed oils are typically extracted through high-heat processing methods that use chemical solvents to pull the oil from the seeds. This process not only strips the oils of nutrients but also damages their molecular structure, making them highly prone to oxidation. Oxidized oils create free radicals in the body, which contribute to oxidative stress, cellular damage, and inflammation. This can accelerate aging, impair immune function, and increase the risk of chronic diseases.

The consumption of oxidized fats also burdens the liver, as it has to work harder to detoxify the body from these harmful byproducts. Long-term intake of oxidized fats, common in seed oils, is associated with atherosclerosis (plaque buildup in the arteries), which heightens cardiovascular risk—ironically the very thing these oils were marketed to prevent.

Risk of Trans Fats and Industrial Processing

To improve the texture and shelf stability of vegetable oils, they are often partially hydrogenated—a process that creates trans fats. Although regulations have limited trans fats in many foods, traces can still be found in processed products, especially in hydrogenated oils. Trans fats are extremely damaging as they interfere with cellular function and raise levels of LDL (bad) cholesterol while lowering HDL (good) cholesterol. This imbalance significantly increases the risk of heart disease.

Given that processed vegan foods frequently rely on these oils to improve texture and taste, even small amounts of trans fats can accumulate over time, posing health risks to those who rely heavily on these products.

Hormonal Disruption and PUFAs

Vegetable and seed oils are rich in polyunsaturated fatty acids (PUFAs), which are less stable than saturated fats due to their multiple double bonds. These PUFAs, when consumed in excess, can disrupt the body's hormone balance. High intake of PUFAs has been shown to impact the function of cell membranes and may disrupt endocrine function by interfering with hormone receptors. This is particularly concerning for vegans who rely on seed oils as their primary fat source and may have elevated PUFA intake compared to those who consume more stable fats from animal products.

Healthier Alternatives for Fat in the Vegan Diet

Replacing vegetable and seed oils with healthier fat sources can make a vegan diet much more health-supportive. Extra virgin olive oil, avocado oil, and coconut oil are more stable options that provide beneficial monounsaturated and saturated fats, which are less prone to oxidation and free radical formation. While these oils still contain some omega-6s, they offer a more balanced profile and are less inflammatory than industrial seed oils.

Moreover, adding whole food fat sources, such as avocados, nuts, seeds (like chia and flax for omega-3s), and even algae-based omega-3 supplements, can provide necessary fats without the same risks associated with processed oils.

There is a hierarchy in which foods are beneficial to the body, much like the outdated food pyramid, but as I have said before, you can thrive on most diets provided that you execute it properly. The diet that you choose should be a combination of what you enjoy, and what does not harm you, or what does the least amount of harm.

Mikhaila Peterson and the Proper Human Diet

Mikhaila Peterson, daughter of psychologist Jordan Peterson, is a prominent advocate for the **Proper Human Diet** (PHD), a diet she believes is aligned with our evolutionary biology and human health needs. Mikhaila has famously transformed her health by following a strict elimination diet that ultimately led her to the carnivore diet— consuming only animal-based foods like beef, lamb, salt, and water. Her experience sheds light on the impact of modern diets filled with processed foods, grains, and sugars, which many people consume daily but may not tolerate well. For Mikhaila, the Proper Human Diet has been a revelation, bringing relief from a lifetime of severe autoimmune conditions, depression, chronic fatigue, and joint pain that conventional treatments failed to address.

Mikhaila's journey began after years of battling autoimmune disorders, including juvenile rheumatoid arthritis, chronic fatigue, and depression. Traditional treatments, including medications and dietary adjustments, provided only temporary relief and often came with additional side effects. Eventually, through her own research and self-experimentation, Mikhaila discovered that certain foods—especially processed carbohydrates, grains, sugars, and even vegetables—exacerbated her symptoms. By gradually eliminating these foods, she found that her symptoms significantly improved. This experience led her to adopt a carnivorous diet, which she describes as a "proper human diet" that aligns with human evolutionary nutrition.

The Proper Human Diet, as Mikhaila describes it, works for her because it eliminates the foods that trigger inflammatory and autoimmune responses in her body. The PHD emphasizes nutrient-dense, animal-based foods that are easily digestible and provide complete proteins, essential fatty acids, vitamins, and minerals without the anti-nutrients found in many plant foods. In Mikhaila's case, even foods traditionally considered "healthy" triggered negative responses. For instance, vegetables, which contain compounds like oxalates and lectins, exacerbated her symptoms. For her, cutting out these plant-based foods and focusing solely on animal products brought substantial health benefits, reinforcing her belief that the human body may not be optimized to process many of the foods commonly consumed in modern diets.

Mikhaila's experience with the Proper Human Diet highlights a growing perspective that today's food environment is incompatible with human biology. Processed foods, high in sugars, seed oils, and artificial ingredients, are a far cry from the ancestral diet humans evolved with. While many can tolerate a variety of foods, there's an increasing understanding that certain individuals, like Mikhaila, may be genetically predisposed to have stronger reactions to these modern foods. By focusing on nutrient-dense, animal-based foods, she is effectively reducing her body's exposure to inflammatory triggers and maintaining a diet closer to what our ancestors consumed. This approach is not only helping her manage her symptoms but has inspired others facing similar health challenges to experiment with their diets in search of relief.

Through her journey, Mikhaila has become an advocate for the Proper Human Diet, sharing her story to demonstrate that what we consider a "normal" diet today may not be suitable for everyone. Her experience exemplifies how eliminating processed foods, sugars, grains, and even certain vegetables can dramatically improve health outcomes for those who struggle with autoimmune and inflammatory conditions. Her case also emphasizes the importance of individualized nutrition and the idea that for some, the most basic, unprocessed animal foods may truly be the optimal fuel.

Mikhaila Peterson's story illustrates how the Proper Human Diet can serve as a reset for the body, reducing the impact of processed and potentially inflammatory foods. Her health transformation is a powerful example of how aligning with a diet closer to human evolution can yield profound benefits for some individuals. Why did this work? Because it's the **PROPER HUMAN DIET.**

The Takeaway

While vegetable and seed oils are widely used in vegan diets, they come with likely health risks due to their omega-6 content, susceptibility to oxidation, and impact on inflammation. Understanding the pitfalls of these oils can encourage individuals to make informed choices, aiming for more balanced fat sources that support long-term health and minimize chronic inflammation. Avoiding highly processed vegan products and opting for whole, nutrient-dense foods can make a vegan diet far healthier and less reliant on these harmful oils.

The 90/5/5 Theory on Health

The **90/5/5 Theory** provides a comprehensive framework for understanding the core drivers of health, positing that **90% of health outcomes are influenced by diet**, with **5% by physical activity** and another **5% by genetics**. While there are undoubtedly various elements that contribute to well-being, this theory emphasizes that the foods we consume are overwhelmingly influential in shaping our health. At its core, the 90/5/5 Theory serves as a reminder that while exercise and genetics play their respective roles, diet is the foundation of health and must be prioritized above all else.

This theory does not suggest a one-size-fits-all model but instead offers a **general guideline**. Within the 90/5/5 framework, each percentage can fluctuate depending on individual lifestyle choices, genetic predispositions, and the quality of one's diet. However, the primary message remains: diet holds the greatest sway over our health, and it cannot be counteracted by other means. Many people believe they can "outrun" a poor diet with intense exercise or rely on favorable genetics to protect them. But according to the 90/5/5 Theory, no amount of physical activity or genetic advantage can fully offset the detrimental effects of a poor diet. This principle is particularly relevant in the modern era, where processed foods, added sugars, and unhealthy fats are ubiquitous and contribute to chronic health issues.

The 90%: Why Diet Holds the Greatest Influence on Health

Diet's impact on health is profound and far-reaching. Our food choices directly influence metabolic processes, inflammatory responses, body composition, and overall wellness. High-quality, nutrient-dense foods provide essential vitamins, minerals, and macronutrients that support cellular function, stabilize blood sugar, reduce inflammation, and bolster the immune system. By contrast, diets high in processed foods, refined sugars, and unhealthy fats can lead to insulin resistance, oxidative stress, and chronic inflammation—all of which are known contributors to conditions like heart disease, diabetes, and obesity.

The 90% figure in this model emphasizes diet's critical role in managing and preventing chronic diseases. A well-balanced diet impacts health on both cellular and hormonal levels, affecting everything from the immune system's function to the body's ability to recover from daily stressors. Whole foods like vegetables, lean proteins, healthy fats, and whole grains are not just calorie sources; they're nutrient powerhouses that help fuel the body's natural processes.

While the 90% is a strong general guideline, it allows for flexibility. The importance of diet can vary depending on individual factors such as food quality, nutrient density, and genetic sensitivities. For instance, a whole-food-based diet may greatly benefit one person, while another individual with specific health concerns might require an even more tailored diet. Nutritional science increasingly supports the idea of personalized nutrition, recognizing that while diet is central to health, individual needs may differ.

Nutrient Density and Dietary Choices

Nutrient density is a crucial factor within the 90% diet component. Foods rich in nutrients, such as leafy greens, cruciferous vegetables, lean proteins, and healthy fats, provide a wealth of vitamins, minerals, and antioxidants that support optimal health. In contrast, highly processed foods are often calorie-dense but nutrient-poor, contributing little to bodily functions while increasing inflammation and impairing metabolic health. This difference in nutrient density can make or break one's health over time. A diet based on nutrient-dense foods offers benefits that go beyond caloric intake, supporting everything from cognitive function and hormonal health to immune response.

By focusing on nutrient-dense foods, individuals are better able to meet their nutritional needs, leading to improved satiety, stable blood sugar levels, and enhanced energy. The result is a body that functions optimally, with better immunity and a more balanced metabolism. Prioritizing whole foods and minimizing processed options is essential within the 90/5/5 model, as it maximizes the impact of diet on overall health.

The Role of Macronutrient Ratios

Another key factor within the 90% diet component is macronutrient composition. Macronutrient ratios, specifically the balance of carbohydrates, fats, and proteins, play an essential role in determining the effectiveness of a diet. Individual needs for these macronutrients vary widely and can depend on factors such as lifestyle, activity level, and metabolic health. For example, a person with insulin resistance may benefit from a low-carbohydrate, high-fat approach to improve glucose management, while someone with higher energy demands might require a moderate carbohydrate intake for optimal performance.

Within the 90/5/5 theory, macronutrient breakdown is flexible and adaptable to individual needs. For example, an athlete may need more carbohydrates to fuel their workouts, whereas someone managing metabolic syndrome might find that a diet lower in carbs and higher in healthy fats supports stable blood sugar levels and reduced inflammation. This flexibility underscores the theory's individualization potential, allowing it to accommodate varying lifestyles and health conditions while keeping diet as the central pillar.

Dietary Consistency Over Time

One often overlooked aspect of the 90% diet factor is the importance of consistency. Occasional indulgences have minimal impact when one's diet is predominantly nutrient-dense and health-focused. However, a diet consistently high in processed foods, sugars, and unhealthy fats can lead to cumulative effects such as chronic inflammation, hormonal imbalance, and metabolic issues.

The 90% theory highlights the importance of sustainable, balanced eating patterns rather than extreme dietary regimens that may not be maintainable. By focusing on whole, unprocessed foods most of the time, individuals can mitigate the effects of occasional dietary lapses, allowing their bodies to recover without long-term health consequences. Consistency in healthy eating supports bodily processes and makes it easier to maintain a balanced metabolism and weight in the long run.

The 5%: Physical Activity's Role in Health

While physical activity plays a smaller role within the 90/5/5 framework, its benefits are undeniable. Exercise supports cardiovascular health, strengthens muscles, improves mood, and increases metabolic rate. It also enhances insulin sensitivity, which can be beneficial for weight management and blood sugar control. However, the 5% allocation reflects the understanding that exercise cannot replace a healthy diet. Exercise serves to complement dietary efforts, not to counteract or "undo" poor eating habits.

Physical activity can vary widely in intensity and form, and different types provide distinct benefits. For example, aerobic activities like walking and running promote cardiovascular fitness, while resistance training supports muscle mass and boosts metabolic rate. Though exercise alone is beneficial, it becomes most effective when combined with a balanced diet. Together, they create a synergy that amplifies their respective benefits, making the 90/5/5 framework a comprehensive approach to health.

Limitations of Exercise Without Dietary Support

One of the misconceptions the 90/5/5 theory addresses is the idea that exercise can "make up for" a poor diet. Many people assume that rigorous physical activity can compensate for unhealthy eating, but research shows that weight loss and metabolic improvements are difficult to achieve through exercise alone. Without proper nutrition, the body lacks the essential nutrients needed to support recovery, maintain metabolic health, and sustain long-term energy.

Within this model, exercise is presented as a supportive measure rather than a primary driver of health. While it's beneficial for well-being, exercise cannot replace the need for nutrient-dense, balanced food intake. This approach underscores the importance of diet as the foundation for health, with exercise serving as an enhancement rather than the main determinant of health outcomes.

The Other 5%: Genetics' Role in Health

The final 5% in the 90/5/5 theory is attributed to genetics, which also play a role in shaping health outcomes but are far less influential than diet and lifestyle. Genetics determine certain predispositions, like the likelihood of developing diabetes, heart disease, or obesity. However, these predispositions are not certainties, as lifestyle choices can significantly influence whether genetic traits manifest in health outcomes.

Research in epigenetics—the study of how lifestyle choices impact gene expression—shows that diet, physical activity, sleep, and stress management can turn certain genes "on" or "off." For example, someone with a family history of heart disease may significantly reduce their risk by following a nutrient-dense, anti-inflammatory diet. The 90/5/5 theory emphasizes that while genetics are a factor, they don't have the final say on health outcomes. Diet, exercise, and lifestyle choices remain more powerful determinants.

Genetic Variation and Nutrient Metabolism

Genetics can influence how individuals metabolize nutrients, respond to certain foods, and tolerate specific macronutrient ratios. For example, some people are genetically predisposed to metabolize fats more effectively, making a low-carb, high-fat diet suitable for them. Others may have a genetic tendency toward increased sensitivity to certain foods, impacting their dietary needs.

179

Even with these variations, the 90/5/5 theory reinforces that diet is the primary factor influencing health. Advances in fields like nutrigenomics, which studies how nutrition interacts with genetics, support personalized dietary recommendations, but diet remains central to health outcomes. This perspective empowers individuals to focus on lifestyle factors that they can control, rather than becoming resigned to genetic predispositions.

The Interplay Between Diet, Exercise, and Genetics

The 90/5/5 theory acknowledges the interplay between diet, exercise, and genetics. While diet is the primary driver, physical activity enhances dietary effects, and genetics provide context for individual variation. Someone with a genetic predisposition to insulin resistance, for example, can offset this risk by following a low-carb diet and engaging in regular physical activity.

This synergy highlights that diet, exercise, and genetics are interconnected in determining health outcomes. A poor diet can still lead to metabolic dysfunction regardless of genetic predisposition, while a balanced diet and consistent exercise can optimize health for those with a genetic tendency toward certain conditions. The 90/5/5 model encourages a holistic view of health that accounts for all factors.

Practical Applications of the 90/5/5 Theory

Implementing the 90/5/5 theory in daily life involves understanding one's unique needs while prioritizing diet as the foundation. By focusing on whole foods, minimizing processed items, and adjusting macronutrients as needed, one can experience significant health improvements. Exercise adds a supportive layer, enhancing metabolic function and complementing dietary efforts.

Practical steps for using the 90/5/5 framework include:

1. **Nutrient Density**: Emphasize whole, nutrient-dense foods to meet nutritional needs.
2. **Individualized Macronutrients**: Tailor protein, fat, and carbohydrate intake based on personal metabolism.
3. **Consistent Exercise**: Engage in regular physical activity to support dietary efforts.
4. **Genetic Awareness**: Understand predispositions but prioritize lifestyle choices.

The 90/5/5 theory provides a comprehensive approach to health, underscoring diet's importance while acknowledging exercise and genetics. It simplifies the complex interplay of health factors, emphasizing that while genetics and exercise contribute to well-being, diet is the foundation. This theory empowers individuals to take control of their health through dietary choices, regular physical activity, and awareness of genetic influences.

By adopting the 90/5/5 framework, people can make informed decisions that support long-term health. This model challenges traditional views that place exercise or genetics as primary factors, refocusing attention on dietary quality and consistency. As lifestyle diseases rise, the 90/5/5 theory serves as a valuable tool for understanding health and promoting a balanced approach to wellness.

Choosing Quality: The Impact of Food Source on Health

In today's food market, not all foods are created equal. When shopping for staples like meat, fish, eggs, and dairy, understanding the differences in how these foods are raised, caught, and processed can significantly impact health. Labels like "wild-caught," "farm-raised," "pasture-raised," and "organic" offer clues about food quality, nutrient content, and environmental impact. In this section, we'll explore these distinctions and why choosing high-quality sources can lead to better health outcomes, support sustainability, and align with a "proper human diet."

Wild-Caught vs. Farm-Raised Fish: Nutritional and Environmental Differences

When it comes to fish and seafood, the terms "wild-caught" and "farm-raised" describe two different methods of obtaining these foods, each with distinct nutritional and environmental implications.

Wild-Caught Fish

Wild-caught fish are sourced directly from their natural habitats, such as oceans, rivers, and lakes. These fish eat a diet based on what they find in the wild, including smaller fish, algae, and plankton, which contributes to a higher nutrient profile. Wild-caught fish tend to have:

- **Higher Omega-3 Levels**: These fish are typically richer in omega-3 fatty acids, which are essential for heart, brain, and overall health. Omega-3s help reduce inflammation and are particularly important for metabolic health.
- **Lower Omega-6 Levels**: Omega-6 fatty acids, often found in farm-raised fish, can contribute to inflammation when consumed in excess. Wild-caught fish have a more balanced omega-3 to omega-6 ratio.
- **Fewer Contaminants**: While wild fish can still contain environmental pollutants, farm-raised fish often have higher levels of toxins due to overcrowded farming conditions and the use of antibiotics and other chemicals.

Farm-Raised Fish

Farm-raised fish are raised in controlled environments like tanks or enclosed areas in bodies of water. While farming can increase fish availability, farm-raised fish often:

- **Contain Higher Omega-6 Levels**: The feed used for farmed fish is usually high in omega-6 oils and processed grains, which increases the omega-6 content and reduces the overall omega-3 to omega-6 balance.
- **Have Higher Levels of Antibiotics and Pesticides**: Farmed fish are often given antibiotics to prevent disease due to close quarters, and pesticides are sometimes used to control parasites. These chemicals can accumulate in the fish and be passed on to consumers.
- **Lower Nutrient Density**: Farm-raised fish may lack the variety of nutrients found in wild fish, as their diet is less diverse and often consists of processed ingredients.

When possible, choosing wild-caught fish is preferable for both nutrient quality and minimizing exposure to contaminants. It also supports more sustainable fishing practices that don't rely on the intensive farming methods required to raise fish in captivity.

Eggs: Conventional, Free-Range, Cage-Free, and Pasture-Raised

Eggs are a nutrient-dense food, packed with protein, healthy fats, vitamins, and minerals. However, the way hens are raised and fed can affect the quality of the eggs they produce. Let's break down the different labels commonly seen on egg cartons.

Conventional Eggs

Conventional eggs come from hens raised in cages with limited space. These are typically fed a diet of grains, and their living conditions are often cramped. Conventional eggs can be affordable, but they're generally lower in nutrients compared to eggs from pasture-raised hens.

Cage-Free and Free-Range Eggs

Cage-free and free-range eggs indicate a slightly better standard of living for hens, though the terms can be misleading:

Cage-Free: Cage-free hens aren't confined to cages, but they are often raised indoors without outdoor access. This setup allows for some movement but does not guarantee improved diets or significant nutritional differences.

Free-Range: Free-range hens have some access to outdoor areas, though this is often limited. The quality of free-range eggs can vary depending on the farming practices used.

Pasture-Raised Eggs

Pasture-raised eggs come from hens that are allowed to roam outdoors on pasture, where they can forage for bugs, grass, and seeds in addition to their regular feed. These eggs typically offer:

- **Higher Omega-3 Content**: Pasture-raised hens produce eggs with a higher omega-3 content, thanks to their varied diet.
- **Better Vitamin Profile**: Studies show that pasture-raised eggs contain more vitamins A, D, and E, as well as antioxidants like lutein and zeaxanthin, which support eye health.
- **Lower Omega-6 Content**: Pasture-raised eggs have a better balance of omega-3 to omega-6 fatty acids, which can help reduce inflammation.

For the highest nutrient density and more humane practices, pasture-raised eggs are the optimal choice. While they may be more expensive, their superior nutritional profile makes them a worthwhile investment in health.

Meat: Conventional, Organic, Grass-Fed, and Pasture-Raised

Choosing quality meat is crucial, as conventional farming practices have altered the nutrient profile and safety of many animal products. Here's a breakdown of the different types of meat available:

Conventional Meat

Conventional meat comes from animals raised in confined spaces, often with limited movement and access to natural diets. These animals are usually fed grains like corn and soy, which are not part of their natural diet. Conventional meat is also more likely to contain:

Hormones and Antibiotics: To promote growth and prevent disease, conventional animals are often given hormones and antibiotics, which can accumulate in their meat.

Higher Omega-6 Content: The grain-heavy diet of conventionally raised animals raises the omega-6 content in the meat, which can contribute to inflammation.

Organic Meat

Organic meat comes from animals raised without the use of synthetic hormones, antibiotics, or GMOs. While organic standards improve the quality of the meat, organic doesn't necessarily mean the animal was raised on pasture or fed a grass-based diet.

Grass-Fed and Grass-Finished Meat

Grass-fed animals are raised primarily on pasture and allowed to eat grass, which aligns with their natural diet. Grass-finished animals, a step further, eat only grass throughout their lives (while grass-fed can sometimes mean they're grain-finished). These meats tend to be:

- **Higher in Omega-3 Fatty Acids**: Grass-fed and grass-finished meats have more omega-3s, which support heart and brain health.
- **Higher in CLA (Conjugated Linoleic Acid)**: CLA is a type of fat that has been linked to improved metabolism and reduced risk of heart disease and cancer.
- **Richer in Vitamins and Antioxidants**: Grass-fed meat often contains more vitamins A and E and other antioxidants that reduce inflammation.

Pasture-Raised Meat

Pasture-raised meat indicates animals that were raised on open pasture, where they could roam and graze naturally. While grass-fed and pasture-raised can overlap, pasture-raised doesn't always mean grass-fed—animals may still be supplemented with grains. However, pasture-raised animals generally live in healthier conditions and tend to produce higher-quality meat.

Conclusion: For optimal nutrition, grass-fed, grass-finished, or pasture-raised meats are superior to conventional meat. They are richer in essential fats, vitamins, and antioxidants, making them a better choice for supporting metabolic health.

Dairy: Conventional, Organic, and Grass-Fed

Dairy products can also vary greatly in quality, depending on how the animals are raised and what they're fed. Here's what to look for when choosing dairy:

- **Conventional Dairy**: Comes from cows raised in confined settings and fed grains, which can impact the nutrient profile of the milk and increase omega-6 levels.
- **Organic Dairy**: Comes from cows raised without synthetic hormones or antibiotics, offering a cleaner product. Organic dairy doesn't necessarily mean grass-fed, so omega-3 content may still be low.
- **Grass-Fed Dairy**: Grass-fed dairy comes from cows that graze on pasture, resulting in higher omega-3 levels, CLA, and fat-soluble vitamins (A, D, E, and K2), which support immune and cardiovascular health.

Grass-fed dairy is the best option for nutrient density, though organic dairy is a step up from conventional in terms of quality.

Organ Meats- The Best of the Best!

Organ meats, often overlooked in modern diets, are some of the most nutrient-dense foods available. Rich in essential vitamins and minerals, they provide a concentrated source of nutrients that are difficult to match with other foods. For example, liver is exceptionally high in vitamin A, B vitamins, iron, and copper, while heart provides a good source of CoQ10, an important compound for cellular energy production. The nutrient profile of organ meats supports overall health, making them a staple in ancestral diets and a highly beneficial addition to modern nutritional practices.

Antiquated Thoughts About Gout and Purines

One of the primary concerns people have when consuming organ meats is their high purine content, which has traditionally been associated with the risk of gout. Gout is a form of arthritis characterized by painful inflammation due to the accumulation of uric acid crystals in the joints. While it is true that organ meats contain more purines than muscle meats, modern research shows that dietary purines alone are not the main culprit in gout development. Instead, the focus should be on the overall metabolic state of the body.

Purines and Metabolic Health

Purines, found in many nutrient-rich foods, are broken down into uric acid in the body. However, the body's ability to manage uric acid levels depends more on other metabolic markers than on dietary purine intake alone. Factors such as insulin resistance, high fructose consumption, obesity, and chronic inflammation can impair the body's ability to excrete uric acid efficiently. When these metabolic markers are under control, moderate consumption of organ meats is unlikely to pose a problem for most individuals.

Balancing Nutrient Intake and Metabolic Health

Incorporating organ meats into a balanced diet can offer profound health benefits due to their rich nutrient profile. The key is to ensure that overall metabolic health is supported through a diet that promotes insulin sensitivity, reduces inflammation, and maintains a healthy body weight. By managing these factors, individuals can enjoy the nutritional advantages of organ meats without undue concern over purine-related issues, such as gout. This modern

186

perspective allows for a more nuanced understanding of how organ meats fit into a healthful diet while challenging outdated notions that have long limited their consumption.

Investing in Quality for Long-Term Health

Choosing foods from wild-caught, pasture-raised, and grass-fed sources may require more effort and a slightly higher investment. However, the health benefits—such as increased nutrient density, better fat balance, and reduced exposure to contaminants—make them worthwhile. Prioritizing quality sources aligns with the principles of a nutrient-dense diet and can support overall health, longevity, and metabolic wellness. By making conscious choices about the foods we consume, we invest not only in our immediate well-being but in our long-term health outcomes as well.

Understanding Fats and Oils: The Misunderstood Nutrients

For decades, fats and oils have been vilified, especially in the context of heart disease, weight gain, and metabolic disorders. However, recent research has redefined our understanding of fats, revealing them as not only essential to health but also as misunderstood nutrients. In this section, we'll explore the different types of fats, their roles in the body, the truth about oils, and how to incorporate healthy fats into a balanced diet.

Types of Fats: Breaking Down the Basics

Fats come in various forms, each with unique chemical structures that determine their behavior in the body. The main categories include:

1. **Saturated Fats**: These fats have no double bonds between carbon molecules, making them solid at room temperature. They are found in animal products like meat, butter, and dairy, as well as some tropical oils such as coconut and palm oil. Despite being linked to heart disease in the past, new research suggests that saturated fats may not be as harmful as once thought when consumed in moderation and within a balanced diet.
2. **Monounsaturated Fats (MUFAs)**: MUFAs contain one double bond in their carbon chain, which makes them liquid at room temperature. They are found in foods like olive oil, avocados, nuts, and seeds. Studies show that MUFAs are

187

beneficial for heart health, inflammation reduction, and improved insulin sensitivity, making them a staple in heart-healthy diets like the Mediterranean diet.

3. **Polyunsaturated Fats (PUFAs)**: PUFAs contain multiple double bonds, which makes them highly flexible but also prone to oxidation. This category includes omega-3 and omega-6 fatty acids, both essential for various bodily functions. Omega-3s, found in fatty fish, flaxseeds, and walnuts, are anti-inflammatory and support brain health. Omega-6s, found in vegetable oils, are necessary but should be consumed in balance with omega-3s to prevent inflammation.

4. **Trans Fats**: These are artificially created fats, commonly found in hydrogenated oils used in processed foods. Trans fats have been strongly linked to heart disease, inflammation, and metabolic disorders and are widely regarded as harmful. Many countries now restrict their use due to these health concerns.

The Role of Fats in the Body

Fats are essential to many bodily functions, and their roles include:

- **Energy Source**: Fats provide a concentrated source of energy, with nine calories per gram, making them more energy-dense than proteins or carbohydrates.
- **Cell Structure and Function**: Fats are integral components of cell membranes, especially phospholipids, which allow cells to function correctly and maintain fluidity.
- **Hormone Production**: Fats are precursors for hormones, including sex hormones like estrogen and testosterone, and adrenal hormones like cortisol.
- **Vitamin Absorption**: Fat-soluble vitamins (A, D, E, and K) require fats for absorption. A low-fat diet can lead to deficiencies in these essential nutrients.
- **Brain Health**: The brain is approximately 60% fat, and healthy fats, especially omega-3 fatty acids, are crucial for cognitive function, mental health, and brain development.

The Truth About Oils: What's Healthy and What's Not

Oils are a concentrated form of fat, and their quality can vary widely based on their source, processing, and nutrient content. Here's a breakdown of commonly used oils and their health implications:

Healthier Oils to Include

1. **Olive Oil**: Known for its high monounsaturated fat content and antioxidants, extra virgin olive oil is one of the healthiest oils available. It has been shown to reduce inflammation, improve heart health, and support metabolic function. However, it has a low smoke point, so it's best used for low-heat cooking or as a dressing.
2. **Coconut Oil**: Rich in medium-chain triglycerides (MCTs), coconut oil is easily digestible and provides quick energy. While it contains saturated fat, the MCTs in coconut oil may benefit brain function and metabolism. It's a versatile cooking oil, especially for higher-heat applications.
3. **Avocado Oil**: Similar to olive oil in its high monounsaturated fat content, avocado oil has a high smoke point, making it suitable for cooking. It also contains beneficial antioxidants like lutein, which supports eye health.
4. **Butter and Ghee**: These are natural animal fats that contain a balanced mixture of saturated and monounsaturated fats. Grass-fed butter and ghee also provide CLA (conjugated linoleic acid) and butyrate, both of which have anti-inflammatory properties. Ghee, a clarified butter, is ideal for high-heat cooking.
5. **Tallow and Lard** : These are traditional animal fats that are considered healthier options for cooking due to their stability at high temperatures and nutrient content. Unlike seed oils, which are often highly processed and can oxidize easily, tallow and lard remain stable when heated, making them less likely to form harmful compounds. Both are rich in healthy saturated and monounsaturated fats, which support hormone production, brain health, and energy levels. Additionally, these fats provide fat-soluble vitamins like vitamin D and K2, essential for bone and cardiovascular health. Because they are minimally processed, tallow and lard align more closely with ancestral diets, offering a natural and nutrient-dense cooking fat that's less likely to contribute to inflammation compared to industrial seed oils.

Oils to Use Very *Very* Sparingly

1. **Vegetable Oils (Canola, Soybean, Corn Oil)**: These oils are high in omega-6 fatty acids and often highly processed. When omega-6s are consumed in excess relative to omega-3s, they contribute to inflammation and may increase the risk of heart disease, obesity, and other chronic conditions.
2. **Sunflower and Safflower Oil**: While these oils are rich in vitamin E, they are also high in omega-6s and prone to oxidation, particularly when used at high temperatures. They should be used sparingly, especially in diets already high in omega-6 fatty acids.
3. **Peanut Oil**: Though it has a moderate amount of monounsaturated fats, peanut oil is also high in omega-6s and may contain harmful aflatoxins, naturally occurring toxins produced by certain fungi found in peanuts.

Oils to Avoid

1. **Partially Hydrogenated Oils (Trans Fats)**: These oils are produced through the hydrogenation process, which makes them solid at room temperature but also creates harmful trans fats. They increase LDL cholesterol, lower HDL cholesterol, and are strongly linked to heart disease and inflammation.
2. **Refined Vegetable Oils**: Refined oils have been processed at high heat, which strips away beneficial nutrients and makes the oil more susceptible to oxidation. This can lead to the formation of harmful compounds and reduce the oil's health benefits.

Fat Quality Matters: Omega-3 to Omega-6 Ratio

The ideal balance between omega-3 and omega-6 fatty acids is around 1:1, but the modern diet often skews toward a 1:20 or even 1:30 ratio in favor of omega-6. This imbalance contributes to chronic inflammation, which is associated with heart disease, diabetes, arthritis, and other inflammatory conditions.

Misconceptions and Myths About Fats

Fats have long been misunderstood, with saturated fats often blamed for heart disease and weight gain. However, recent research suggests that natural fats, particularly when unprocessed, are not inherently harmful. In fact, studies show that diets high in healthy fats can improve cholesterol levels, enhance brain function, and even aid in weight management.

Low-Fat Diets Are Not Always Healthier

Low-fat diets surged in popularity during the 1980s and 1990s as fat was widely considered the main dietary cause of heart disease and weight gain. However, the trend had unintended consequences: in many cases, food manufacturers replaced fats with refined carbohydrates and added sugars to make low-fat products more palatable. This shift led to foods that, while low in fat, were high in quickly digestible carbs, causing spikes in blood sugar and insulin. Elevated insulin levels drive fat storage and can lead to insulin resistance over time, a condition linked to obesity, diabetes, and other metabolic disorders.

The result was an increase in obesity and metabolic health issues, contrary to the original intention of promoting a healthier population. Low-fat diets can lack essential nutrients and satiating qualities that healthy fats provide, often leaving people hungry and more likely to overeat. Today, research emphasizes that quality fats, such as those from avocados, nuts, and olive oil, are beneficial to heart and metabolic health. Moving away from blanket low-fat recommendations, current dietary guidelines now encourage a balanced intake of healthy fats, which support everything from brain health to hormone balance and provide lasting energy.

Saturated Fats and Heart Disease: Rethinking the Connection

Although saturated fats were once demonized and linked to heart disease, recent studies and comprehensive reviews reveal that there was never a strong, scientifically substantiated connection between saturated fats and heart disease. In fact, the original research that suggested such a link has been criticized for methodological flaws and selective data interpretation, often excluding countries and populations that didn't fit the hypothesis.

Today, a growing body of evidence suggests that moderate intake of saturated fats from whole food sources, such as meat, eggs, and dairy, is not only safe but can be beneficial when part of a balanced diet. These foods provide essential nutrients and support functions

191

like cell membrane integrity, hormone production, and energy. The real culprits behind heart disease are increasingly recognized to be processed foods, refined carbohydrates, and inflammatory seed oils—factors that drive insulin resistance, inflammation, and other metabolic dysfunctions.

By focusing on whole, nutrient-dense sources of saturated fat, individuals may even improve heart health and overall well-being. Rather than being harmful, saturated fats, especially those from natural sources, contribute to a stable energy supply and support the body's structural needs. This shift in perspective encourages a more nuanced understanding of dietary fats, challenging outdated paradigms and underscoring the importance of diet quality over simplistic fat classifications.

The Role of Fats in Weight Management and Metabolic Health

Healthy fats can play an essential role in managing weight and supporting metabolic health. Fats are more satiating than carbs, which can help reduce overall calorie intake by keeping you full for longer. Diets higher in healthy fats, such as the Mediterranean and ketogenic diets, are associated with weight loss, improved blood sugar levels, and reduced inflammation.

Ketogenic Diet and Fat Adaptation

The ketogenic diet is a high-fat, low-carb diet that encourages the body to enter a state of ketosis, where it primarily burns fat for energy. This shift from glucose to fat as a fuel source has been shown to improve insulin sensitivity, reduce inflammation, and support cognitive health. Fat adaptation, or the body's ability to efficiently use fat for fuel, can also lead to sustained energy levels without the crashes associated with high-carb diets.

Practical Tips for Incorporating Healthy Fats

1. **Choose Whole Foods Over Processed Fats**: Opt for natural sources of fat such as nuts, seeds, avocados, and fatty fish rather than processed oils or trans fats found in packaged foods.
2. **Cook with Stable Oils**: Use oils with high smoke points, like coconut oil or avocado oil, for high-heat cooking, and reserve oils like olive oil for dressings and low-heat cooking to preserve their nutrients.

3. **Prioritize Omega-3s**: Increase intake of omega-3-rich foods like salmon, sardines, flaxseeds, and walnuts. This can help balance the omega-3 to omega-6 ratio and reduce inflammation.
4. **Limit Omega-6 Oils**: Reduce consumption of vegetable oils high in omega-6 fatty acids. Instead, focus on monounsaturated fats and omega-3 sources to support anti-inflammatory pathways.
5. **Embrace Whole-Food Fats**: Enjoy eggs, grass-fed meats, and full-fat dairy, as they offer a complete nutrient profile that includes vitamins, minerals, and fatty acids essential for health.

Redefining Fats and Oils for Health

Fats are essential to human health and well-being, providing necessary nutrients, supporting cellular function, and aiding in hormone production. By choosing quality fats and balancing omega-3 and omega-6 fatty acids, we can harness their benefits and promote a healthier, more balanced lifestyle. Embracing healthy fats while avoiding processed oils and trans fats is a simple but impactful change that can lead to lasting health improvements.

Chapter 9 Your Path to a Healthier Future

I get it, reversing the dietary mess we're in, with carbs and processed foods everywhere, is easier said than done. We're not going to see everyone magically switching to a strict carnivore diet anytime soon. But we can still take steps to minimize the damage and support our health, one choice at a time.

If you can go carnivore, great, it's one of the cleanest, most nutrient-dense options out there. But if that's not feasible, you can still make solid choices with fruits and vegetables, just being mindful of things like phytochemicals and anti-nutrients that might impact digestion or cause inflammation. Choosing low-inflammatory foods is another powerful move: steering clear of processed seed oils, refined sugars, and high-glycemic carbs can do wonders for stabilizing blood sugar and managing inflammation.

Finding balance with omega-6 and omega-3 fatty acids is also key, as this ratio can seriously influence inflammation levels. And adding a few key supplements can be a game-changer. CoQ10, D-ribose, magnesium, and L-carnitine, for example, give your cells a much-needed energy boost, support muscle health, and help protect the heart, especially if our diet isn't always perfect. So even if we can't change the whole food system overnight, there's still a lot we can do, day by day, to make smarter choices that really make a difference.

Dr. Robert Lustig, a prominent figure in metabolic health and endocrinology, has developed a philosophy that resonates with health professionals and enthusiasts alike: "Protect the Liver, Feed the Gut." This simple yet profound mantra encapsulates the essential elements of maintaining metabolic health by focusing on two critical areas in our bodies. As an avid believer in Dr. Lustig's work, I've come to view this approach as transformative for anyone seeking to improve their well-being and reverse or prevent chronic health conditions. This section will explore how protecting the liver and feeding the gut can optimize overall health, diving into the mechanisms and reasoning behind this philosophy.

The Role of the Liver: Why Protection is Essential

The liver is a vital organ responsible for numerous metabolic processes, including the detoxification of chemicals, the production of proteins for blood clotting, and, importantly, the regulation of blood glucose. It is the body's main organ for processing and distributing nutrients. However, with the modern diet often high in refined sugars, processed foods, and trans fats, the liver frequently faces overwork and damage. Dr. Lustig emphasizes that protecting the liver means preventing it from being overwhelmed by unnecessary or harmful substances. When the liver is forced to process excessive amounts of sugars and refined fats, it can lead to a cascade of metabolic dysfunction, resulting in conditions like insulin resistance, fatty liver disease, and metabolic syndrome.

Sugar and Fructose Overload

One of the key stressors for the liver is an excess of fructose. Unlike glucose, which every cell in the body can metabolize, fructose must be processed by the liver. When we consume foods high in refined sugars, the liver becomes overwhelmed with fructose, leading to a process called de novo lipogenesis (DNL), where excess sugars are converted into fat. This accumulation of fat in the liver can eventually lead to non-alcoholic fatty liver disease (NAFLD), a condition that is now affecting children as well as adults.

Dr. Lustig has been particularly vocal about the dangers of sugar, specifically fructose, in our diet. He describes it as a "poison" to the liver because, unlike other carbohydrates, it places a disproportionate load on this organ, triggering inflammatory processes and setting the stage for insulin resistance. Protecting the liver, therefore, requires reducing or eliminating added sugars, particularly high-fructose corn syrup and other forms of concentrated fructose, from our diets.

Alcohol's Impact on Liver Health

Another major contributor to liver disease is alcohol, which, like fructose, undergoes extensive processing in the liver. Even moderate alcohol consumption can exacerbate liver stress, especially in individuals already consuming a high-sugar diet. Lustig emphasizes that protecting the liver also means understanding the cumulative effects of alcohol and fructose. Both contribute to liver fat accumulation and damage, leading to inflammation and impaired liver function over time.

By focusing on protecting the liver, Dr. Lustig underscores that limiting both sugar and alcohol is crucial. A diet free from these stressors allows the liver to function optimally, improving overall metabolic health and lowering the risk of chronic diseases.

Feeding the Gut: The Importance of Gut Health

"Feeding the gut" refers to nourishing the microbiome, the collection of trillions of bacteria residing in our intestines. These bacteria play a vital role in digestion, immune function, and even mood regulation. Dr. Lustig's philosophy emphasizes that a healthy gut is central to preventing inflammation, maintaining metabolic health, and ensuring that nutrients are effectively absorbed. In fact, poor gut health has been linked to numerous health issues, from obesity and diabetes to mental health disorders like depression and anxiety.

The Role of Fiber in Gut Health

To "feed the gut," Dr. Lustig advocates for a diet rich in dietary fiber, particularly from fruits, vegetables, and whole grains. Fiber serves as food for the beneficial bacteria in the gut, known as probiotics. When fiber is fermented by these bacteria, it produces short-chain fatty acids (SCFAs) such as butyrate, which have anti-inflammatory effects and promote a healthy gut lining. This is crucial, as a compromised gut lining can lead to conditions like leaky gut syndrome, where harmful substances leak into the bloodstream, triggering inflammation.

By prioritizing fiber intake, we support a balanced microbiome and prevent the overgrowth of harmful bacteria that thrive on sugars and processed foods. Dr. Lustig highlights the need for fiber-rich diets not just for weight loss, but for comprehensive metabolic health, explaining that a well-fed microbiome can positively impact everything from insulin sensitivity to mental health.

Avoiding Processed Foods and Artificial Additives

Dr. Lustig's philosophy also warns against processed foods, which often contain additives, preservatives, and artificial sweeteners that can disrupt the gut microbiome. Artificial sweeteners, in particular, have been shown to alter gut bacteria, potentially contributing to insulin resistance and glucose intolerance. These findings underscore the importance of feeding the gut with whole, natural foods that nourish rather than harm our microbiota.

In his philosophy, Lustig stresses that feeding the gut well goes beyond just eating more fruits and vegetables. It involves eliminating foods that may damage the microbiome, such as processed foods and sugars, while focusing on a diet rich in prebiotics and probiotics, which help sustain beneficial bacteria.

The Interplay Between Liver and Gut Health

One of the unique aspects of Dr. Lustig's philosophy is its focus on the interplay between liver and gut health. The health of these organs is intricately connected, as a healthy gut microbiome can directly impact liver function, and vice versa. For example, when the gut is inflamed or leaky, it can send inflammatory signals to the liver, compounding the liver's stress and leading to a cycle of inflammation and dysfunction. Likewise, when the liver is overworked and inflamed, it can negatively impact the gut, further throwing the microbiome out of balance.

This interplay is crucial in understanding why protecting the liver and feeding the gut simultaneously can lead to profound health improvements. By supporting the liver through dietary changes, we reduce its inflammatory burden, making it easier to process nutrients without generating excess fat. Concurrently, feeding the gut with fiber and avoiding toxins allows the microbiome to flourish, aiding in the digestion and absorption of essential nutrients.

Practical Steps to Protect the Liver and Feed the Gut

Incorporating Dr. Lustig's philosophy into daily life requires actionable steps that focus on whole foods, fiber, and a reduction in harmful substances. Here are a few strategies based on his recommendations:

1. **Reduce Sugar and Processed Foods**: Limit added sugars and refined carbohydrates, as these stress the liver and contribute to insulin resistance. Focus on whole food sources of carbohydrates, like vegetables and low-sugar fruits, which don't place an excessive burden on the liver.
2. **Increase Fiber Intake**: Aim for at least 25-30 grams of fiber per day, primarily from vegetables, nuts, seeds, and low-sugar fruits. This not only feeds the gut but also helps stabilize blood sugar, reducing the liver's workload.
3. **Limit Alcohol Consumption**: Minimize or avoid alcohol, especially if already consuming a high-sugar diet. This

reduces the liver's toxic burden, allowing it to focus on essential metabolic functions without the added stress of detoxifying alcohol.

4. **Incorporate Probiotic-Rich Foods**: Foods like yogurt, kefir, sauerkraut, and kimchi introduce beneficial bacteria to the gut, supporting a balanced microbiome that aids in digestion and immune function.

5. **Avoid Artificial Sweeteners and Additives**: Opt for natural, whole foods over processed options, as additives and artificial sweeteners can disrupt the microbiome and promote insulin resistance.

Why "Protect the Liver, Feed the Gut" Matters for Overall Health

Dr. Lustig's mantra is especially powerful because it targets the root of many chronic diseases rather than merely addressing symptoms. By protecting the liver and feeding the gut, we create a foundation for metabolic health that can prevent or reverse conditions like diabetes, obesity, and cardiovascular disease.

Through this philosophy, Lustig has highlighted how the modern diet has veered far from what our bodies are designed to handle, with its heavy reliance on sugar, processed foods, and artificial ingredients. By shifting our focus to whole foods, fiber, and a reduction in toxic substances, we can support the liver and gut, thus improving not only our physical health but also our mental and emotional well-being.

As an avid supporter of Dr. Lustig's work, I believe that the "Protect the Liver, Feed the Gut" approach is one of the most practical and impactful ways to achieve lasting health in today's world. This philosophy serves as a reminder that small, sustainable dietary changes can yield significant benefits, empowering individuals to take control of their health from the inside out.

Eating for longevity differs significantly from eating to lose fat, or to manage disease. While weight loss and disease management often focus on specific dietary strategies to meet immediate goals, longevity-focused eating is about building a foundation for sustained, optimal health over the long term. In my view, a well-executed carnivore diet, emphasizing nutrient-dense animal foods, offers one of the best approaches for fat loss, health optimization, and longevity. However, like any diet, it requires fine-tuning to meet each individual's unique needs and goals.

The Carnivore Diet for Longevity: Nutrient Density and Low Toxicity

In the quest for longevity, diet plays a central role, as the foods we consume profoundly impact our health, vitality, and aging process. While many dietary strategies aim to promote health, the carnivore diet—focused solely on nutrient-dense animal products—presents a unique approach to enhancing longevity through its high nutrient density and low toxicity. By centering on foods like high-quality meats, organ meats, and animal fats, the carnivore diet supplies essential nutrients in bioavailable forms while avoiding plant-based anti-nutrients that can impair absorption or cause inflammation. This makes it an excellent choice for those looking to optimize health over the long term, preventing disease and fostering resilience against the physical and mental challenges of aging.

Nutrient Density: The Foundation of Longevity

One of the most compelling arguments for the carnivore diet in promoting longevity lies in its unparalleled nutrient density. Unlike plant foods, which often contain anti-nutrients like oxalates, lectins, and phytates that hinder nutrient absorption, animal-based foods provide vitamins, minerals, and amino acids in forms that are easily absorbed by the body. This bioavailability ensures that each nutrient is effectively utilized, supporting optimal bodily functions, cellular repair, and immune resilience—factors critical to both health and longevity.

Animal-based foods are rich sources of essential nutrients like B vitamins, vitamin D, and heme iron, as well as omega-3 fatty acids, all of which play a role in reducing inflammation, promoting cognitive health, and supporting the cardiovascular system. Organ meats, often referred to as "nature's multivitamin," are particularly nutrient-dense and provide concentrated amounts of vitamins A, B12, and folate, as well as minerals like zinc, copper, and selenium. These nutrients are indispensable in the maintenance of cellular health and in protecting the body from oxidative damage—a key factor in aging. Vitamin A, for instance, is crucial for maintaining skin health and vision, while B vitamins are essential for cellular energy production and neurological function, supporting mental acuity and reducing the risk of age-related cognitive decline.

Omega-3 Fatty Acids: Anti-Inflammatory Powerhouses

Animal-based foods, particularly fatty fish, eggs, and grass-fed meats are excellent sources of omega-3 fatty acids, which are essential for heart and brain health. Omega-3s, specifically EPA and DHA, have strong anti-inflammatory effects that protect against chronic inflammation—a significant contributor to aging and age-related diseases like cardiovascular disease, arthritis, and neurodegenerative conditions. Studies suggest that omega-3s improve cognitive function, support heart health, and can even help extend lifespan. The omega-3 content found in animal foods is in its most effective form, unlike the ALA found in plant sources like flaxseeds, which the body converts inefficiently to usable EPA and DHA.

The anti-inflammatory effects of omega-3s are crucial for reducing the burden of low-grade inflammation, which accelerates cellular aging by damaging tissues and impairing immune function. By regularly consuming foods rich in omega-3s, the carnivore diet helps mitigate this inflammatory process, promoting not only a longer lifespan but also a healthier, more active life well into old age.

Vitamin D: A Critical Nutrient for Aging Well

Vitamin D, often called the "sunshine vitamin," plays a pivotal role in maintaining immune health, bone strength, and mental wellness—all critical for aging gracefully. Animal foods, particularly fatty fish and egg yolks, provide bioavailable vitamin D, ensuring adequate levels without reliance on supplementation or UV exposure. Maintaining optimal vitamin D levels is especially important as we age since deficiencies are associated with a higher risk of osteoporosis, cognitive decline, and compromised immunity.

Vitamin D facilitates calcium absorption, supporting bone density and reducing the risk of fractures and osteoporosis, conditions that often limit mobility and quality of life in older adults. Furthermore, vitamin D is known for its role in modulating the immune response, which becomes increasingly important as immune function tends to decline with age. By including vitamin D-rich foods in the diet, the carnivore approach provides a steady supply of this essential nutrient, supporting immune resilience and protecting against infections and autoimmune issues.

Avoiding Anti-Nutrients: The Low-Toxicity Advantage

The carnivore diet's exclusive reliance on animal foods inherently avoids plant-based anti-nutrients, which are compounds that plants produce to protect themselves from predators. While these compounds are beneficial for the plant, they can pose challenges for humans. Anti-nutrients like oxalates, lectins, and phytates interfere with nutrient absorption and can irritate the digestive system, contributing to inflammation—a key driver of many age-related diseases.

For example, oxalates found in leafy greens and some nuts can bind to calcium in the body, forming kidney stones and depleting calcium stores that would otherwise support bone health. Lectins, which are found in legumes and grains, can damage the gut lining, leading to a condition known as "leaky gut" and allowing inflammatory compounds to enter the bloodstream. Over time, this can weaken immune function, compromise nutrient absorption, and fuel chronic inflammation.

By focusing on animal-based foods, the carnivore diet circumvents these anti-nutrients, allowing the body to absorb nutrients more effectively and reducing inflammatory triggers. This low-toxicity approach helps to maintain cellular integrity, supports digestive health, and ultimately reduces the risk of chronic conditions, paving the way for a longer, healthier life.

Insulin Regulation and Blood Sugar Stability

One of the most significant benefits of the carnivore diet for longevity is its ability to regulate insulin and stabilize blood sugar. Carbohydrates, particularly refined sugars and grains, are known to cause spikes in blood glucose, which in turn leads to a rise in insulin—a hormone that plays a role in storing fat and managing blood sugar. Constantly high insulin levels are associated with insulin resistance, a key factor in metabolic syndrome, diabetes, and obesity, all of which are risk factors for chronic diseases and shortened lifespan.

The carnivore diet's low-carb nature minimizes blood sugar spikes, reducing the demand on the pancreas to produce insulin and promoting insulin sensitivity over time. This metabolic stability is crucial for longevity, as it prevents the cellular damage that occurs from glycation, a process in which excess sugar binds to proteins, creating harmful compounds known as Advanced Glycation End-products (AGEs). AGEs contribute to oxidative stress, tissue damage, and accelerated aging. By reducing insulin spikes, the carnivore diet helps to prevent the formation of AGEs, slowing down the aging process and reducing the risk of age-related diseases.

Gluconeogenesis: A Steady Fuel Source

One of the unique aspects of the carnivore diet is its reliance on gluconeogenesis, a metabolic process in which the liver converts protein into glucose. This process provides a steady, controlled source of glucose without the need for dietary carbohydrates. By producing glucose only when needed, gluconeogenesis prevents the blood sugar fluctuations that come with carbohydrate consumption, promoting energy stability, mental clarity, and a balanced metabolism. This slow-release mechanism supports longevity by maintaining metabolic efficiency and reducing stress on the body's insulin system.

Mental Clarity and Cognitive Health

Brain health is paramount to longevity, and diet has a profound impact on cognitive function. The carnivore diet, rich in essential fats, proteins, and micronutrients, provides the building blocks necessary for a healthy brain. The brain thrives on ketones—an alternative fuel source produced from fat when carbohydrate intake is low. Ketones are not only an efficient energy source for the brain but are also associated with neuroprotective effects, reducing oxidative stress and inflammation in brain cells.

Additionally, essential nutrients like B vitamins, omega-3 fatty acids, and choline found in animal foods are integral to brain health. Choline, found abundantly in egg yolks, is a precursor to acetylcholine, a neurotransmitter involved in memory and learning. Omega-3s, particularly DHA, support neuronal health and reduce the risk of cognitive decline. The carnivore diet, by providing these nutrients in optimal amounts, helps preserve cognitive function, potentially delaying or preventing neurodegenerative conditions such as Alzheimer's and Parkinson's disease.

Physical Vitality and Muscle Maintenance

Maintaining muscle mass is crucial for longevity, as sarcopenia, or age-related muscle loss, is associated with a decrease in physical function, increased risk of falls, and lower quality of life. The carnivore diet, with its emphasis on high-quality protein sources, provides the amino acids necessary for muscle synthesis and repair. By consuming sufficient protein, individuals on a carnivore diet can preserve lean muscle mass, support metabolic health, and maintain strength as they age.

Amino acids like leucine, found in animal products, are particularly effective at stimulating muscle protein synthesis, helping to counteract sarcopenia. Furthermore, the carnivore diet's nutrient density ensures that the body receives adequate vitamins and minerals to support muscle function, such as magnesium, potassium, and calcium. This focus on muscle preservation not only enhances physical resilience but also supports metabolic rate and insulin sensitivity, creating a positive feedback loop for health and longevity.

Mitochondrial Health and Cellular Energy

Longevity depends on the health of our cells, particularly the mitochondria—the "powerhouses" of our cells that generate energy. The nutrient-rich profile of animal foods on the carnivore diet supports mitochondrial function by providing essential cofactors such as Coenzyme Q10 (CoQ10), creatine, and carnitine, which play a role in cellular energy production. CoQ10, found in meat and organ meats, is crucial for mitochondrial health and has been shown to reduce oxidative stress within cells, supporting cellular energy and protecting against age-related decline.

Carnitine, another nutrient abundant in red meat, facilitates the transport of fatty acids into the mitochondria, where they are oxidized for energy. This process is essential for maintaining energy levels, promoting fat metabolism, and supporting cellular repair. By enhancing mitochondrial function and energy production, the carnivore diet contributes to cellular health and resilience, key factors for longevity.

Summary: The Carnivore Diet as a Foundation for Longevity

Incorporating a carnivore diet focused on nutrient density and low toxicity offers a powerful strategy for promoting longevity and maintaining health over the long term. The diet's nutrient-rich composition provides essential vitamins, minerals, and fatty acids that support vital bodily functions, from muscle maintenance and brain health to immune resilience and cellular energy. By avoiding anti-nutrients and maintaining metabolic stability, the carnivore diet reduces the risk of chronic inflammation, insulin resistance, and oxidative stress—conditions that accelerate aging and limit quality of life.

While the carnivore diet offers a unique approach to longevity, individual needs and tolerances vary, and dietary choices should align with one's specific health goals and metabolic requirements. For those seeking a foundational diet that minimizes inflammatory triggers and maximizes nutrient absorption, the carnivore diet presents a viable and effective option. With proper execution, it fosters a state of health that not only counters the effects of aging but also empowers individuals to live a vibrant, active life well into their later years.

Tailoring Diet for Individual Needs and Goals

Creating an effective diet is not about following a universal plan; it's about understanding individual needs, goals, and unique metabolic responses. Diets that work for one person may not work for another due to differences in genetics, lifestyle, activity level, health conditions, and personal goals. Tailoring dietary choices allows for a more personalized, sustainable approach that supports both short-term wellness and long-term health. Whether one's goals are weight management, muscle gain, mental clarity, or disease prevention, an individualized diet provides the foundation for achieving these outcomes.

Recognizing Unique Genetic and Metabolic Differences

Everyone's body responds differently to food due to genetic variation. Some people are genetically predisposed to metabolize certain macronutrients, like fats and carbohydrates, more efficiently. For example, individuals with a certain gene variant in the FTO gene may be more prone to weight gain with a high-carb diet, while others thrive on carbohydrates and struggle with high-fat foods. Genetic testing can provide insights into how your body responds to specific macronutrients, helping to shape a diet that minimizes inflammation, balances blood sugar, and promotes metabolic health.

The Role of Gut Health in Dietary Response

Another crucial factor in tailoring a diet is gut health. The microbiome, or the trillions of microorganisms living in our digestive tract, influences how we digest and absorb nutrients. For example, some people may have bacteria that produce more enzymes to digest fiber, while others may lack them, making high-fiber diets uncomfortable or even counterproductive. Additionally, gut health impacts how well we absorb micronutrients like vitamin B12 and iron. Tailoring the diet to support gut health by including fermented foods, low-inflammatory fiber sources, and avoiding problematic foods is essential for those who have digestive sensitivities or chronic gastrointestinal issues.

Identifying Clear, Realistic Goals

When tailoring a diet, it's essential to set clear, achievable goals. The type of diet and macronutrient distribution may vary significantly depending on whether the primary goal is weight loss, muscle gain, enhanced cognitive function, or managing a specific health condition.

1. **Weight Management**: For weight loss, a low-carb or ketogenic approach may help stabilize insulin levels and reduce hunger by promoting satiety. Alternatively, intermittent fasting may work well for individuals who benefit from periods without caloric intake, as it naturally reduces calorie consumption and promotes fat burning. Including sufficient protein and healthy fats in the diet can prevent muscle loss and support metabolism during weight loss.
2. **Muscle Gain and Athletic Performance**: For muscle gain and athletic performance, a higher protein intake is often necessary, along with sufficient carbohydrates to fuel high-intensity workouts. Carbohydrates are beneficial for replenishing glycogen stores, which are essential for recovery and energy. However, some athletes thrive on a low-carb or ketogenic approach if their sports are endurance-focused, as it allows their bodies to efficiently use fat as a fuel source.
3. **Enhanced Mental Clarity**: For those focused on improving cognitive function, a high-fat, low-carb approach that promotes ketone production may be effective. Ketones are an alternative energy source for the brain and can promote mental clarity and reduce brain fog. Omega-3 fatty acids

205

from fatty fish or fish oil are particularly beneficial for brain health. Some individuals may also benefit from limiting high-sugar foods and avoiding foods with inflammatory effects, as these can disrupt focus and contribute to mental fatigue.

4. **Managing Chronic Conditions**: Specific dietary adjustments can support individuals managing chronic conditions such as diabetes, autoimmune diseases, or cardiovascular issues. For instance, a low-carb diet is often effective in managing Type 2 diabetes by reducing the demand for insulin and stabilizing blood sugar levels. Those with autoimmune conditions may benefit from an elimination diet that avoids foods known to cause inflammation, like gluten, dairy, and certain nightshades. Personalized supplementation may also be necessary to address nutrient deficiencies that are common in specific conditions.

Balancing Macronutrients for Optimal Health

Different goals and health conditions require varied macronutrient ratios. While the ideal diet for one person may be high in fats and low in carbs, another person may require more carbohydrates, particularly if they have high energy demands or struggle with low blood sugar.

1. **Protein**: Protein is essential for muscle maintenance, immune function, and overall cellular health. It provides the amino acids necessary for tissue repair and hormone production. Aiming for 1.2-2 grams of protein per kilogram of body weight is generally sufficient for most individuals, though athletes and bodybuilders may require more. Protein can be adjusted based on specific goals, such as muscle gain or weight loss, where higher protein intake can aid in preserving muscle mass.
2. **Fat**: Healthy fats are crucial for cellular structure, hormone production, and energy. For those who thrive on a higher-fat diet, such as those on a ketogenic plan, fats become the primary energy source, replacing carbohydrates. Sources like avocados, olive oil, grass-fed butter, and fatty fish provide omega-3 fatty acids and are beneficial for reducing inflammation. For others, too much dietary fat can lead to weight gain if not carefully managed with activity levels.

3. **Carbohydrates**: Carbohydrates can be tailored based on individual insulin sensitivity and activity level. For individuals with insulin resistance, a low-carb approach may help stabilize blood sugar, while active people or athletes may require moderate to high carbohydrate intake to support their energy needs. Whole-food sources like vegetables, fruits, and occasionally grains provide some vitamins and fiber. For sedentary individuals or those looking to lose weight, lowering carbohydrates can prevent insulin spikes and support fat metabolism.

Rethinking Calcium: Why It's Not as Essential as We Once Thought

For decades, calcium has been touted as the cornerstone of bone health and overall wellness, with recommendations to consume dairy or calcium-rich foods regularly. However, recent insights reveal that calcium alone may not be as beneficial as once believed—and without proper nutrient balance, it can even be harmful. The true key to bone health and calcium's role in the body lies in ensuring a synergy with other nutrients, especially **vitamin K2** and **magnesium**.

Calcium Without Vitamin K2 and Magnesium: When calcium is consumed without adequate levels of vitamin K2, it may not be directed where it's needed most—into the bones and teeth. Instead, calcium can accumulate in soft tissues, leading to calcification in areas like arteries and kidneys, which may increase the risk of cardiovascular issues and kidney stones. Vitamin K2 is essential because it activates proteins, such as osteocalcin, which bind calcium and direct it into the bone matrix. This means that without vitamin K2, dietary or supplemental calcium is far less effective and may even pose health risks by depositing in soft tissues.

Rethinking Calcium's Necessity: Interestingly, the body maintains a steady level of calcium in the blood, often pulling calcium from bones when levels are low. However, this process doesn't require large, constant external sources of calcium, especially in the presence of other bone-supportive nutrients like magnesium and vitamin D. Cultures that consume little to no dairy but emphasize a diet rich in vegetables, animal products with vitamin K2, and other micronutrients often experience lower rates of osteoporosis. This suggests that calcium is not the sole determinant of bone health, and its intake can be minimized without risking bone integrity if the diet is balanced.

Whole Food Sources of K2 and Balanced Nutrients: Foods rich in vitamin K2, such as organ meats, egg yolks, grass-fed butter, and fermented foods like natto, help direct calcium into the bones. Magnesium, found in leafy greens, seeds, and nuts, also supports bone health by aiding in vitamin D metabolism, which indirectly regulates calcium levels. When calcium intake is balanced with these other nutrients, the need for high levels of dietary calcium diminishes. This approach supports bone health more naturally, without risking calcification or relying heavily on calcium supplements.

Implications for Bone Health: The focus on calcium supplements and high dairy intake as the primary defense against osteoporosis and bone fractures is now being questioned. The body doesn't simply need calcium but requires a balanced intake of minerals and vitamins to maintain strong bones and proper cellular function. Calcium, without adequate co-factors like vitamin K2 and magnesium, is less effective and may contribute to health problems rather than prevent them. Supporting bone health with a holistic diet rich in these balancing nutrients may be a far better approach than simply loading up on calcium.

In summary, while calcium plays a role in the body, it is not the standalone solution for bone health and is not as essential as commonly believed. Ensuring adequate levels of vitamin K2, magnesium, and other supporting nutrients is key to preventing the misguided deposition of calcium in soft tissues and promoting true bone strength. This shift in perspective challenges traditional calcium recommendations and emphasizes the need for a balanced approach that supports the body's natural processes for utilizing and managing minerals effectively.

Micronutrient Focus: Beyond Macronutrient Ratios

Tailoring a diet for optimal health involves ensuring sufficient intake of key micronutrients and other vital compounds that support cellular energy, muscle function, and overall wellness. Nutrients like magnesium, zinc, potassium, and vitamins D and K2 play essential roles in maintaining health, yet many individuals are deficient in these due to modern dietary patterns, lifestyle factors, or limited sun exposure. Adding compounds such as CoQ10, D-ribose, and L-carnitine can further enhance energy production and metabolic resilience.

Magnesium: Involved in over 300 biochemical reactions, magnesium is essential for muscle function, nerve signaling, and blood glucose regulation. Foods rich in magnesium, such as leafy greens, seeds, and fish, can help meet daily needs, although supplementation may benefit those experiencing chronic stress or frequent muscle cramps.

Vitamin D and K2: These vitamins work together to manage calcium in the body, with vitamin D aiding calcium absorption and vitamin K2 ensuring it's directed to bones rather than soft tissues, where it could lead to calcification. People who consume dairy or leafy greens often meet calcium needs, but K2, found in animal-based foods like egg yolks and liver, is critical for bone health and calcium balance.

Iron and B12: Crucial for red blood cell production and sustained energy, iron and B12 are especially important for individuals with low energy levels or anemia. Foods such as red meat, liver, and eggs provide bioavailable sources of these nutrients, which are often more effective for those who struggle with plant-based iron sources.

CoQ10: This antioxidant is essential for cellular energy production and supports heart health by assisting mitochondria in generating energy. CoQ10 is naturally found in organ meats, fatty fish, and muscle meats, but supplementation may be beneficial, especially for those on statin medications, which can lower CoQ10 levels.

D-Ribose: D-ribose is a sugar that forms the backbone of ATP, the energy molecule our cells use. It's particularly beneficial for those with energy deficits or metabolic concerns, as it supports quick energy replenishment and may help improve muscle recovery, especially in active individuals.

L-Carnitine: This amino acid derivative is critical for transporting fatty acids into cells to be burned for energy, making it especially useful for heart health and fat metabolism. Found in red meat and fish, L-carnitine can support endurance and exercise recovery, and supplementation may benefit those with specific metabolic or energy needs.

Together, these nutrients and compounds form a comprehensive approach to diet optimization, addressing not only foundational health needs but also supporting cellular energy and metabolic flexibility.

Adjusting for Lifestyle and Activity Levels

The diet of a highly active individual, such as an athlete or manual laborer, will differ significantly from that of someone with a sedentary lifestyle. Physical activity not only affects energy requirements but also impacts nutrient needs and macronutrient distribution.

High Activity Levels: Those with active lifestyles need more energy and may benefit from a higher carbohydrate intake for performance and recovery. Post-workout nutrition is crucial for replenishing glycogen stores, which carbohydrates help restore. Protein timing also matters, as consuming protein after exercise aids in muscle repair. Active individuals may require more hydration and electrolytes, particularly in hot climates or during high-intensity workouts.

Sedentary Lifestyles: For those who spend much of their day sitting, a lower-calorie intake may be necessary to maintain a healthy weight. Lower carbohydrate intake can prevent unnecessary insulin spikes, which are less likely to be burned off through physical activity. Protein and healthy fats can provide satiety and stable energy, preventing energy crashes associated with high-sugar foods.

Stress Management: Chronic stress impacts dietary needs, particularly for nutrients like magnesium and B vitamins, which can become depleted during periods of prolonged stress. People under high stress may benefit from foods that help modulate cortisol, like fatty fish for omega-3s, or adaptogenic herbs like ashwagandha. Additionally, a nutrient-dense diet rich in vitamins C and E can support immune resilience, which can become compromised under chronic stress.

Practical Application: Finding What Works for You

An individualized approach may involve trial and error to find the optimal macronutrient distribution, meal frequency, and food choices. Some people thrive on three meals a day with no snacks, while others benefit from smaller, more frequent meals. Intermittent fasting can be a helpful tool for some, while others may find it negatively affects their energy levels or focus.

Self-Monitoring: Keeping a food journal or using an app to track meals, energy levels, and mood can provide valuable insights into how different foods and meal timing affect well-being.

Testing and Feedback: Regular blood tests can provide insights into how well a diet is supporting health markers, such as blood sugar, *insulin levels*, cholesterol levels, and inflammatory markers. Adjustments can be made based on these results, ensuring the diet remains aligned with health goals.

Consulting with a Health Professional: For those with complex health conditions, working with a knowledgeable nutritionist, dietitian, or healthcare provider can ensure a safe, tailored approach. Professionals can help fine-tune diets based on individual needs, provide guidance on portion sizes, and recommend any necessary supplements.

Adapting Over Time: Evolving with Your Health Needs

Lastly, it's important to recognize that dietary needs change over time. What works for an individual in their 20s may not be effective in their 40s, as hormonal shifts, changes in metabolism, and evolving health goals come into play. For instance, an individual may thrive on a low-carb diet for years but may need to incorporate more carbohydrates later in life to support thyroid function or hormone balance. Staying flexible and responsive to the body's feedback is key to maintaining a diet that promotes long-term health.

Creating a diet tailored to individual needs is an empowering way to take control of health, avoid fad diets, and make sustainable lifestyle choices. A one-size-fits-all approach is rarely effective because each person has unique needs, genetic predispositions, and lifestyle factors. By focusing on nutrient density, macronutrient balance, and adjusting for specific health goals, individuals can find an approach that truly supports their well-being.

In today's society, it's common to hear that weight gain is an inevitable part of aging, an expectation that leads many people to view gradual health decline as a natural part of getting older.

However, the reality is that many of these age-related health issues, especially weight gain, are not inevitable. Instead, they are often the result of growing insulin resistance and poor metabolic health, influenced by modern lifestyles and dietary habits. In fact, as generations progress, we are witnessing an increase in insulin resistance and related health conditions, from Type 2 diabetes and heart disease to various forms of metabolic syndrome. Rather than a foregone conclusion of aging, these trends highlight the importance of examining our relationship with food, lifestyle, and the ways society conditions us to accept poor health as a given.

The Myth of "Age-Related" Weight Gain

One of the most pervasive myths is that weight gain is simply a natural part of getting older. This notion is reinforced by cultural norms, where jokes about "middle-aged spread" and "dad bod" normalize the belief that weight gain, lower energy, and declining health are unavoidable as we age. People often attribute this to a slowing metabolism, believing that it's only natural to pack on a few pounds with each passing decade. This mindset can lead to complacency, where people accept weight gain as inevitable rather than seeing it as something they can address and even prevent.

However, research indicates that the metabolic slowdown often cited as the culprit for age-related weight gain is overstated. While our resting metabolic rate may slightly decrease with age, studies have shown that this decline is minimal until we reach our senior years, particularly around age 60. Most of the so-called "metabolic slowdown" observed in middle age is actually linked to lifestyle changes. As we grow older, people tend to become less active, often due to increased work responsibilities, family commitments, and less time dedicated to physical activity. This decrease in movement, combined with the high-calorie, processed diets that dominate today's food landscape, leads to an imbalance between energy intake and expenditure—fueling weight gain.

Insulin Resistance: The Real Culprit Behind Midlife Weight Gain

If a slowing metabolism isn't primarily to blame, then what is? A growing body of evidence points to insulin resistance as the root cause of most age-related weight gain and chronic illness. Insulin is a hormone produced by the pancreas that regulates blood sugar levels and helps store glucose for future energy needs. However, when we consume diets high in refined carbohydrates and sugars, our bodies produce more insulin to manage the spike in blood sugar. Over time, this constant demand on the pancreas to release insulin leads to a condition called insulin resistance, where cells become less responsive to insulin's effects. As a result, blood sugar levels remain elevated, leading the body to produce even more insulin in an attempt to maintain balance.

This cycle creates a "high insulin environment," where the body is continuously in a state of energy storage, prioritizing fat storage over fat burning. This chronic insulin elevation disrupts other metabolic processes, leading to increased hunger, fat accumulation, and inflammation. Insulin resistance not only promotes weight gain but also contributes to the development of various diseases, including Type 2 diabetes, hypertension, and cardiovascular disease. While insulin resistance can develop at any age, its effects become more pronounced as we get older, especially if left unaddressed.

The increasing rates of insulin resistance among today's population are not just personal health issues; they represent a generational health crisis. Unlike past generations, today's society has greater access to highly processed foods, sedentary lifestyles, and increased exposure to stressors, all of which contribute to insulin resistance. As a result, conditions that were once rare, like Type 2 diabetes, are now appearing at younger ages. This shift underscores the urgent need to recognize insulin resistance as a significant factor in age-related weight gain and health decline.

Society's Role in Normalizing Weight Gain and Declining Health

Cultural norms and media messaging play a powerful role in shaping our beliefs about health and aging. Advertisements, for instance, promote fast food, sugary drinks, and convenience snacks, reinforcing a lifestyle that prioritizes immediate satisfaction over long-term health. Similarly, the weight-loss industry often promotes quick fixes rather than sustainable lifestyle changes, which can further obscure the role of insulin resistance and metabolic health.

Moreover, many healthcare providers inadvertently reinforce these norms. It's not uncommon for doctors to tell patients that gaining weight in their 30s, 40s, and beyond is normal. Rather than addressing underlying factors like insulin resistance, dietary habits, and lifestyle choices, medical advice often focuses on symptom management. As a result, patients may be prescribed medications for high blood pressure, cholesterol, or blood sugar without being encouraged to make the lifestyle changes that could address the root causes of these issues.

The societal acceptance of weight gain as an inevitable part of aging has led many people to ignore or overlook the warning signs of insulin resistance. Common symptoms like fatigue, sugar cravings, and weight gain, especially around the abdomen, are often dismissed as normal parts of aging. However, these symptoms are red flags that signal a deeper issue with metabolic health. When ignored, these signs can escalate, leading to the onset of chronic illnesses that require more intensive medical intervention.

The Generational Impact: From Baby Boomers to Gen Z

Each generation seems to experience declining health earlier than the previous one. Baby Boomers were the first generation to experience widespread access to processed and convenience foods, and rates of obesity, diabetes, and cardiovascular disease increased alongside this dietary shift. Millennials and Gen Z are now following suit but at an accelerated pace. With increased exposure to high-sugar, high-fat, processed foods, these younger generations are developing insulin resistance, obesity, and Type 2 diabetes at rates that are unprecedented.

The generational impact of these trends is far-reaching, affecting not only individuals but also families, communities, and healthcare systems. Families are experiencing the financial and emotional burdens of chronic illness earlier in life. Communities are facing public health crises as they grapple with rising rates of preventable diseases. Meanwhile, healthcare systems are overwhelmed with the demands of managing chronic conditions that could have been prevented with earlier intervention and lifestyle changes. As generations progress, the cost of this health decline continues to rise, impacting society as a whole.

Addressing Insulin Resistance for Long-Term Health and Longevity

While aging may bring certain inevitable changes to the body, weight gain and poor metabolic health are not a given. By addressing insulin resistance through dietary choices, physical activity, and lifestyle changes, we can mitigate many of the so-called "age-related" health declines. Prioritizing whole foods, reducing refined carbohydrates, and increasing physical activity can have a profound impact on insulin sensitivity.

Intermittent fasting, for example, has shown promise in reducing insulin resistance by giving the pancreas a break from constant insulin production. Physical activity, especially resistance training, can improve insulin sensitivity by increasing muscle mass and promoting glucose uptake in the muscles. Incorporating healthy fats and proteins into the diet also helps balance blood sugar levels, reducing the need for high insulin output. By making these lifestyle adjustments, individuals can support their metabolic health, maintain a healthy weight, and improve their overall quality of life as they age.

The Need for Education and Awareness

Breaking free from the societal conditioning that promotes weight gain and poor health as a natural part of aging requires education and awareness. People need to understand the role of insulin resistance in weight gain and chronic illness and learn how to make choices that support metabolic health. Schools, workplaces, and healthcare providers all have a role to play in promoting awareness and providing resources for healthier living.

Furthermore, policy changes can help shift cultural norms around food and health. Tax incentives for healthy foods, restrictions on advertising unhealthy foods to children, and educational campaigns about the benefits of whole foods can all contribute to a healthier society. Additionally, employers can support health and wellness programs that encourage regular physical activity and stress management, both of which play a role in preventing insulin resistance.

Reclaiming Health and Redefining Aging

By challenging the myth that aging and weight gain go hand in hand, we can begin to redefine what it means to age well. Instead of viewing each decade as a period of decline, we can embrace it as an opportunity to optimize health and vitality. With the right dietary choices, exercise, and lifestyle habits, individuals can maintain their metabolic health, avoid unnecessary weight gain, and reduce the risk of chronic diseases.

Ultimately, understanding the role of insulin resistance in age-related weight gain empowers individuals to take control of their health. Rather than accepting poor health as a consequence of aging, we can see it as a signal to make positive changes. In doing so, we can break the cycle of generational health decline and build a foundation of health and vitality for future generations.

Chapter 10 Flipping the Script on Diseases and Disorders

In our modern world, the prevalence of chronic diseases and disorders has escalated dramatically, with many individuals and communities suffering from conditions once considered rare. However, there is a growing body of evidence suggesting that a return to a "proper human diet" one that emphasizes nutrient-dense, unprocessed, and evolutionarily consistent foods — could potentially eliminate or at least reduce the incidence and severity of many of these conditions. Let's dive into some of the most prevalent diseases and disorders that may be profoundly impacted by diet. Note that some information is repeated here, but it should serve as a reinforcement for understanding the importance of pathophysiology.

Cancer: Rethinking the Metabolic Roots

Cancer is often considered a genetic disease, but there's increasing support for the idea that it may, in fact, be more fundamentally a metabolic disorder. Cancer cells exhibit abnormal energy production, relying heavily on glucose through a process known as the Warburg effect. Unlike normal cells, which use oxygen for energy production, cancer cells often prefer a fermentation process, even in the presence of oxygen. This metabolic dysfunction may be fueled by diets high in sugar and refined carbohydrates, which consistently spike blood glucose and insulin levels, providing a readily available fuel source for these abnormal cells.

Recent studies suggest that adopting a low-carb or ketogenic diet may starve cancer cells by depriving them of their primary fuel source: glucose. This type of diet forces the body to burn fat for energy, producing ketones that cancer cells cannot efficiently use. The metabolic theory of cancer, pioneered by researchers like Dr. Thomas Seyfried, posits that reducing glucose availability through diet may help slow or even stop the progression of certain cancers. While more research is needed, adopting a diet that minimizes processed sugars and emphasizes healthy fats and proteins shows promise as an adjunct to traditional treatments, potentially reducing the burden of this devastating disease.

Here are some of the key points that support the metabolic theory of cancer:

Warburg Effect: In the 1920s, Otto Warburg discovered that cancer cells prefer to produce energy through glycolysis (fermentation) even in the presence of oxygen, a phenomenon known as the "Warburg effect." This shift to inefficient energy production suggests that cancer cells are metabolically compromised, relying heavily on glucose and producing lactic acid as a byproduct.

Mitochondrial Dysfunction: The metabolic theory argues that damaged or dysfunctional mitochondria may trigger cells to shift to glycolysis. This metabolic change could lead to mutations as a secondary effect rather than the primary cause, as genetic mutations are a hallmark of cancer but may occur due to mitochondrial stress or damage rather than being the initial cause.

Dietary and Metabolic Influences: The metabolic theory posits that factors such as insulin resistance, chronic inflammation, obesity, and diet may create conditions that support cancer growth. Cancer cells thrive on glucose and, in some cases, glutamine, suggesting that restricting these fuels (e.g., through ketogenic diets, fasting) might starve cancer cells, limiting their growth.

New Treatment Approaches: Treatments that focus on cancer metabolism, such as dietary interventions, hyperbaric oxygen therapy, and metabolic drugs like metformin, show promising results in some cases. These treatments target the unique metabolic needs of cancer cells rather than focusing solely on genetic targets.

However, this doesn't mean that genetic factors are irrelevant; rather, it suggests a more integrated view where genetic mutations may be a result of or contribute to metabolic dysfunction. Many researchers believe that a combined approach, addressing both genetic and metabolic factors, may be more effective for understanding and treating cancer.

Alzheimer's and Dementia

Alzheimer's disease, often referred to as "Type 3 diabetes," is increasingly being understood as a condition with deep metabolic roots. Like other metabolic disorders, it involves the body's inability to process energy effectively, particularly in the brain. In Alzheimer's, the brain's cells gradually lose their ability to utilize glucose, leading to a range of symptoms, including memory loss, cognitive decline, and behavioral changes. This condition, along with other forms of dementia, affects millions worldwide, with cases increasing each year. But what if diet could play a role in reducing the risk or slowing the progression?

A major contributor to Alzheimer's may be insulin resistance. The brain is highly dependent on glucose for energy, and insulin plays a crucial role in allowing brain cells to absorb this glucose. When insulin resistance occurs in the brain, it creates an energy deficit that can impair cognitive function. Over time, this dysfunction is believed to contribute to the accumulation of amyloid plaques and tau tangles, hallmarks of Alzheimer's pathology. By adopting a diet that minimizes insulin resistance — low in refined carbohydrates and sugars and rich in healthy fats — we can potentially protect brain cells and support cognitive function over the long term.

Ketones: An Alternative Fuel for the Brain

When glucose metabolism falters, as it does in Alzheimer's, ketones can offer an alternative fuel source. Ketogenic diets, which limit carbohydrate intake and encourage the production of ketones from fat, may help bypass the brain's impaired glucose metabolism. The ketones produced in a state of ketosis can cross the blood-brain barrier and provide energy for neurons that are starved for glucose, potentially improving cognitive function. Clinical studies have shown promise in the use of ketogenic diets for managing symptoms and slowing the progression of cognitive decline, although more research is needed to confirm the long-term benefits.

Chronic Inflammation and Oxidative Stress

Chronic inflammation and oxidative stress are other key factors in the development of Alzheimer's. Diets high in processed foods, sugars, and unhealthy fats tend to fuel inflammation and oxidative damage, which can worsen brain health. By contrast, diets rich in antioxidants, healthy fats (like those from fish and olive oil), and anti-inflammatory foods may help reduce these effects. Nutrients like omega-3 fatty acids, found in fatty fish, and antioxidants from berries, leafy greens, and other colorful vegetables can support brain health by reducing inflammation and protecting neurons from oxidative damage.

Gut-Brain Axis and Microbiome

Another emerging area of research is the link between gut health and brain health, known as the gut-brain axis. Our gut microbiome — the diverse community of bacteria in our digestive tract — plays a significant role in regulating inflammation, immune function, and even neurotransmitter production. A diet that supports a healthy gut microbiome, emphasizing whole foods, fiber, and fermented foods, may therefore also benefit cognitive health. Conversely, diets high in sugar, refined carbohydrates, and processed foods can disrupt the microbiome, potentially contributing to inflammation that reaches the brain.

The Role of Lifestyle and Diet in Prevention

While there's currently no cure for Alzheimer's, lifestyle changes offer a promising route for prevention and potentially slowing the disease's progression. Combining a low-carb, nutrient-dense diet with regular exercise, quality sleep, and stress management can create a holistic approach to brain health. Emphasizing foods that stabilize blood sugar, reduce inflammation, and support metabolic health is likely our best defense against Alzheimer's and dementia.

In summary, Alzheimer's and dementia may not be purely genetic or inevitable consequences of aging. By addressing the metabolic and inflammatory contributors through diet and lifestyle, we can take proactive steps to protect our cognitive health and reduce the risk of these devastating conditions.

Multiple Sclerosis: The Metabolic and Dietary Connection

Multiple sclerosis (MS) is a chronic autoimmune disease that affects the central nervous system, leading to inflammation and damage to the protective myelin sheath that surrounds nerve fibers. This results in communication breakdowns between the brain and the body, causing a wide range of symptoms like fatigue, muscle weakness, and coordination issues. While the exact cause of MS remains unknown, growing evidence suggests that metabolic and dietary factors can influence disease progression and symptom severity.

Inflammation and Autoimmunity in MS

MS is characterized by chronic inflammation, which leads to the immune system attacking the myelin sheath. Diets high in processed foods, sugars, and omega-6-rich seed oils can exacerbate inflammation, potentially worsening MS symptoms. By reducing inflammatory triggers through diet, individuals may be able to alleviate some of the disease's symptoms and slow its progression.

Role of Fatty Acids: Omega-3 vs. Omega-6

Research highlights the importance of achieving a balanced intake of omega-3 and omega-6 fatty acids in autoimmune diseases like MS. Omega-3s, found in fatty fish and flaxseed, are known for their anti-inflammatory effects, while an excess of omega-6s, common in vegetable oils and processed foods, promotes inflammation. A 1:1 ratio of omega-6 to omega-3 is ideal for reducing inflammation, but modern diets often reach ratios as high as 20:1. By increasing omega-3 intake through fatty fish or supplements and reducing omega-6-heavy processed foods, those with MS may experience a reduction in inflammation and an improvement in symptom management.

A ketogenic diet, which is high in fats and low in carbohydrates, has shown promise in managing MS symptoms. The reduction in carbohydrates lowers blood glucose and insulin levels, reducing inflammation. Furthermore, ketones, the alternative fuel produced in a ketogenic state, may provide a neuroprotective effect, supporting brain function and reducing oxidative stress. Research is still ongoing, but initial findings suggest that the ketogenic diet may help manage fatigue and improve cognitive function, two common challenges for individuals with MS.

Gut Health and the Immune System

The gut microbiome plays a crucial role in regulating the immune system, and imbalances in gut bacteria have been associated with autoimmune diseases like MS. Diets high in fiber, probiotics, and prebiotics can promote a healthy microbiome, potentially reducing autoimmune activity. Conversely, processed foods, high-sugar diets, and certain artificial additives may disrupt gut health and worsen inflammation. By supporting a balanced microbiome with a nutrient-dense, whole-food diet, individuals with MS may positively influence immune function and inflammation levels.

Vitamin D is essential for immune function, and its deficiency has been linked to an increased risk of developing MS and worsening symptoms. While dietary sources of vitamin D are limited, supplementation or adequate sunlight exposure can help maintain optimal levels. For those living in regions with limited sunlight, especially in winter months, vitamin D supplementation may be critical for managing MS and promoting overall immune health.

MS remains a complex and challenging disease, but dietary and lifestyle modifications offer a promising approach to symptom management. By focusing on an anti-inflammatory diet, optimizing omega-3 intake, considering ketogenic approaches, and supporting gut health, individuals with MS may find relief and potentially slow disease progression.

Other well-known common diseases are linked to misconceived dietary choices. Osteoporosis also can be considered a metabolic disease. It is often categorized as a *metabolic bone disorder* because it involves abnormalities in bone metabolism. Osteoporosis is primarily characterized by decreased bone mass and density, leading to fragile bones that are more susceptible to fractures.

Key factors linking osteoporosis to metabolic disease include:

1. **Bone Remodeling and Calcium Metabolism**: Bone is constantly being remodeled through the actions of osteoblasts (which build bone) and osteoclasts (which break down bone). In osteoporosis, this balance is disrupted, often due to hormonal changes, insufficient intake of critical nutrients, or metabolic dysfunction, leading to bone resorption outpacing bone formation.
2. **Insulin Resistance and Metabolic Syndrome**: Research suggests that metabolic syndrome and insulin resistance may increase the risk of osteoporosis. People with insulin resistance often have chronic low-grade inflammation, which can disrupt the bone remodeling process.
3. **Hormonal Imbalances**: Osteoporosis is closely linked to hormonal changes, especially those involving estrogen in women and testosterone in men. Since metabolic health influences hormone production and regulation, poor metabolic health can accelerate bone loss.
4. **Vitamin D and Calcium Absorption**: Again, poor metabolic health can impair nutrient absorption, including calcium and vitamin D, which are essential for bone health. Low vitamin D levels are common in people with metabolic disorders and can exacerbate osteoporosis.

5. **Advanced Glycation End-products (AGEs)**: Accumulated AGEs, often resulting from poor metabolic health and high blood sugar levels, can weaken the structural integrity of bones and contribute to osteoporosis.

Osteoporosis has strong ties to metabolic health, and addressing metabolic factors—such as improving diet, managing blood sugar levels, and ensuring hormonal balance—can help reduce osteoporosis risk and support better bone health.

There are too many metabolic diet related issues to name here. The best thing to do is clean up your diet, step by step, and make yourself a plan to start making better choices with the food that you consume. It makes all the difference in the world.

Coenzyme Q10 (CoQ10)

If we're talking about disease and disease prevention, I have to include a section on supplementation and beneficial *nutrients*. Nutritional supplements can fill gaps in our diets, support cellular function, and provide essential vitamins, minerals, and compounds that help our bodies thrive, especially when natural levels decline with age or under specific health conditions. Supplements such as antioxidants, essential fatty acids, vitamins, and coenzymes—like CoQ10—play significant roles in mitigating risk factors and enhancing resilience against disease.

For instance, omega-3 fatty acids support heart health and reduce inflammation, while vitamin D enhances immune function and supports bone health. Magnesium aids in muscle and nerve function, vitamin C boosts immune defense, and B vitamins support energy production and cognitive health. Incorporating these supplements alongside a balanced diet can fortify the body's natural defenses, providing an additional layer of protection and promoting long-term health.

Coenzyme Q10, or CoQ10, is a vital antioxidant that plays a central role in cellular energy production and offers substantial health benefits, particularly for cardiovascular health. Naturally occurring in the mitochondria of our cells, CoQ10 assists in ATP (adenosine triphosphate) synthesis, the process that powers cell function. Given that energy demand is high in organs like the heart, liver, and kidneys, CoQ10 is especially crucial for these areas. As we age, CoQ10 levels diminish, which can impact energy production and increase oxidative stress, factors implicated in a wide range of health conditions, especially cardiovascular disease.

The Basics of CoQ10 and Cellular Energy Production

CoQ10 is an essential component of the electron transport chain within mitochondria, where it facilitates the transfer of electrons between molecules, a process fundamental to ATP synthesis. ATP serves as the cell's primary energy currency, required for nearly all cellular processes. This energy production is especially important for high-energy-demand organs like the heart, where any disruption in ATP synthesis can lead to compromised function.

In addition to its role in energy production, CoQ10 has antioxidant properties that protect cells from damage caused by free radicals, which are unstable molecules generated during ATP synthesis. Free radicals, in excess, can damage cellular structures, DNA, and proteins, accelerating aging and contributing to the development of various chronic diseases. As a lipid-soluble antioxidant, CoQ10 can protect cell membranes from oxidative damage, particularly in the mitochondria where reactive oxygen species are most abundant.

Cardiovascular Health Benefits of CoQ10

CoQ10 has garnered significant attention in cardiovascular health, given its dual roles in energy production and antioxidation. Cardiovascular diseases, including hypertension, heart failure, and atherosclerosis, are associated with oxidative stress, inflammation, and diminished cellular energy — areas where CoQ10 provides critical support.

1. **Heart Failure and CoQ10 Supplementation**: Clinical studies have shown that CoQ10 supplementation can be beneficial for individuals with heart failure, a condition characterized by the heart's inability to pump blood efficiently. Heart failure is associated with mitochondrial dysfunction and reduced CoQ10 levels, leading to energy deficiencies in heart cells. Supplementing with CoQ10 has been shown to improve symptoms, exercise tolerance, and overall quality of life in patients with heart failure, helping

restore the energy production that is necessary for optimal heart function.

2. **Reduction of Hypertension**: CoQ10 has been studied for its effects on blood pressure. High blood pressure, or hypertension, is a major risk factor for heart disease and stroke. Research indicates that CoQ10 supplementation can help lower systolic and diastolic blood pressure, potentially by improving mitochondrial function in blood vessels, enhancing nitric oxide production, and reducing oxidative stress. These effects contribute to the relaxation and dilation of blood vessels, which can reduce blood pressure.

3. **Protection Against Atherosclerosis**: Atherosclerosis, the buildup of plaque within arteries, is driven by oxidative damage to LDL cholesterol, which becomes more dangerous when oxidized. As an antioxidant, CoQ10 helps reduce the oxidation of LDL cholesterol, thereby lowering the risk of plaque buildup and promoting healthier arteries. This property makes CoQ10 an important consideration in the prevention of atherosclerosis and the reduction of heart disease risk.

4. **Improvement in Lipid Profiles**: CoQ10 may positively influence lipid profiles by increasing HDL cholesterol (the "good" cholesterol) and potentially reducing levels of LDL cholesterol (the "bad" cholesterol). Studies suggest that CoQ10, through its antioxidant effects, can protect HDL particles from oxidative damage, supporting their cholesterol-clearing functions and reducing inflammation in the arteries. This dual action on lipid oxidation and HDL support further positions CoQ10 as beneficial for heart health.

Antioxidant and Anti-Inflammatory Properties of CoQ10

Beyond cardiovascular health, CoQ10's antioxidant role is essential for protecting cells throughout the body. Oxidative stress is a significant factor in aging and the development of various chronic diseases, including cancer, neurodegenerative diseases, and metabolic syndrome. By neutralizing free radicals, CoQ10 protects cells from oxidative damage and reduces inflammation, contributing to healthier aging and a lower risk of chronic disease.

- **Reduction of Oxidative Stress in Mitochondria**: Mitochondria are both the primary producers and primary targets of oxidative stress. CoQ10's location within the

225

mitochondrial membrane enables it to directly counteract reactive oxygen species where they are generated, protecting mitochondrial DNA and reducing the risk of mutations and mitochondrial dysfunction.

- **Neuroprotective Benefits**: CoQ10's antioxidant effects extend to brain health. Neurodegenerative diseases such as Alzheimer's and Parkinson's are associated with oxidative damage and mitochondrial dysfunction. Research indicates that CoQ10 may offer neuroprotective effects by mitigating oxidative stress in neurons and supporting mitochondrial function, potentially slowing the progression of these conditions.

Supporting Metabolic Health

Given its role in energy production, CoQ10 also influences metabolic health, impacting insulin sensitivity and inflammation — both crucial factors in conditions like metabolic syndrome and type 2 diabetes. Studies have shown that CoQ10 supplementation can improve insulin sensitivity, helping to regulate blood sugar levels and reduce the risk of diabetes-related complications. This effect may be linked to CoQ10's role in protecting cells from oxidative stress, which is a known factor in insulin resistance.

1. **Improved Blood Sugar Control**: By enhancing mitochondrial function and reducing oxidative stress in cells, CoQ10 can improve cellular response to insulin, helping to maintain stable blood sugar levels. For those with insulin resistance or metabolic syndrome, this can be a valuable addition to their nutritional regimen.
2. **Decreased Inflammation in Adipose Tissue**: Inflammatory cytokines are often elevated in people with obesity and type 2 diabetes, contributing to insulin resistance. CoQ10's anti-inflammatory properties help reduce these cytokines, particularly in adipose (fat) tissue, thereby promoting better insulin sensitivity and metabolic health.

Aging and Cellular Health

As people age, natural CoQ10 levels decrease, particularly in high-energy organs like the heart, brain, and liver. This decline can contribute to lower energy levels, reduced cellular function, and increased susceptibility to chronic diseases. Supplementing with CoQ10 may help counteract age-related declines in mitochondrial function, enhancing overall energy levels, cognitive function, and physical performance in older adults.

1. **Enhanced Physical Performance**: Athletes and older adults alike may benefit from CoQ10 supplementation to support endurance and recovery. CoQ10 has been shown to improve muscle energy production and reduce muscle fatigue, enhancing exercise tolerance and performance. This effect is particularly valuable for aging individuals, as it helps counteract the natural decline in physical capacity.
2. **Support for Cognitive Function**: Brain cells are highly dependent on energy, making them vulnerable to mitochondrial dysfunction. Research indicates that CoQ10 supplementation may improve cognitive function in older adults, particularly in areas related to memory and mental clarity, by supporting mitochondrial health and reducing oxidative stress in brain cells.

Sources and Supplementation

CoQ10 is found in various foods, with organ meats (such as liver and kidney), fatty fish (like salmon, sardines, and mackerel), and some plant-based sources like spinach, broccoli, and cauliflower being particularly rich. However, dietary sources may not provide sufficient CoQ10 to significantly impact health, especially for individuals with health conditions or those on medications that deplete CoQ10 levels.

As a supplement, CoQ10 is available in two forms: ubiquinone and ubiquinol. Ubiquinol is the active antioxidant form, and studies indicate it may be more bioavailable, particularly in older adults whose bodies may not efficiently convert ubiquinone to ubiquinol. While CoQ10 is generally safe, it's recommended to take it with a meal containing fat, as it is fat-soluble and requires dietary fats for optimal absorption.

CoQ10's role in energy production and its potent antioxidant properties make it a valuable component in supporting cardiovascular health, cellular health, and metabolic function. From heart health to exercise performance and cognitive function, CoQ10 addresses a variety of health concerns by optimizing mitochondrial function and reducing oxidative stress. For individuals at risk of heart disease, those on statin medications, or anyone experiencing low energy, supplementing with CoQ10 may offer considerable benefits.

The significance of CoQ10 in the body underscores the need to maintain adequate levels for health and longevity. Given its broad range of benefits and crucial roles in cellular health, CoQ10 can be a cornerstone of a holistic approach to wellness, particularly in a modern world where chronic stress, poor diet, and aging take a toll on mitochondrial function and cellular resilience.

Given this book's stance on health and nutrition, emphasizing a carnivore-based diet and fasting, it's likely that most essential nutrients can be obtained through nutrient-dense animal foods. However, even with this approach, there can be times when supplements can help bridge potential gaps or optimize health. Here are some beneficial supplements and minerals to consider, especially if certain nutrient sources are limited or if health goals require additional support:

D-ribose

D-ribose is a naturally occurring sugar molecule that plays a critical role in the production of adenosine triphosphate (ATP), the primary energy carrier in cells. Found in every cell of the human body, D-ribose is essential for cellular energy metabolism and the synthesis of nucleotides. While the body can produce D-ribose on its own, supplementation can be particularly beneficial for individuals with conditions that impair energy production or lead to chronic fatigue, such as fibromyalgia, chronic fatigue syndrome, and cardiovascular diseases.

One of the most significant benefits of D-ribose supplementation lies in its ability to support heart health. Research suggests that D-ribose can enhance the heart's energy reserve, especially following conditions that cause ischemia or insufficient blood flow, which can deplete ATP levels in heart muscle cells. By replenishing ATP levels more efficiently, D-ribose aids in the recovery of myocardial function and reduces fatigue, making it a useful supplement for individuals with heart disease, heart failure, or angina. Some studies indicate that D-ribose can improve heart muscle function and contribute to better overall cardiac performance.

Athletes and individuals who engage in high-intensity physical activities may also benefit from D-ribose supplementation due to its potential to support faster recovery and reduce post-exercise fatigue. By accelerating the restoration of ATP levels, D-ribose helps muscles recover more efficiently, minimizing soreness and improving endurance. This can be especially beneficial in scenarios where energy demand exceeds the body's natural ATP production rate.

In addition to its applications for heart health and athletic recovery, D-ribose may have a role in reducing oxidative stress and supporting general energy production within the body. By improving ATP synthesis, it ensures that cells maintain their energy balance, which is particularly important for individuals with metabolic or mitochondrial dysfunction. Overall, D-ribose supplementation provides a targeted approach to supporting cellular energy metabolism, enhancing recovery, and promoting overall cardiovascular health.

Vitamin D

Vitamin D is a fat-soluble vitamin essential for maintaining overall health and plays a critical role in various bodily functions. One of its primary functions is to facilitate the absorption of calcium and phosphorus in the intestines, which helps in the development and maintenance of strong bones and teeth. Adequate levels of vitamin D are essential to prevent rickets in children, a condition characterized by weakened and deformed bones, and osteomalacia in adults, which results in bone pain and muscle weakness. Additionally, sufficient vitamin D intake can reduce the risk of osteoporosis and fractures, particularly in older adults.

Beyond its role in bone health, vitamin D has significant benefits for the immune system. It modulates both the innate and adaptive immune responses, helping the body defend against infections. Research has shown that individuals with adequate vitamin D levels are less likely to suffer from acute respiratory infections and may have a lower risk of developing autoimmune diseases such as multiple sclerosis and rheumatoid arthritis. Vitamin D's immune-regulating properties are especially relevant in the context of seasonal illnesses and overall immune health, as it helps reduce inflammation and enhance the pathogen-fighting effects of monocytes and macrophages.

Emerging evidence also links vitamin D to heart health and chronic disease prevention. Vitamin D receptors are found in many tissues throughout the body, including the heart and blood vessels, suggesting its role in cardiovascular function. Studies have indicated that low levels of vitamin D may be associated with an increased risk of hypertension, heart disease, and stroke. Additionally, there is ongoing research exploring the potential connection between vitamin D and reduced risks of developing certain types of cancers, type 2 diabetes, and neurodegenerative diseases. The anti-inflammatory properties of vitamin D contribute to its potential in supporting overall metabolic health, which can positively influence conditions such as obesity and insulin resistance.

In summary, vitamin D is crucial not just for bone health but also for immune support, heart health, and chronic disease prevention. Given that many people are at risk of deficiency due to limited sun exposure, especially in higher latitudes or during the winter months, supplementation or dietary intake through fortified foods and fatty fish may be necessary to maintain optimal vitamin D levels. Ensuring adequate vitamin D levels can have a far-reaching impact on both physical and metabolic health, underscoring its importance in a comprehensive health and wellness strategy.

L-Carnitine

L-carnitine is a naturally occurring amino acid derivative that plays a critical role in energy production and metabolic health. Found primarily in animal-based foods like red meat, fish, and dairy, L-carnitine is also produced by the body, but often not in large enough quantities to meet all its demands, especially in certain individuals or under specific health conditions. It's particularly valued for its role in transporting fatty acids into the mitochondria, the energy-producing centers of cells, where they can be burned for energy. This process makes L-carnitine especially beneficial for heart health, exercise performance, and overall energy levels.

Energy Production and Fat Metabolism: L-carnitine is essential for transporting long-chain fatty acids into the mitochondria, where they're oxidized to produce ATP, the primary energy currency of the body. This process not only provides energy but also helps reduce fat stores, making L-carnitine beneficial for individuals seeking improved body composition and metabolic health. For people following a high-fat or ketogenic diet, L-carnitine supports the body's fat-burning processes, making it an ideal supplement for those looking to maximize the metabolic benefits of these diets.

Heart Health: The heart is a highly energy-demanding muscle that relies heavily on fatty acids for fuel. L-carnitine's role in transporting fats into the heart's mitochondria makes it particularly supportive of cardiovascular health. Studies have shown that L-carnitine can improve heart function, especially in individuals with heart conditions, by enhancing energy production and reducing oxidative stress in heart cells. It has been linked to improvements in heart muscle function and reduced symptoms in people with conditions like angina and heart failure.

Exercise Performance and Recovery: Athletes and active individuals benefit from L-carnitine due to its ability to support energy production and enhance endurance. By optimizing fatty acid transport and utilization, L-carnitine helps reduce glycogen depletion, allowing athletes to exercise for longer periods. It also reduces the buildup of lactic acid, which can delay the onset of fatigue and improve recovery. Additionally, L-carnitine has been found to reduce muscle soreness and oxidative stress following intense exercise, making it a useful tool for both performance and recovery.

Cognitive Health and Brain Function: L-carnitine, particularly its acetylated form (acetyl-L-carnitine or ALCAR), crosses the blood-brain barrier and supports cognitive health by providing the brain with energy and supporting neurotransmitter function. ALCAR has been studied for its potential benefits in enhancing memory, focus, and mental clarity, especially in older adults. It also acts as an antioxidant in the brain, protecting neurons from oxidative damage and potentially slowing cognitive decline.

Natural Sources and Supplementation: While L-carnitine is present in red meat, fish, and poultry, those who follow a plant-based diet, have certain medical conditions, or are older may have lower levels of L-carnitine and benefit from supplementation. L-carnitine supplements come in several forms, including L-carnitine tartrate (for physical performance) and acetyl-L-carnitine (for cognitive health), allowing individuals to choose based on their specific needs.

Magnesium

Magnesium is an essential mineral that plays a critical role in over 300 biochemical reactions within the body, making it indispensable for optimal health. One of its most well-known benefits is its support for muscle and nerve function. Magnesium helps regulate muscle contractions and prevents cramping and spasms by counteracting calcium, which promotes muscle contractions. This balance is crucial for athletes, individuals who engage in regular physical activity, and those who suffer from muscle cramps. Additionally, magnesium is involved in the transmission of nerve impulses, ensuring the proper functioning of the nervous system.

Beyond muscle and nerve health, magnesium is integral to heart health and maintaining a stable cardiovascular system. It acts as a natural calcium channel blocker, helping relax blood vessels and maintain healthy blood pressure levels. Adequate magnesium intake has been linked to a reduced risk of hypertension, arrhythmias, and other cardiovascular conditions. Its anti-inflammatory properties can also help decrease systemic inflammation, which plays a significant role in the development of heart disease. By supporting the electrical conduction system of the heart, magnesium helps regulate a steady heartbeat and reduce the risk of arrhythmias.

Magnesium is also essential for bone health and energy production. It works in synergy with calcium and vitamin D to support bone density and prevent osteoporosis. Magnesium is a component of the bone matrix and assists in the conversion of vitamin D into its active form, which in turn helps regulate calcium absorption. Furthermore, magnesium plays a key role in ATP (adenosine triphosphate) production, which is the energy currency of cells. This function makes magnesium vital for combating fatigue and maintaining overall energy levels. Deficiencies in magnesium can result in chronic fatigue, muscle weakness, and impaired exercise performance.

Emerging research highlights the connection between magnesium and mental health, emphasizing its potential role in reducing symptoms of depression and anxiety. Magnesium modulates neurotransmitters that are associated with mood regulation, including serotonin. Low levels of magnesium have been associated with an increased risk of depression and other mood disorders, as magnesium deficiency can lead to disrupted nerve function and heightened stress response. Its calming effect on the nervous system can also promote better sleep quality, as it helps regulate the production of melatonin, the hormone that controls the sleep-wake cycle.

Overall, magnesium's benefits are extensive, ranging from supporting muscular and cardiovascular health to boosting bone density, energy production, and mental well-being. Given that many people do not meet the recommended dietary intake of magnesium due to factors such as poor diet and soil depletion, supplementation or magnesium-rich foods—such as leafy green vegetables, nuts, seeds, and whole grains—may be necessary to ensure adequate levels.

Electrolytes (Sodium, Potassium, and Calcium)

Electrolytes are minerals that carry an electric charge and are vital for many essential processes in the body. These include sodium, potassium, calcium, magnesium, chloride, phosphate, and bicarbonate. Electrolytes help regulate fluid balance, nerve function, muscle contractions, and maintain the body's pH level. Each electrolyte has a specific role, and an appropriate balance is crucial for optimal health and bodily function.

Sodium is one of the primary electrolytes that helps maintain fluid balance in the body. It plays a key role in transmitting nerve impulses and enabling muscle contractions. While it is essential for many bodily functions, too much sodium can lead to high blood pressure and fluid retention. Sodium loss can occur during intense exercise or through excessive sweating, which is why replenishing sodium is crucial, especially for athletes and individuals engaged in heavy physical activity.

Potassium works closely with sodium to regulate fluid balance and maintain proper muscle and nerve function. It is particularly important for heart health, as it helps regulate heartbeats and prevents conditions such as arrhythmias. Potassium also plays a role in controlling blood pressure by counteracting the effects of sodium. Low potassium levels, or hypokalemia, can lead to muscle weakness, cramping, and even irregular heart rhythms.

Calcium is widely recognized for its essential role in building and maintaining strong bones and teeth, but it also plays a critical role in other bodily functions, including blood clotting, muscle contractions, and nerve signaling. Together with magnesium, calcium helps control muscle function, allowing muscles to contract and relax smoothly. When calcium levels are imbalanced, individuals may experience muscle twitching or spasms, and, over time, bone health can also be affected.

However, recent insights emphasize that if you choose to supplement with calcium, pairing it with vitamin K2 is crucial to prevent calcium deposits from accumulating in soft tissues rather than in bones where it is needed. Vitamin K2 directs calcium to bones and teeth while helping prevent calcification in the arteries and other soft tissues. This combination helps to balance calcium's benefits, ensuring it supports skeletal health without posing a risk to cardiovascular health.

Electrolytes work synergistically to maintain the body's fluid balance. Proper hydration is not just about drinking water; it involves maintaining a balance of water and electrolytes. This balance ensures that cells function properly and prevents dehydration or overhydration, both of which can have severe health implications. An imbalance of electrolytes can lead to symptoms such as fatigue, dizziness, irregular heartbeat, muscle weakness, and confusion.

For those engaging in high-intensity workouts or prolonged physical activities, electrolyte supplements or sports drinks can help replenish lost electrolytes and maintain performance. Similarly, people who experience frequent dehydration, whether due to hot climates, illness, or certain medications, can benefit from paying closer attention to their electrolyte intake. Foods such as bananas, oranges, spinach, yogurt, and avocados are natural sources rich in key electrolytes like potassium and magnesium.

In summary, electrolytes play a fundamental role in the body's day-to-day functions, from maintaining fluid balance and supporting nerve and muscle activity to aiding energy production and bone health. Ensuring that the body receives an adequate and balanced intake of electrolytes is crucial for maintaining overall health and preventing potential complications associated with electrolyte imbalances.

Vitamin K2

Vitamin K2, a lesser-known form of vitamin K, is crucial for a variety of bodily functions, particularly those involving bone health and cardiovascular health. Unlike vitamin K1, which is mainly involved in blood clotting and is found in green leafy vegetables, vitamin K2 is found in animal-based and fermented foods, such as natto (fermented soybeans), certain cheeses, egg yolks, and organ meats. It exists in several subtypes, the most notable being MK-4 and MK-7, which vary in their absorption and half-life in the body.

One of the most significant benefits of vitamin K2 is its role in calcium metabolism. It acts as a cofactor for the proteins osteocalcin and matrix Gla-protein (MGP). Osteocalcin is essential for binding calcium to the bone matrix, which enhances bone density and reduces the risk of fractures. Without sufficient vitamin K2, osteocalcin remains inactive and unable to bind calcium effectively, leading to weaker bones. This is particularly important for individuals at risk of osteoporosis or those looking to improve bone health as they age.

In addition to its impact on bone health, vitamin K2 plays a critical role in cardiovascular health by preventing the calcification of arteries. Calcification occurs when calcium deposits build up in the arteries, leading to hardening and an increased risk of cardiovascular diseases such as atherosclerosis. Vitamin K2 activates matrix Gla-protein (MGP), which helps prevent calcium from being deposited in the arterial walls and instead directs it to the bones where it belongs. Research has shown that higher intakes of vitamin K2 are associated with a reduced risk of coronary artery disease, emphasizing its importance for heart health.

Another compelling aspect of vitamin K2 is its synergy with vitamin D. Vitamin D enhances the absorption of calcium in the intestines, but without sufficient vitamin K2, this calcium may end up in soft tissues rather than being directed to the bones. The combined action of vitamin D and K2 ensures that calcium is optimally utilized in the body, supporting both bone and cardiovascular health. This synergy is why some health experts recommend supplementing with both vitamins to achieve the best outcomes for bone strength and heart protection.

Emerging evidence also suggests that vitamin K2 may have broader health benefits, such as supporting dental health, improving insulin sensitivity, and potentially aiding in the prevention of certain types of cancer. Its role in modulating calcium metabolism may contribute to better dental health by aiding in the remineralization of teeth and preventing tooth decay. There is also preliminary research indicating that vitamin K2 could play a role in metabolic health by supporting insulin function, which can be beneficial for those managing conditions like type 2 diabetes.

Given the limited dietary sources of vitamin K2 and its significant benefits for bone and cardiovascular health, many people may benefit from supplementation, particularly those who do not regularly consume fermented foods or animal products. Ensuring adequate intake of vitamin K2 can be an essential part of a comprehensive approach to maintaining strong bones and a healthy cardiovascular system.

Zinc and Copper

Importance: Zinc supports immune function, wound healing, and protein synthesis, while copper is essential for energy production and iron metabolism. Both minerals need to be balanced.

Sources: Red meat and shellfish are good sources, but if intake is limited, a supplement can help, especially since zinc and copper work together in immune and metabolic functions.

Iodine

Iodine is an essential trace mineral that plays a vital role in the production of thyroid hormones, which regulate various bodily functions, including metabolism, growth, and development. The thyroid gland uses iodine to produce two main hormones: thyroxine (T4) and triiodothyronine (T3). These hormones are critical for energy production, maintaining body temperature, and supporting the proper function of organs and tissues. Without sufficient iodine, the thyroid cannot synthesize adequate amounts of these hormones, leading to potential imbalances and disorders.

One of the most well-known benefits of iodine is its role in preventing thyroid-related issues such as goiter and hypothyroidism. A goiter, an enlarged thyroid gland, occurs when the gland works overtime to compensate for insufficient iodine. Hypothyroidism, characterized by fatigue, weight gain, and cold intolerance, can develop when the thyroid is unable to produce enough hormones due to iodine deficiency. Ensuring adequate iodine intake can help prevent these conditions and maintain healthy thyroid function, which is essential for metabolic health.

Iodine is also crucial for brain development, especially during pregnancy and early childhood. A deficiency in iodine during pregnancy can lead to serious consequences, including impaired brain development and cognitive function in the fetus, resulting in conditions like cretinism, which is associated with severe physical and mental developmental delays. Even mild iodine deficiency during critical periods of development can lead to lower IQ levels in children. For this reason, pregnant and breastfeeding women are encouraged to maintain sufficient iodine levels to support their own health and that of their baby.

Beyond thyroid health, iodine possesses antimicrobial properties and is sometimes used topically as an antiseptic to clean wounds and prevent infections. In the context of public health, iodine's role in preventing iodine deficiency disorders (IDD) has been widely recognized, leading to the fortification of table salt with iodine in many countries. This measure has greatly reduced the prevalence of IDD worldwide and remains an important strategy for ensuring population-level intake.

Dietary sources of iodine include seafood, seaweed, dairy products, eggs, and iodized salt. Seaweed, such as kelp and nori, is particularly rich in iodine and can provide more than the recommended daily amount. However, for individuals who do not consume enough iodine-rich foods, supplementation may be necessary to avoid deficiency. The recommended daily intake of iodine varies by age and life stage, with adults generally needing about 150 micrograms per day, while pregnant and breastfeeding women require higher amounts.

While maintaining adequate iodine levels is crucial, it's also important not to consume excessive amounts, as too much iodine can lead to thyroid dysfunction. Excessive iodine intake may cause hyperthyroidism, characterized by an overactive thyroid, or can exacerbate autoimmune thyroid conditions like Hashimoto's disease. Therefore, it's essential to strike the right balance, either through a diet rich in iodine-containing foods or careful supplementation if needed.

Iodine is essential for healthy thyroid function, metabolic regulation, and proper brain development. It plays a preventive role against thyroid disorders, supports cognitive health, and is crucial during pregnancy for fetal development. With its limited but vital role in the diet, ensuring sufficient iodine intake through balanced nutrition or appropriate supplementation can significantly impact overall health and well-being.

Collagen or Gelatin

Collagen and gelatin are proteins that play a key role in supporting various aspects of health, particularly related to skin, joint, and gut

237

health. Both are derived from the same source—animal connective tissue—and have similar amino acid profiles, but they differ in their structure and how they are used in the body. Understanding their benefits can help in making informed dietary and supplementation choices.

Collagen is the most abundant protein in the human body, found in skin, bones, muscles, tendons, and ligaments. It acts as the structural framework that helps keep tissues firm and resilient. As we age, natural collagen production decreases, leading to common signs of aging such as wrinkles, joint discomfort, and decreased skin elasticity. Supplementing with collagen can help counteract these effects by providing the body with the amino acids it needs to support and rebuild its natural collagen supply. Collagen peptides, which are hydrolyzed for better absorption, are particularly popular as they dissolve easily in liquids and are highly bioavailable.

The benefits of collagen supplementation extend beyond skin health. Studies have shown that regular collagen intake can improve joint health by reducing pain and improving mobility, especially in those with joint conditions like osteoarthritis. Collagen helps support cartilage repair and maintenance, which is essential for joint function. It also contributes to muscle recovery and maintenance, as it is rich in glycine and proline—amino acids that play a role in muscle repair and energy production.

Gelatin is a form of cooked collagen and shares many of its health benefits, but with some unique properties of its own. When collagen is heated, it breaks down into gelatin, which can then be used as a gelling agent in foods like jellies, soups, and desserts. Gelatin is also a rich source of the amino acids glycine and proline, which contribute to its anti-inflammatory properties and support for gut health. Glycine, in particular, has been studied for its potential to improve digestive health by enhancing the integrity of the gut lining and reducing intestinal permeability (often referred to as "leaky gut").

Both collagen and gelatin are known to support skin health by promoting hydration, elasticity, and wound healing. Collagen has been found to stimulate the body's natural production of collagen, which helps maintain a youthful appearance and reduces the formation of wrinkles. Gelatin, due to its ability to absorb water, may help keep the skin plump and hydrated.

In addition to joint, skin, and gut benefits, collagen and gelatin have roles in overall body repair and metabolic health. Collagen's high glycine content supports metabolic processes, contributes to better sleep, and aids in the body's natural detoxification pathways. Gelatin, with its gel-forming capabilities, can promote satiety and support digestive function, making it useful for those looking to manage weight or improve digestion.

Dietary sources of collagen and gelatin include bone broth, slow-cooked meats with connective tissue, and certain animal parts like chicken skin and fish skin. For those looking for a convenient option, collagen supplements in the form of collagen peptides or powders are widely available. Gelatin can also be found in powdered form, which can be used in cooking to create gelatin-rich dishes.

Overall, collagen and gelatin are valuable proteins that contribute to various health benefits, from skin rejuvenation and joint support to gut health and muscle recovery. Including these proteins in the diet, whether through natural food sources or supplements, can help maintain the structure and function of connective tissues, support overall well-being, and promote a healthier aging process.

Selenium

Selenium is an essential trace mineral that plays a critical role in numerous bodily processes, primarily due to its powerful antioxidant properties. It is an integral component of selenoproteins, which are involved in DNA synthesis, thyroid hormone metabolism, immune function, and protection against oxidative damage. Although only required in small amounts, selenium is vital for maintaining overall health and preventing chronic diseases.

One of selenium's most important roles is its function as an antioxidant. Selenium helps combat oxidative stress by supporting the production of glutathione peroxidase, a key antioxidant enzyme that protects cells from damage caused by free radicals. By neutralizing these unstable molecules, selenium helps prevent cellular damage that can lead to chronic inflammation and diseases such as cancer and cardiovascular conditions. Research has shown that adequate selenium intake is associated with a reduced risk of certain types of cancer, including prostate, lung, and colorectal cancers.

Selenium is also essential for proper thyroid function. The thyroid gland contains higher concentrations of selenium than any other organ in the body. Selenium contributes to the synthesis and metabolism of thyroid hormones by facilitating the conversion of thyroxine (T4) into its active form, triiodothyronine (T3). This process is crucial for maintaining a healthy metabolism and supporting energy production. Selenium deficiency can impair thyroid function, leading to hypothyroidism or an increased risk of developing autoimmune thyroid conditions such as Hashimoto's thyroiditis. Ensuring adequate selenium intake helps promote balanced thyroid function and overall metabolic health.

Immune system support is another significant benefit of selenium. This mineral aids in the modulation of the immune response, helping the body defend itself against infections. Studies have indicated that selenium supplementation can enhance immune function, particularly in individuals with compromised immune systems. For example, selenium has been shown to boost the activity of immune cells and support the body's ability to respond to viral infections, potentially reducing the severity and duration of illnesses.

Cardiovascular health is also impacted by selenium levels. Some research suggests that selenium helps reduce the risk of heart disease by preventing oxidative damage to blood vessel walls and lowering inflammation. Additionally, selenium's role in reducing oxidative stress contributes to the prevention of atherosclerosis, a condition in which plaque builds up in the arteries, potentially leading to heart attacks or strokes.

Dietary sources of selenium include Brazil nuts, seafood, organ meats, and whole grains. Brazil nuts are particularly rich in selenium, with just one or two nuts providing more than the recommended daily allowance. Other good sources include tuna, sardines, eggs, and sunflower seeds. However, the selenium content in plant-based foods can vary widely depending on the soil in which they are grown, as selenium levels in the soil influence the mineral content of crops.

It is important to balance selenium intake, as both deficiency and excessive intake can have adverse effects. Selenium deficiency is rare in developed countries but can lead to Keshan disease (a heart condition) and Kashin-Beck disease (a type of osteoarthropathy) in areas with selenium-poor soil. Conversely, selenium toxicity, known as selenosis, can occur if intake significantly exceeds recommended levels and can cause symptoms such as hair loss, nail brittleness, and, in severe cases, neurological damage. The recommended dietary allowance (RDA) for adults is 55 micrograms per day, with the upper intake limit set at 400 micrograms per day to avoid potential toxicity.

In summary, selenium is a crucial mineral that supports antioxidant defense, thyroid health, immune function, and cardiovascular protection. Ensuring adequate selenium intake through diet or, if necessary, supplementation can promote overall health and help prevent chronic disease. However, moderation is key to reaping its benefits while avoiding the risks associated with excessive consumption.

Final Note

While a carnivore or low-carb, nutrient-dense diet provides most necessary nutrients, these supplements offer targeted support when specific needs arise. Balancing nutrients—especially fat-soluble vitamins and electrolytes—is key to thriving on any diet, and supplementation may optimize health when particular nutrients are difficult to obtain through food alone.

The Science of Nutrition: An Introduction

Nutrition is more than simply consuming food; it is a complex biochemical process that impacts every system in the human body. At the core of the science of nutrition is an understanding of how nutrients are processed, how they influence health, and how deficiencies or excesses contribute to disease. The fields of biochemistry, pathophysiology, and endocrinology each provide essential insights into how food and nutrients affect our bodies at the molecular level. Together, they reveal the intricate processes that dictate energy production, cellular repair, hormonal balance, and more.

Biochemistry of Nutrition: The Foundation of Health

Biochemistry is the study of chemical processes within living organisms, and it forms the foundation of nutritional science. Biochemistry serves as the bridge between nutrition and health, allowing us to understand how the foods we consume influence the body's cellular and systemic functions. Every nutrient we eat undergoes a series of chemical transformations, beginning with digestion and absorption in the digestive tract. From there, these nutrients are transported through the bloodstream to cells, where they participate in biochemical pathways that power various bodily processes. These pathways are responsible for generating ATP (adenosine triphosphate), the primary energy currency of the cell, and for synthesizing proteins, DNA, and other vital molecules. In short, biochemistry reveals the fundamental mechanisms by which nutrients fuel cellular activities, support growth, repair tissues, and maintain metabolic balance.

Macronutrients—carbohydrates, proteins, and fats—serve as the body's main energy sources, each with unique biochemical roles. Carbohydrates are primarily broken down into glucose, which enters cells and undergoes glycolysis, the citric acid cycle, and oxidative phosphorylation to generate ATP. Proteins are broken down into amino acids, which serve as building blocks for new proteins, enzymes, and hormones, and can also be used as an energy source when necessary. Fats, once broken down into fatty acids and glycerol, provide a highly efficient source of energy through beta-

242

oxidation and ketogenesis, particularly in low-carbohydrate or fasting states. Fats are also crucial for building cell membranes and producing signaling molecules like hormones. These macronutrients not only provide energy but also contribute structural components that support cellular integrity and functionality.

Micronutrients, vitamins and minerals, are equally essential in biochemistry, acting as co-factors and coenzymes in enzymatic reactions. For example, B vitamins are integral to energy metabolism as they enable enzymes to perform crucial steps in processes like glycolysis and the citric acid cycle. Vitamin C is necessary for collagen synthesis, while vitamin K plays a key role in blood clotting. Minerals like magnesium, calcium, and potassium are involved in nerve signaling, muscle contraction, and cellular communication. Though required in smaller amounts, these micronutrients are indispensable; without them, the body's biochemical pathways would fail, leading to deficiencies, compromised immune function, and decreased metabolic efficiency.

Biochemistry also highlights the intricate interplay between nutrients and hormones in regulating metabolism. For instance, insulin, a hormone produced by the pancreas, facilitates the uptake of glucose into cells for energy production and signals the liver to store excess glucose as glycogen. Hormones such as leptin and ghrelin regulate hunger and satiety, interacting with nutrient levels in the blood to control appetite. Nutrient status and biochemical signals also affect gene expression through processes like methylation, further underscoring the importance of nutrition in modulating health at a molecular level.

In essence, biochemistry allows us to understand the critical importance of a balanced diet. Proper intake of macronutrients and micronutrients fuels biochemical pathways that sustain energy, repair tissues, support immunity, and regulate metabolism. Nutritional biochemistry provides a scientific foundation for dietary recommendations and helps clarify how specific nutrients and dietary patterns impact overall health, from cellular function to long-term disease prevention. This understanding equips us to make informed food choices that support metabolic health and optimize the body's natural resilience.

The Role of Macronutrients in Biochemistry

Macronutrients serve as the primary source of energy and building blocks for cellular structures. Each macronutrient has a unique biochemical role and undergoes specific metabolic pathways.

Carbohydrates: The Body's Quick Energy Source

Carbohydrates are one of the most readily accessible sources of energy, especially for the brain and muscles. When we consume carbohydrates, they are broken down into simple sugars, primarily glucose, through a process called digestion. Once absorbed into the bloodstream, glucose travels to cells and tissues, where it enters a metabolic pathway called glycolysis.

Glycolysis: Glycolysis occurs in the cytoplasm of cells, breaking down one molecule of glucose into two molecules of pyruvate while generating a net gain of two ATP (adenosine triphosphate) molecules, which are the cell's energy currency. Glycolysis does not require oxygen, making it an anaerobic process suitable for short bursts of energy.

Krebs Cycle and Electron Transport Chain: If oxygen is available, pyruvate from glycolysis is further oxidized in the mitochondria through the Krebs cycle (also known as the citric acid cycle). This cycle produces additional ATP, NADH, and $FADH_2$, which are used in the electron transport chain to generate more ATP through oxidative phosphorylation. This aerobic process provides a more sustained energy release than glycolysis alone.

Glycogen Storage: Excess glucose that is not immediately needed for energy is stored as glycogen in the liver and muscles. During fasting or physical activity, glycogen can be broken down into glucose for energy. When glycogen stores are full, excess carbohydrates are converted into fat for long-term storage.

Proteins: Building Blocks and Functional Molecules

Proteins are composed of amino acids, which serve as building blocks for various structural and functional components in the body. Unlike carbohydrates, proteins are not primarily used as an energy source; instead, they play essential roles in muscle repair, enzyme function, immune response, and more.

Amino Acid Metabolism: When dietary proteins are consumed, they are broken down into individual amino acids, which are absorbed into the bloodstream. Amino acids can be used to synthesize new proteins, repair tissues, or serve as precursors for neurotransmitters and hormones.

Gluconeogenesis: In times of prolonged fasting or low carbohydrate intake, the body can produce glucose from non-carbohydrate sources, such as certain amino acids, through a process called gluconeogenesis. This process occurs mainly in the liver and provides glucose to tissues that rely on it, such as the brain and red blood cells.

Nitrogen Balance: Proteins contain nitrogen, which differentiates them from carbohydrates and fats. The body maintains a nitrogen balance by excreting excess nitrogen through urea. This balance is crucial for optimal health, as both excess and deficiency of nitrogen can disrupt cellular function.

Fats: Energy Storage and Cellular Structure

Fats, or lipids, are dense sources of energy, providing 9 kcal per gram compared to 4 kcal per gram for carbohydrates and proteins. Fats are also essential for building cell membranes, producing hormones, and absorbing fat-soluble vitamins (A, D, E, and K).

1. **Fatty Acid Oxidation**: Dietary fats are broken down into fatty acids and glycerol. Fatty acids undergo beta-oxidation in the mitochondria, where they are broken down into acetyl-CoA, which enters the Krebs cycle to produce ATP. This process is highly efficient and provides a sustained energy supply during fasting or low-intensity activities.
2. **Ketogenesis**: In the absence of carbohydrates, such as during fasting or a ketogenic diet, the liver converts fatty acids into ketone bodies (acetone, acetoacetate, and beta-hydroxybutyrate). Ketones can serve as an alternative fuel source, particularly for the brain, which normally relies on glucose.
3. **Cholesterol and Hormone Synthesis**: Fats play a role in the synthesis of cholesterol, which is a precursor to steroid hormones like cortisol, estrogen, and testosterone. Cholesterol is also essential for maintaining cell membrane integrity and is involved in the production of bile acids that aid in fat digestion.

The Role of Micronutrients: Catalysts of Biochemical Reactions

Micronutrients, including vitamins and minerals, are essential for various biochemical processes but are required in smaller quantities. Unlike macronutrients, micronutrients do not provide energy directly, but they act as co-factors or coenzymes in metabolic reactions, enabling enzymes to function optimally.

Vitamins: Essential Organic Compounds

Here's a closer look at the biochemical processes involving each vitamin group and their essential roles in the body:

1. B Vitamins: Essential Coenzymes in Energy Metabolism

The B-complex vitamins are coenzymes that assist enzymes in catalyzing metabolic reactions essential for energy production, DNA synthesis, and more.

Vitamin B1 (Thiamine): As part of the coenzyme thiamine pyrophosphate (TPP), vitamin B1 is crucial in the decarboxylation of alpha-keto acids, such as pyruvate, during glycolysis and the citric acid cycle. It helps convert pyruvate to acetyl-CoA, enabling glucose metabolism and energy production.

Vitamin B2 (Riboflavin): Riboflavin is a precursor for FAD (flavin adenine dinucleotide) and FMN (flavin mononucleotide), coenzymes involved in redox reactions in cellular respiration. FAD acts as an electron carrier in the citric acid cycle and the electron transport chain, helping produce ATP.

Vitamin B3 (Niacin): Vitamin B3 is converted into NAD^+ (nicotinamide adenine dinucleotide) and $NADP^+$ (nicotinamide adenine dinucleotide phosphate), essential electron carriers in redox reactions. NAD^+ accepts electrons during glycolysis and the citric acid cycle, passing them to the electron transport chain to generate ATP. $NADP^+$, in turn, is vital for biosynthetic pathways, including fatty acid and cholesterol synthesis.

Vitamin B5 (Pantothenic Acid): Pantothenic acid is a component of coenzyme A (CoA), which is necessary for the synthesis and oxidation of fatty acids and the production of acetyl-CoA, which feeds into the citric acid cycle.

Vitamin B6 (Pyridoxine): The active form of vitamin B6, pyridoxal phosphate (PLP), serves as a coenzyme in amino acid metabolism, facilitating transamination reactions that produce non-essential amino acids and neurotransmitters like serotonin and dopamine.

Vitamin B7 (Biotin): Biotin is a coenzyme for carboxylation reactions, such as in the conversion of pyruvate to oxaloacetate in gluconeogenesis and fatty acid synthesis. Biotin's role in carboxylase enzymes is crucial for synthesizing glucose and fatty acids.

Vitamin B9 (Folate): Folate is converted to tetrahydrofolate (THF), a coenzyme involved in transferring single carbon units in DNA and RNA synthesis, as well as amino acid metabolism. This process is crucial for cell division and proper development.

Vitamin B12 (Cobalamin): Vitamin B12 functions in two main biochemical reactions. It acts as a coenzyme for methionine synthase in the synthesis of methionine and tetrahydrofolate, essential for DNA synthesis. It also plays a role in the conversion of methylmalonyl-CoA to succinyl-CoA in the citric acid cycle, aiding in energy production.

2. Vitamin C: Antioxidant and Collagen Synthesis

Antioxidant Role: Vitamin C (ascorbic acid) is a potent electron donor and neutralizes reactive oxygen species (ROS) by donating electrons. This antioxidant action protects cellular structures, proteins, and DNA from oxidative damage by ROS and free radicals.

Collagen Synthesis: Vitamin C acts as a cofactor for prolyl hydroxylase and lysyl hydroxylase, enzymes involved in hydroxylating proline and lysine residues in collagen precursors. These hydroxylations stabilize the collagen triple helix, supporting the structural integrity of connective tissues, skin, and blood vessels.

Immune Function: Vitamin C enhances immune cell activity, particularly that of white blood cells (leukocytes), by increasing chemotaxis, phagocytosis, and the generation of reactive oxygen species to combat pathogens.

3. Fat-Soluble Vitamins (A, D, E, and K)

Each fat-soluble vitamin plays a unique role in biochemical pathways critical for vision, bone health, antioxidant defense, and blood clotting.

Vitamin A: The active form of vitamin A, retinol, is converted into retinal and retinoic acid. Retinal combines with the protein opsin to form rhodopsin in the retina, a molecule essential for low-light vision. Retinoic acid acts as a signaling molecule, influencing gene expression and cellular differentiation, particularly in skin and immune cells.

Vitamin D: In its active form, calcitriol (1,25-dihydroxyvitamin D), vitamin D binds to the vitamin D receptor (VDR) in the nucleus, acting as a transcription factor that regulates calcium and phosphate homeostasis. It promotes the synthesis of calcium-binding proteins in the intestines, enhancing calcium and phosphate absorption for bone mineralization and remodeling.

Vitamin E: Vitamin E (alpha-tocopherol) is a lipid-soluble antioxidant that integrates into cell membranes, where it protects polyunsaturated fatty acids from lipid peroxidation. By donating electrons to neutralize lipid radicals, vitamin E prevents oxidative damage to cell membranes, supporting cellular stability and reducing oxidative stress.

Vitamin K: Vitamin K serves as a cofactor for gamma-glutamyl carboxylase, an enzyme that catalyzes the carboxylation of glutamic acid residues on specific proteins. This process is critical for activating proteins involved in blood coagulation (e.g., prothrombin) and bone metabolism (e.g., osteocalcin), enabling calcium binding for proper blood clotting and bone formation.

Minerals: Inorganic Elements with Diverse Functions

Minerals are inorganic elements required for various structural and regulatory roles in the body.

1. **Calcium and Phosphorus**: Both are essential for bone health and also play roles in cellular signaling and muscle contraction.
2. **Iron**: A critical component of hemoglobin, iron allows red blood cells to transport oxygen. Iron deficiency can lead to anemia, affecting oxygen delivery to tissues.

3. **Electrolytes (Sodium, Potassium, and Magnesium)**: These minerals help maintain fluid balance, nerve transmission, and muscle contraction. Potassium, for example, is crucial for heart health, while magnesium is involved in over 300 enzymatic reactions, including energy production.

Key Biochemical Pathways in Nutrition

Nutritional biochemistry encompasses several essential pathways that dictate how nutrients are metabolized, processed, and utilized by the body to maintain health. Each of these pathways has a specific function in energy production, biosynthesis, and the regulation of metabolic balance, enabling the body to respond dynamically to various physiological needs.

Glycolysis and the Citric Acid Cycle: Glycolysis is the pathway that breaks down glucose, the primary carbohydrate in our diet, into pyruvate, producing ATP and NADH as energy sources. Pyruvate then enters the citric acid cycle (also known as the Krebs or TCA cycle) in the mitochondria, where it undergoes further oxidation. This cycle produces additional NADH and FADH$_2$, which carry electrons to the electron transport chain, generating ATP through oxidative phosphorylation. Together, glycolysis and the citric acid cycle form the cornerstone of cellular respiration and are pivotal in converting glucose into usable energy.

Beta-Oxidation and Ketogenesis: Fatty acids, derived from dietary fats, are broken down through a process called beta-oxidation. In the mitochondria, fatty acids are sequentially oxidized, producing acetyl-CoA, NADH, and FADH$_2$, which feed into the citric acid cycle and electron transport chain to produce ATP. During periods of low carbohydrate intake or fasting, acetyl-CoA is also converted into ketone bodies in the liver, a process known as ketogenesis. These ketone bodies, such as beta-hydroxybutyrate, provide an alternative fuel source for the brain and muscles, underscoring the body's metabolic flexibility.

Protein Catabolism and Amino Acid Metabolism: Proteins are broken down into amino acids, which serve as building blocks for new proteins, enzymes, and hormones, and participate in a range of biochemical processes. Some amino acids are glucogenic, meaning they can be converted into glucose through gluconeogenesis, while others are ketogenic, producing ketone bodies for energy. The urea cycle, another critical pathway, processes excess nitrogen from amino acid breakdown into urea for safe excretion, maintaining nitrogen balance in the body.

Lipid and Cholesterol Synthesis: Beyond serving as an energy source, fats are crucial for building cell membranes and synthesizing cholesterol, which is essential for hormone production and cell structure. Lipogenesis is the process of converting excess carbohydrates into fatty acids, which are then stored as triglycerides in adipose tissue. The liver also synthesizes cholesterol, which is used to produce steroid hormones, vitamin D, and bile acids necessary for fat digestion. Proper regulation of lipid and cholesterol synthesis is essential for metabolic health.

Pentose Phosphate Pathway (PPP): This pathway operates alongside glycolysis, breaking down glucose to produce NADPH and ribose-5-phosphate. NADPH is a reducing agent used in biosynthetic reactions, such as fatty acid and cholesterol synthesis, and in maintaining antioxidant defenses. Ribose-5-phosphate, meanwhile, is a precursor for nucleotide and DNA/RNA synthesis, making the PPP crucial for cellular repair, growth, and immune function.

Gluconeogenesis: This process occurs primarily in the liver and allows the body to produce glucose from non-carbohydrate sources, such as lactate, glycerol, and amino acids. Gluconeogenesis is essential during fasting, prolonged exercise, or carbohydrate-restricted diets, providing a steady glucose supply for tissues that rely on glucose, such as the brain and red blood cells.

Each of these pathways contributes to a dynamic and complex metabolic network that ensures the body can adapt to different energy sources and environmental conditions. Nutritional biochemistry helps us understand how these pathways interact, reinforcing the importance of balanced nutrition to support these critical functions and maintain optimal health.

Metabolic Flexibility and Nutritional Balance

The body's ability to switch between fuel sources—glucose and fatty acids—is known as metabolic flexibility, an important indicator of metabolic health. A well-balanced diet that includes a variety of macronutrients and micronutrients supports metabolic flexibility, allowing the body to efficiently use glucose during periods of high energy demand and shift to fat oxidation during fasting or low-intensity activity.

Metabolic flexibility is the body's remarkable ability to switch seamlessly between fuel sources—primarily glucose and fat—and it is essential for optimal health and longevity. In an age dominated by high-carbohydrate diets, many people's metabolisms have become rigid, relying almost exclusively on glucose. This inflexibility can lead to energy crashes, insulin resistance, and a dependence on frequent meals to sustain energy. Achieving metabolic flexibility, however, enables the body to tap into its fat stores when glucose is low, utilizing ketones as an efficient, clean fuel source. Ketones, produced during fat metabolism, particularly in low-carb or fasting states, are an ideal energy source for the brain and muscles. Unlike glucose, which can cause rapid fluctuations in blood sugar, ketones provide a steady, long-lasting fuel that stabilizes energy levels and avoids the spikes and crashes associated with a high-glucose diet.

This reliance on ketones offers profound health benefits. For one, it improves insulin sensitivity by lowering the body's need for insulin to manage frequent glucose intake. This helps protect against insulin resistance, a major factor in conditions like obesity, diabetes, and metabolic syndrome. Moreover, ketones themselves have anti-inflammatory properties, generating fewer reactive oxygen species (ROS) compared to glucose metabolism. This reduction in oxidative stress benefits those with chronic inflammation and is advantageous for managing conditions like metabolic disorders and autoimmune diseases. The brain, too, thrives on ketones, as they efficiently cross the blood-brain barrier and provide a consistent fuel source. When the body is in ketosis, people often experience enhanced mental clarity, focus, and mood stability, as ketones prevent the mental fluctuations seen with glucose.

For physically active individuals, metabolic flexibility enables greater endurance and performance. Athletes with the ability to burn fat and ketones can tap into stored fat during prolonged activity, enhancing stamina and reducing the need to replenish glycogen stores continually. This adaptability supports sustained physical performance and faster recovery, as the body is less likely to hit an energy "wall." Additionally, metabolic flexibility supports weight management by utilizing fat stores, which naturally aids in fat loss and helps control appetite. By shifting to a metabolic state where ketones are efficiently utilized, the body can stabilize hunger and energy levels, making it easier to manage calorie intake and avoid overeating.

To cultivate metabolic flexibility in a high-carb world, practices like intermittent fasting, low-carb or ketogenic diets, and periodic prolonged fasting can help retrain the body to access fat stores. These approaches encourage the body to adapt to fat and ketone utilization, reducing reliance on glucose and unlocking the metabolic benefits of ketones. As more people embrace metabolic flexibility, they discover improved energy, enhanced cognitive function, reduced inflammation, and better metabolic health—demonstrating the body's natural potential when it can efficiently shift between fuel sources for optimal performance and resilience.

An imbalance in nutrient intake, such as excessive carbohydrate consumption or a lack of essential vitamins, can impair metabolic flexibility. For example, high sugar intake may lead to insulin resistance, reducing the body's ability to access stored fat. Similarly, vitamin deficiencies can disrupt enzyme function, affecting energy production and other vital processes.

The Power of Biochemistry in Nutrition

The biochemistry of nutrition reveals that food is not merely fuel but a complex interplay of molecules that impact nearly every function in the body. By understanding the roles of macronutrients and micronutrients, as well as the biochemical pathways they support, we can appreciate the profound effects of diet on health. Nutritional biochemistry underscores the importance of a balanced, nutrient-dense diet in supporting cellular function, energy production, and overall wellness.

The science of nutrition reminds us that the quality and balance of what we eat have far-reaching implications, from energy levels to disease prevention. In a world of processed foods and nutrient-deficient diets, returning to whole, unprocessed foods can help ensure we meet our biochemical needs, empowering us to live healthier, more resilient lives.

The Role of Endocrinology in Nutrition: How Hormones Regulate Metabolic Health

In the field of nutrition, endocrinology provides critical insights into how hormones regulate appetite, energy balance, nutrient storage, and metabolism. Hormones are powerful chemical messengers produced by endocrine glands, and they play an essential role in how the body processes food and maintains homeostasis. A healthy balance of hormones allows for effective digestion, absorption, and utilization of nutrients, while hormonal imbalances can contribute to metabolic disorders, weight gain, and chronic diseases.

In this section, we'll explore how key hormones, including insulin, glucagon, leptin, ghrelin, cortisol, thyroid hormones, and sex hormones, interact with nutrition to influence metabolic health. By understanding these hormonal processes, we gain insights into how diet affects not only our energy levels but also our long-term health.

Insulin and Glucagon: Managing Blood Sugar and Energy Storage

Insulin: Storing and Regulating Energy

Insulin is a hormone produced by the pancreas in response to rising blood glucose levels after eating, particularly when consuming carbohydrates. Its primary role is to lower blood glucose by promoting the uptake of glucose into cells, where it can be used for immediate energy or stored as glycogen in the liver and muscles. When insulin levels are elevated, the body enters a state that favors energy storage.

- **Role in Fat Storage**: Insulin also plays a key role in fat storage, as high insulin levels suppress lipolysis (the breakdown of fat). This is why frequent spikes in insulin from a high-carb, high-sugar diet can contribute to weight gain, as insulin promotes lipogenesis (the storage of fat). Maintaining balanced insulin levels through moderate carbohydrate intake helps to prevent excessive fat storage and promotes metabolic health.
- **Insulin Resistance and Its Implications**: Prolonged periods of high insulin due to frequent high-sugar intake can lead to insulin resistance, a condition where cells no longer respond effectively to insulin. This forces the pancreas to produce more insulin, setting up a cycle that ultimately contributes to type 2 diabetes, obesity, and metabolic syndrome. Managing insulin sensitivity through a balanced diet is essential for preventing these conditions.

Glucagon: The Counter-Hormone to Insulin

Glucagon, also produced by the pancreas, works in opposition to insulin. When blood glucose levels fall between meals or during fasting, glucagon is released to increase blood glucose by stimulating the liver to break down glycogen into glucose. This process, known as glycogenolysis, helps stabilize blood sugar levels and provides a steady energy supply.

- **Gluconeogenesis and Fat Breakdown**: In addition to glycogenolysis, glucagon stimulates gluconeogenesis, where the liver converts amino acids into glucose. Glucagon also promotes lipolysis, allowing stored fat to be used as energy, especially during fasting or carbohydrate restriction. By alternating between periods of insulin and glucagon dominance, the body maintains energy balance and metabolic flexibility, shifting between using glucose and fat as fuel sources.

Leptin and Ghrelin: Hormones of Appetite and Satiety

Leptin: The Satiety Hormone

Leptin is a hormone produced by fat cells that signals the brain when energy stores are sufficient, reducing hunger and promoting a sense of fullness. It is a key regulator of appetite and energy balance, helping to prevent overeating. The more body fat one has, the higher the leptin levels, as the body interprets this as a signal that it has adequate energy reserves.

- **Leptin Resistance in Obesity**: In individuals with obesity, leptin resistance can develop, meaning the brain no longer responds effectively to leptin's satiety signals. This leads to a continuous feeling of hunger and increased food intake despite adequate or excessive energy stores. Managing leptin sensitivity through a balanced diet, regular physical activity, and minimizing processed foods can support effective weight management.

Ghrelin: The Hunger Hormone

Ghrelin is produced in the stomach and is responsible for stimulating appetite. Ghrelin levels rise before meals, signaling hunger, and decrease after eating. Diets high in processed foods and sugars can disrupt ghrelin levels, leading to increased hunger and cravings, which can contribute to overeating. This is an important hormone to be aware of, because you can avoid spiking ghrelin when you need to.

- **Managing Hunger through Diet**: Diets rich in protein, fiber, and healthy fats are associated with lower ghrelin levels and prolonged satiety. Foods high in fiber slow digestion, which helps manage ghrelin levels by promoting a feeling of fullness. Balancing these hormones by selecting nutrient-dense foods can prevent overeating and support healthy weight maintenance.

Cortisol: The Stress Hormone and Its Effect on Nutrition

Cortisol, a hormone produced by the adrenal glands, plays a crucial role in regulating metabolism, blood sugar, and immune function. Known as the "stress hormone," cortisol is released during times of physical or emotional stress to provide an immediate energy boost, enabling the body to respond quickly to challenges. This hormone supports various body functions, including maintaining blood pressure, reducing inflammation, and focusing the mind during short-term stress. While beneficial in acute situations, prolonged or chronic elevation of cortisol due to ongoing stress can negatively impact health.

When cortisol remains consistently high, it can lead to increased appetite and fat storage, particularly around the abdomen. It can also suppress immune function, making the body more vulnerable to infections and slowing the healing process. Elevated cortisol levels often disrupt sleep by interfering with melatonin production, leading to poor sleep quality, which further heightens stress and inflammation. Over time, these effects increase the risk of developing metabolic issues such as insulin resistance, hypertension, and heart disease. High cortisol also affects mental health, contributing to mood disorders, anxiety, and depression due to its influence on neurotransmitters like serotonin. To protect against the damaging effects of chronic cortisol elevation, stress management techniques, regular exercise, quality sleep, and a balanced diet are essential. Together, these approaches can help maintain cortisol at healthy levels and support overall well-being, reducing the impact of prolonged stress on the body.

Impact on Blood Sugar and Fat Storage

During stressful situations, cortisol promotes gluconeogenesis, ensuring that glucose is available to fuel the body. While beneficial in short bursts, chronic stress leads to consistently elevated cortisol levels, which can disrupt metabolism and lead to blood sugar imbalances. Elevated cortisol also promotes visceral fat storage, particularly around the abdomen, which is linked to increased risk for heart disease and metabolic syndrome.

- **Dietary Implications for Cortisol**: Consuming balanced meals that include protein, fiber, and healthy fats can help manage cortisol levels by stabilizing blood sugar and preventing spikes and crashes. Reducing caffeine intake and eating foods rich in magnesium, such as leafy greens and nuts, can also help lower cortisol and reduce stress.

Thyroid Hormones: Regulating Metabolism and Energy Expenditure

The thyroid gland produces hormones—primarily T3 (triiodothyronine) and T4 (thyroxine)—that regulate metabolic rate and energy expenditure. Thyroid hormones are crucial for determining how quickly the body burns calories, impacting weight, energy levels, and overall metabolic health.

Influence on Metabolism: Thyroid hormones stimulate metabolic processes, increasing the rate of ATP production in cells. When thyroid hormones are balanced, they maintain a stable metabolic rate, supporting normal growth, development, and cellular repair.

Hypothyroidism and Weight Gain: An underactive thyroid, or hypothyroidism, slows down metabolism, leading to weight gain, fatigue, and sensitivity to cold. Iodine, selenium, and zinc are essential for thyroid hormone synthesis, and a deficiency in these nutrients can impair thyroid function, resulting in hypothyroid symptoms.

Hyperthyroidism and Weight Loss: Conversely, an overactive thyroid, or hyperthyroidism, leads to an accelerated metabolic rate, causing weight loss, anxiety, and muscle weakness. Dietary management and adequate nutrient intake can support thyroid health, helping to prevent both underactive and overactive thyroid issues.

Sex Hormones: Estrogen, Testosterone, and Nutritional Influence

Sex hormones, including estrogen, testosterone, and progesterone, play a significant role in body composition, fat distribution, and muscle mass. These hormones fluctuate throughout life and are influenced by diet and lifestyle.

Estrogen and Metabolism

Estrogen, produced predominantly in the ovaries, influences fat distribution and metabolic processes. It promotes insulin sensitivity and helps regulate glucose and lipid metabolism. During menopause, when estrogen levels decline, many women experience weight gain, increased abdominal fat, and higher risk of insulin resistance.

- **Dietary Impact on Estrogen Levels**: Foods rich in phytoestrogens, like flaxseeds and soy, may support estrogen balance in women, particularly during menopause. A diet high in whole grains, fruits, and vegetables can help maintain healthy estrogen levels and support metabolic health.

Testosterone and Muscle Mass

Testosterone, produced in the testes and in smaller amounts in women, supports muscle growth and fat loss. Testosterone's role in metabolism is significant as it promotes lean muscle mass, which increases basal metabolic rate (BMR) and supports weight management.

- **Dietary Support for Testosterone**: Nutrients like zinc, healthy fats, and lean proteins are essential for testosterone production. Foods high in zinc, such as shellfish, nuts, and seeds, support testosterone synthesis, while healthy fats like omega-3s provide essential building blocks for hormone production.

Hormonal Balance and Metabolic Health

Maintaining hormonal balance is key to metabolic health. Hormones work in harmony to regulate appetite, fat storage, energy production, and cellular repair. Here are some dietary strategies that can help maintain hormonal balance:

Avoid Processed Foods: Processed foods, particularly those high in sugar and unhealthy fats, can disrupt hormone balance by causing spikes in insulin and cortisol. A diet centered around whole foods helps prevent hormonal imbalances that contribute to weight gain and metabolic disorders.

Support Nutrient Intake: Vitamins and minerals like B vitamins, magnesium, and antioxidants play a role in hormone synthesis and regulation. For instance, magnesium helps reduce cortisol, while vitamin D supports immune and endocrine function.

Balance Macronutrients: Protein, fats, and fiber support stable blood sugar and help prevent excessive insulin release. Diets rich in these macronutrients help regulate insulin, ghrelin, and leptin, promoting a sense of fullness and balanced energy levels.

Limit Endocrine Disruptors: Chemicals found in plastics, pesticides, and some personal care products can interfere with hormone production. Limiting exposure to endocrine disruptors and choosing organic foods can support healthier hormone levels.

The Interconnectedness of Nutrition and Endocrinology

The field of endocrinology reveals how deeply interconnected our hormones are with nutrition and metabolic health. Hormones like insulin, leptin, ghrelin, cortisol, and thyroid hormones respond to dietary choices, impacting our energy levels, hunger, metabolism, and long-term health. By understanding the role of these hormones and making mindful dietary choices, we can support optimal hormonal balance, improve metabolic health, and reduce the risk of chronic disease. Ultimately, a balanced diet rich in whole foods, lean proteins, healthy fats, and essential nutrients is essential for maintaining hormonal harmony and promoting lifelong wellness.

Scientific Processes in Nutrition: Beyond Metabolism

Nutrition involves a vast network of biochemical processes and physiological mechanisms beyond basic metabolism. These processes work together to ensure that nutrients are digested, absorbed, transported, and utilized efficiently in the body. Here, we explore advanced scientific processes that underpin nutritional health, such as cellular signaling, nutrient transport mechanisms, detoxification pathways, the gut microbiome, and epigenetics. Each of these processes sheds light on how nutrients interact with the body at a molecular level to support health and longevity.

1. Cellular Signaling Pathways in Nutrient Sensing

One of the critical aspects of nutrition is how cells sense and respond to nutrients. Cellular signaling is a complex communication process that allows cells to detect and react to nutrient availability, thereby regulating growth, energy production, and cellular repair.

mTOR Pathway: Regulating Growth and Metabolism

The mammalian target of rapamycin (mTOR) pathway is a central regulator of cell growth and metabolism in response to nutrient availability, particularly amino acids. When protein intake is high, amino acids stimulate the mTOR pathway, promoting protein synthesis, cell growth, and muscle repair. This pathway is critical for tissue maintenance but also has implications for aging and metabolic health.

- **Nutrient Availability and mTOR Activation**: Excessive activation of mTOR, especially through constant high protein intake, may contribute to accelerated aging and certain diseases, as it encourages cell proliferation. By contrast, periodic fasting and balanced protein intake can help modulate mTOR activity, supporting cellular longevity and autophagy, the body's process of clearing damaged cells.

AMPK Pathway: Energy Sensing and Fat Oxidation

AMP-activated protein kinase (AMPK) is another crucial cellular energy sensor activated during low energy states, such as fasting or physical activity. When cellular energy levels are low, AMPK promotes energy-conserving processes and activates fat oxidation for fuel, helping the body maintain energy balance.

259

- **AMPK and Nutrient Restriction**: AMPK activation helps the body shift toward burning stored fat during periods of low energy intake. Nutritional strategies like intermittent fasting, calorie restriction, and consuming foods that support AMPK (e.g., green tea, berberine) can activate this pathway, enhancing fat burning and supporting metabolic health.

2. Nutrient Absorption Mechanisms in the Digestive System

Once ingested, nutrients must be efficiently broken down and absorbed to be used by the body. Absorption involves specific mechanisms tailored to different nutrients, each of which has unique pathways in the gastrointestinal (GI) tract.

Carbohydrate Absorption

Carbohydrates are broken down into monosaccharides (simple sugars) like glucose, fructose, and galactose by digestive enzymes in the small intestine. These monosaccharides are absorbed via active transport or facilitated diffusion, a process that relies on specific transport proteins.

SGLT1 and GLUT2 Transporters: Glucose and galactose are transported into cells via the sodium-glucose linked transporter (SGLT1), which uses a sodium gradient to facilitate glucose uptake. Fructose is absorbed by facilitated diffusion through GLUT5 transporters and enters the bloodstream via GLUT2. This efficient transport system ensures that glucose is readily available for energy production.

Protein Absorption

Proteins are broken down into amino acids and smaller peptides by proteolytic enzymes (e.g., pepsin, trypsin). Amino acids are absorbed through active transport mechanisms involving amino acid-specific transporters.

PEPT1 Transporter: The PEPT1 transporter plays a vital role in absorbing dipeptides and tripeptides in the intestine. Once inside cells, these peptides are broken down into amino acids, which enter the bloodstream for distribution to tissues.

Fat Absorption and Transport

Dietary fats are emulsified by bile acids and broken down into free fatty acids and monoglycerides, which are absorbed by enterocytes (intestinal cells) in the small intestine. Once inside enterocytes, fatty acids are reassembled into triglycerides and packaged into chylomicrons, lipoprotein particles that transport fats through the lymphatic system and into the bloodstream.

Chylomicrons and Lipoproteins: Chylomicrons deliver triglycerides to tissues for energy use or storage. Smaller fats, like medium-chain triglycerides (MCTs), are absorbed directly into the bloodstream without needing chylomicrons, providing a rapid source of energy.

3. Nutrient Transport and Cellular Uptake

Once nutrients are absorbed, they must be transported to cells and tissues for utilization. The bloodstream serves as the primary transport route, carrying nutrients bound to specific carrier proteins or within lipoproteins.

Glucose Transport and Insulin Regulation

The transport of glucose into cells is regulated by insulin, which binds to receptors on cell membranes, signaling glucose transporters (GLUT4) to move glucose from the bloodstream into cells. This insulin-dependent transport is especially important in muscle and fat cells.

GLUT4 Transporter: The GLUT4 transporter is sensitive to insulin and helps regulate blood glucose levels by promoting cellular glucose uptake. Physical activity can increase GLUT4 expression in muscle cells, improving glucose uptake and insulin sensitivity even in the absence of insulin.

Amino Acid Transport and Protein Synthesis

Amino acids circulate in the bloodstream and are taken up by cells based on demand. They are transported across cell membranes by various amino acid-specific transporters and used to build proteins, enzymes, and other functional molecules.

mTOR and Protein Synthesis: The presence of amino acids, particularly leucine, activates the mTOR pathway, signaling cells to initiate protein synthesis. This process is essential for muscle repair, immune function, and cellular growth.

4. Detoxification Pathways in the Liver

Detoxification is a vital biochemical process by which the liver neutralizes and removes toxins from the body. This process is essential for maintaining metabolic health and preventing the accumulation of harmful substances.

Phase I and Phase II Detoxification

The liver detoxifies substances in two phases. Phase I involves breaking down toxins into intermediate compounds, often through oxidation, reduction, or hydrolysis. Phase II involves conjugation, where intermediate compounds are bound to molecules like glutathione, sulfate, or glucuronic acid, making them water-soluble for excretion.

Cytochrome P450 Enzymes in Phase I: These enzymes are responsible for oxidizing toxins to make them more water-soluble. However, Phase I reactions can produce free radicals, so they are tightly regulated to prevent oxidative stress.

Conjugation Pathways in Phase II: Phase II reactions use compounds like glutathione to neutralize toxins, allowing them to be excreted through urine or bile. Consuming cruciferous vegetables, rich in sulfur compounds, can support Phase II detoxification by enhancing glutathione levels.

5. Gut Microbiome and Nutrient Interactions

The gut microbiome, a community of trillions of bacteria in the intestines, plays an essential role in nutrient metabolism, immune function, and even mood regulation. These microorganisms help break down complex carbohydrates, synthesize certain vitamins, and protect against pathogens.

Fermentation of Fiber

Dietary fiber, particularly soluble fiber, is fermented by gut bacteria to produce short-chain fatty acids (SCFAs) like butyrate, acetate, and propionate. SCFAs serve as energy sources for colon cells and help regulate inflammation and insulin sensitivity.

Butyrate and Colon Health: Butyrate is especially beneficial for colon health, as it provides energy to colonocytes (cells in the colon) and has anti-inflammatory properties. A fiber-rich diet promotes butyrate production, supporting gut health and reducing inflammation.

Vitamin Synthesis by Gut Bacteria

Certain gut bacteria synthesize vitamins, such as vitamin K2 and some B vitamins, which contribute to the host's nutrient pool. These bacteria-derived vitamins can be absorbed by the body, making the gut microbiome an essential contributor to overall nutrient status.

6. Epigenetics: Nutritional Influence on Gene Expression

Epigenetics is the study of changes in gene expression without altering the DNA sequence. Nutrients can affect epigenetic modifications, influencing how genes are turned on or off, thereby impacting health outcomes.

DNA Methylation

Methylation is an epigenetic mechanism in which a methyl group is added to DNA, usually silencing gene expression. Nutrients like folate, B vitamins, and choline provide methyl groups for DNA methylation, influencing gene expression patterns related to aging, disease susceptibility, and metabolism.

- **Methylation and Aging**: Diets rich in methyl donors, such as leafy greens, eggs, and fish, support healthy methylation patterns, which may slow aging and reduce the risk of chronic diseases.

Histone Modification

Histones are proteins that help package DNA within the cell nucleus. Chemical modifications, such as acetylation, can change the structure of histones, making genes more or less accessible for transcription. Nutrients, including polyphenols from fruits and vegetables, can influence histone modifications, potentially affecting inflammation and cancer risk.

- **Polyphenols and Anti-Inflammatory Effects**: Certain plant compounds like curcumin and resveratrol can inhibit pro-inflammatory gene expression by modulating histone acetylation. This demonstrates how diet can influence epigenetic markers that impact inflammation and disease risk.

Integrating Scientific Processes for Nutritional Health

The science of nutrition extends beyond digestion and metabolism, encompassing complex cellular signaling, nutrient transport, detoxification, microbiome interactions, and epigenetic modifications. By understanding these processes, we gain deeper insights into how nutrients impact health at a molecular level. Supporting these processes through balanced nutrition and lifestyle choices can enhance cellular function, metabolic health, and longevity, reinforcing the role of nutrition as a cornerstone of wellness.

Chapter 12 Additional Relevant Information

Nutritional Anthropology: Case Studies of Ancestral Diets Across Cultures

When examining diets across different cultures, it's important to recognize that dietary needs and adaptations are deeply rooted in the historical, geographical, and cultural contexts in which these diets evolved. If you're living in the United States, you are likely exposed to an integration of global influences alongside modern challenges, including widespread access to processed foods and artificial ingredients that contribute to the health issues underlying the standard American diet. This is one of the primary reasons for this book's focus on dietary awareness and improvement.

While this book emphasizes that carbohydrates are not essential for human survival, readers might observe that many traditional diets around the world include carbohydrates—often in seemingly large quantities. However, it's essential to put this into perspective. For example, traditional diets have often remained unchanged over centuries, allowing people to adapt to certain carbohydrate-rich foods through evolution and lifestyle. These communities consume whole, unprocessed foods that are free from the artificial sugars, preservatives, and refined ingredients common in the Western diet. Carbohydrates in traditional diets are also frequently paired with nutrient-dense foods that support metabolic health, and their sources—like tubers, vegetables, or fermented grains—are vastly different from the processed carbs commonly consumed in modern Western diets.

In many of these cultures, physical activity levels are higher, and the social and environmental stressors differ from those in industrialized societies, all of which can impact how these populations metabolize and benefit from carbohydrates. For example, a traditional high-carb diet in a rural area often consists of fiber-rich, slow-digesting carbohydrates from whole foods, which affect blood sugar and insulin levels differently than the refined sugars and starches prevalent in the standard American diet. Additionally, people from these cultures may have genetic adaptations that enable them to thrive on specific local foods, which is a key factor to consider when assessing diets outside our own environment.

Thus, while some traditional diets may include higher carbohydrate intake, the context is everything. These diets evolved in environments where whole foods were the only option, and processed foods were absent. What works in one part of the world may not be universally beneficial, especially when processed foods and modern eating habits distort the nutrient quality and balance. In other words, just because certain populations consume carbohydrates doesn't mean all carbs are appropriate or necessary, especially in a context where modern foods have skewed our natural dietary needs.

Examining the diets of ancestral populations provides invaluable insights into the role of traditional foods in health and longevity. Nutritional anthropology studies these ancient dietary practices across various cultures, highlighting how regional differences in food availability, climate, and cultural practices shaped unique eating patterns. Despite their diversity, these diets share a common thread: they are rooted in natural, minimally processed foods that align closely with human physiology. By studying these diets, we gain a deeper understanding of how traditional food practices supported the health and resilience of our ancestors and how modern diets can be adapted to harness similar benefits.

In this chapter, we explore three distinct ancestral diets—the Inuit, Maasai, and Okinawan diets—each of which reflects a unique adaptation to the local environment. We will examine the core components of these diets, their health implications, and what modern populations can learn from these enduring food traditions.

The Inuit Diet: Survival on Animal Fat and Protein in the Arctic

The Inuit people of the Arctic region have thrived for thousands of years in one of the harshest climates on Earth, where plant-based food sources are extremely limited. Their traditional diet consists primarily of fatty marine mammals, fish, and other cold-water animals, along with occasional seasonal berries. This high-fat, low-carbohydrate diet is a striking contrast to modern Western diets, which are typically carbohydrate-heavy. The Inuit's reliance on animal foods provides a fascinating case study in how humans can adapt to a diet that is nearly devoid of plant foods.

Key Components of the Inuit Diet

1. **Marine Mammals**: The Inuit consume seal, whale, and walrus, all of which provide high levels of omega-3 fatty

acids and fat-soluble vitamins (A, D, and E). These nutrients support brain health, cardiovascular function, and immune resilience, which are essential for survival in extreme cold.

2. **Fish**: Arctic fish, such as salmon and char, are rich in protein and essential fatty acids, both critical for maintaining energy levels and cellular repair.

3. **Raw and Fermented Foods**: Due to limited cooking resources, the Inuit often consume raw or fermented foods, which preserve heat-sensitive nutrients and maintain beneficial bacteria for gut health.

Health Implications of the Inuit Diet

The Inuit's high-fat diet leads to a state of metabolic ketosis, where the body relies on fat-derived ketones for energy instead of glucose. This metabolic state provides a steady and sustainable energy supply, essential for long periods without food in the Arctic. Studies of the Inuit population have shown low rates of heart disease, despite high-fat intake, likely due to their consumption of omega-3 rich foods, which counteract inflammation and support heart health. Additionally, the nutrient density of their diet helps prevent deficiencies, maintaining strong immune defenses in a challenging environment.

The Maasai Diet: A Carnivorous, High-Dairy Diet in East Africa

The Maasai, a semi-nomadic people of East Africa, have traditionally consumed a diet centered around cattle, which are their primary source of sustenance. The Maasai diet includes fresh milk, meat, and blood from their livestock, which together provide a complete nutrient profile suited to their active lifestyle. This diet is notably high in saturated fat and low in carbohydrates, challenging common dietary guidelines that promote low-fat, high-carb eating patterns.

Key Components of the Maasai Diet

1. **Milk and Blood**: The Maasai consume fresh milk and blood regularly, both of which are rich in protein, healthy fats, and minerals such as calcium, iron, and potassium. Milk provides lactic acid bacteria, which support gut health, while blood offers a source of heme iron, critical for oxygen transport.

2. **Meat**: Meat is consumed less frequently but provides a concentrated source of nutrients, including essential amino acids, B vitamins, and bioavailable minerals.
3. **Medicinal Herbs**: The Maasai also use a variety of herbs to treat illnesses and aid digestion, adding an element of plant-based nutrition and medicinal value to their diet.

Health Implications of the Maasai Diet

Research on the Maasai population has found that they experience low rates of heart disease, hypertension, and diabetes, despite their high intake of saturated fat. This may be attributed to the nutrient density of their animal-based diet and their active lifestyle, which helps maintain cardiovascular health. The Maasai's diet is also low in processed sugars and refined grains, two modern dietary components associated with metabolic disorders. The Maasai demonstrate how a high-fat, low-carb diet can support health, especially when it is paired with physical activity and minimal intake of processed foods.

The Okinawan Diet: Plant-Rich, Low-Calorie Diet in a Subtropical Climate

The Okinawan diet, followed by the indigenous population of Okinawa, Japan, is renowned for its role in promoting longevity and reducing chronic diseases. Okinawa is one of the world's "Blue Zones," where people frequently live beyond 100 years in good health. The Okinawan diet is low in calories but rich in plant-based foods, including sweet potatoes, vegetables, legumes, and small amounts of fish and pork. This diet emphasizes nutrient-dense, low-calorie foods that promote satiety and metabolic health.

Key Components of the Okinawan Diet

1. **Sweet Potatoes**: A staple food in Okinawa, sweet potatoes are a complex carbohydrate rich in fiber, vitamins (especially vitamin A), and antioxidants. They provide sustained energy and support gut health.
2. **Soy Foods**: Tofu, miso, and other soy products are excellent sources of plant-based protein and contain phytoestrogens, which may play a role in reducing the risk of hormone-related diseases.
3. **Sea Vegetables and Fish**: Seaweed provides iodine, which supports thyroid health, and fish offers omega-3 fatty acids

for cardiovascular health. These foods contribute important minerals often lacking in land-based diets.

4. **Herbs and Medicinal Plants**: The Okinawan diet includes a variety of herbs like turmeric and mugwort, which have anti-inflammatory properties and support overall health.

Health Implications of the Okinawan Diet

The Okinawan diet's low-calorie, nutrient-dense nature contributes to the population's long lifespan and low incidence of chronic diseases such as cancer, heart disease, and diabetes. Rich in antioxidants and anti-inflammatory compounds, this diet helps counteract oxidative stress and inflammation, two processes associated with aging and chronic illness. Additionally, the emphasis on plant foods provides fiber and phytonutrients that support gut health and reduce the risk of metabolic diseases.

Note on the "Blue Zones"

The concept of **Blue Zones**—regions where people reportedly live longer and healthier lives—has been popularized by Dan Buettner's research and books. While it offers inspiration for adopting healthier lifestyles, it has also been met with significant critiques. Here are some of the key criticisms:

1. Questionable Data Accuracy

- **Birth Records and Longevity Claims**: In some Blue Zones, such as Sardinia and Ikaria, the accuracy of birth records has been questioned. Poor or incomplete record-keeping may exaggerate claims of extreme longevity. Some critics argue that data manipulation or errors in historical documentation could inflate the number of centenarians.
- **Survivor Bias**: In regions with historically high infant mortality rates, those who survive into adulthood may naturally skew the average lifespan upward, creating a false impression of unusually long lifespans for the population as a whole.

2. Retrospective Selection Bias

- Blue Zones were identified after the fact, meaning researchers selected regions with high observed longevity and then examined their lifestyles to find commonalities.

This retrospective approach risks cherry-picking data and ignoring regions with similar lifestyles but no notable longevity patterns.

3. Over-Simplification of Complex Factors

- **Dietary Narratives**: Blue Zones often emphasize plant-based diets as a cornerstone of longevity, but this oversimplifies dietary patterns. For example, Sardinians consume significant amounts of dairy, and Okinawans traditionally ate pork and lard in addition to vegetables.
- **Genetic Factors**: The Blue Zones framework largely ignores the role of genetics in longevity. Populations in isolated regions may share genetic predispositions that contribute to their long lifespans, independent of lifestyle factors.
- **Socioeconomic and Healthcare Systems**: Longevity in Blue Zones could also be influenced by access to healthcare, low levels of industrial pollution, or socioeconomic stability—factors that may not be transferable to other populations.

4. Cultural and Environmental Context

- **Non-Replicability**: The unique environmental, cultural, and social conditions of Blue Zones are difficult, if not impossible, to replicate elsewhere. For instance, the communal lifestyles, stress-reduction practices, and local diets of these regions are deeply tied to their specific histories and geographies.
- **Modernization and Change**: Many Blue Zones are now undergoing significant modernization, with younger generations adopting Westernized diets and lifestyles. This raises questions about whether their longevity trends will persist in the future.

5. Lack of Scientific Rigor

- **Correlation vs. Causation**: Blue Zones research often identifies correlations between lifestyle factors and longevity but fails to establish causation. For example, while social connections and low stress are linked to better health, it's unclear if they directly cause longer life spans or are simply associated with other factors like socioeconomic stability.

- **Inconsistent Methodology**: Critics argue that the methodologies used in identifying and studying Blue Zones lack the scientific rigor required for reliable conclusions. For example, the criteria for defining a Blue Zone are not always transparent or consistent.

6. Overemphasis on Plant-Based Diets

- While plant-based diets are often touted as a primary factor in Blue Zone longevity, this ignores other critical aspects of their diets, such as high-quality fats, moderate animal protein consumption, or fermentation practices. Some argue this focus is overly influenced by popular diet trends rather than balanced, evidence-based nutrition science.

7. Commercialization

- **Branding and Marketing**: Critics have pointed out that the Blue Zones concept has been heavily commercialized, including partnerships with cities to create "Blue Zones projects." These efforts often prioritize profit and marketing over scientific accuracy and measurable health outcomes.
- **Simplistic Health Recommendations**: The "secrets" of Blue Zones are often presented as universal solutions, which may oversimplify or misrepresent the complex interplay of factors contributing to longevity.

While Blue Zones offer valuable insights into healthy living—such as the importance of community, movement, and unprocessed foods—the concept is not without flaws. Data accuracy issues, selection bias, and oversimplifications undermine its credibility as a scientific model for longevity. Readers and policymakers should approach Blue Zones with a critical eye, recognizing its strengths while remaining cautious about overgeneralized conclusions.

Lessons from Ancestral Diets for Modern Health

The study of ancestral diets reveals that while traditional diets differ widely across cultures, they share several fundamental principles. Here are some lessons that modern readers can draw from these case studies:

1. **Nutrient Density**: Ancestral diets prioritize nutrient-dense foods, providing essential vitamins, minerals, and healthy

271

fats. Focusing on whole, unprocessed foods in the modern diet can help mimic this nutrient density.

2. **Low Sugar and Refined Carbohydrates**: Traditional diets were naturally low in refined sugars and processed carbohydrates, which are now known to contribute to obesity, diabetes, and other chronic conditions. Reducing intake of these modern foods can benefit metabolic health.

3. **Adaptation to Environment**: Each diet is adapted to the natural environment, using available resources to meet nutritional needs. This approach encourages seasonal and local eating, aligning with our evolutionary history and supporting sustainable practices.

4. **Emphasis on Quality Fats**: High-fat diets, like those of the Inuit and Maasai, challenge the low-fat dietary dogma often promoted in modern guidelines. Including high-quality fats—such as those found in fish, dairy, and grass-fed meats—can support satiety, hormone balance, and cellular function.

5. **Incorporating Medicinal Foods**: The use of medicinal herbs and plants for their health-promoting properties is common in ancestral diets. Incorporating spices and herbs with known health benefits, like turmeric, garlic, and ginger, can enhance the nutritional quality of the diet.

6. **Intermittent Fasting and Natural Caloric Restriction**: Traditional diets often include natural periods of fasting or caloric restriction, either due to seasonal scarcity or lifestyle patterns. Incorporating intermittent fasting can support metabolic flexibility, a trait valued in ancestral eating practices.

Applying Ancestral Wisdom to Modern Diets

Ancestral diets offer a valuable framework for understanding human nutritional needs and the impact of diet on health. While our environments and lifestyles have changed dramatically, the principles underlying these diets remain relevant. By drawing on the lessons from traditional diets like those of the Inuit, Maasai, and Okinawans, we can develop a more holistic approach to eating that respects our evolutionary roots and promotes lasting health.

This exploration of ancestral diets underscores the value of diverse food traditions, nutrient density, and the balance between animal and plant-based foods. As we look to the past, we find guidance on how to navigate modern dietary challenges, equipping ourselves with knowledge that bridges history and science for a healthier future.

The Concept of Nutritional Resilience: Adapting to Modern Stressors

In today's fast-paced and often stressful world, building resilience is critical—not only mentally but also physically. Nutritional resilience is the concept of fortifying the body through diet to better withstand stressors, whether they are environmental toxins, psychological stress, physical challenges, or nutritional deficiencies. Unlike survival-based resilience, which prepares the body for immediate survival in difficult environments, nutritional resilience emphasizes long-term health and the ability to thrive despite modern lifestyle challenges.

This chapter explores the dietary approaches and strategies that foster resilience. We look at foods, nutrients, and lifestyle practices that support the body's ability to manage stress, maintain metabolic flexibility, and enhance immune response.

1. The Basis of Nutritional Resilience: Adaptability and Balance

Nutritional resilience begins with the concept of adaptability—the body's ability to respond to and recover from stress. The human body has remarkable mechanisms to cope with adverse conditions, from physical injuries to psychological trauma. However, the chronic stressors of modern life can overwhelm these systems, particularly when diets are low in essential nutrients.

- **Metabolic Flexibility**: One of the foundations of resilience is metabolic flexibility, the ability to switch between using carbohydrates and fats for energy. Diets high in processed carbohydrates and sugars often hinder this flexibility, creating an overreliance on glucose as a fuel source. A resilient diet encourages metabolic flexibility, allowing the body to efficiently use fat as an energy source, which is essential during fasting or in times of stress.
- **Balance of Macronutrients**: Consuming a balanced ratio of macronutrients (proteins, fats, and carbohydrates) provides the body with a steady supply of energy and building blocks for cellular repair. High-quality proteins support muscle maintenance and immune function, while healthy fats stabilize energy levels and support cellular health.

273

2. Antioxidants and Anti-Inflammatory Nutrients

Resilience against environmental stressors, including pollution, chemicals, and free radicals, largely depends on the body's ability to neutralize oxidative damage. Antioxidants are compounds that combat free radicals, reducing cellular stress and inflammation. Chronic inflammation, linked to many modern diseases, can be mitigated by incorporating anti-inflammatory foods into the diet.

- **Antioxidant-Rich Foods**: Berries, dark leafy greens, nuts, and seeds are rich in antioxidants like vitamins C and E, flavonoids, and carotenoids. These compounds protect cells from oxidative stress, enhancing resilience against environmental pollutants and metabolic stress.
- **Omega-3 Fatty Acids**: Omega-3 fatty acids, found in fatty fish, flaxseeds, and walnuts, play a powerful anti-inflammatory role. They help regulate the body's inflammatory response, which is essential for resilience, as chronic inflammation is linked to conditions such as heart disease, arthritis, and autoimmune disorders.
- **Polyphenols**: Found in foods like green tea, dark chocolate, and grapes, polyphenols are plant compounds that also act as antioxidants and may support healthy aging. They reduce oxidative stress and inflammation, supporting resilience at a cellular level.

3. Adaptogens: Natural Stress Resilience Aids

Adaptogens are natural substances, primarily herbs and mushrooms, that help the body adapt to stress. They work by modulating the adrenal glands and supporting the body's stress response, reducing the negative effects of chronic stress. Although adaptogens are not replacements for nutrients, they complement a nutrient-dense diet by enhancing resilience to both mental and physical stressors.

- **Ashwagandha**: Known for its calming effects, ashwagandha helps reduce cortisol levels and manage anxiety. It can support sleep, balance energy levels, and improve focus, making it valuable in today's high-stress environment.
- **Rhodiola Rosea**: This herb is known for its ability to improve endurance and reduce fatigue. Rhodiola supports mental clarity and physical stamina, benefiting individuals facing intense physical or mental demands.

- **Reishi Mushroom**: Often called the "mushroom of immortality," reishi enhances immune resilience and reduces stress by regulating inflammatory pathways. It supports sleep quality and is particularly beneficial for maintaining a calm, steady energy.

4. Gut Health as a Foundation for Nutritional Resilience

The gut microbiome—trillions of bacteria and microorganisms living in the digestive tract—plays a crucial role in nutrient absorption, immunity, and mental health. A balanced microbiome is essential for resilience, as it affects everything from digestion to stress tolerance.

- **Fiber and Prebiotics**: Fiber-rich foods like fruits, vegetables, and whole grains feed beneficial gut bacteria, supporting a healthy microbiome. Prebiotics (found in foods like garlic, onions, and bananas) specifically nourish probiotics, which contribute to immune resilience.
- **Probiotic Foods**: Fermented foods like yogurt, kefir, sauerkraut, and kimchi contain probiotics that enhance gut diversity. A diverse microbiome improves digestion, boosts immunity, and produces neurotransmitters that influence mood and stress response.
- **Reducing Gut Inflammatory Triggers**: Avoiding highly processed foods, refined sugars, and artificial additives can reduce gut inflammation and support a resilient microbiome. A healthy gut is better able to manage the stressors of modern diets and lifestyles.

5. Nutrients for Immune Resilience

The immune system is the body's primary defense against infection, but modern lifestyles, poor diets, and stress can compromise immune resilience. Certain nutrients are essential for maintaining a robust immune response.

- **Vitamin D**: Vitamin D, often obtained from sun exposure, plays a vital role in immune health. It helps modulate immune responses, reducing the risk of infections and autoimmune diseases. Dietary sources include fatty fish, fortified dairy products, and supplements, especially in regions with limited sunlight.
- **Zinc**: This mineral is crucial for immune cell production and function. Zinc-rich foods include shellfish, beef, pumpkin

seeds, and lentils. Regular intake supports immune resilience, particularly during cold and flu season.
- **Vitamin C**: Known for its antioxidant properties, vitamin C supports immune resilience by reducing oxidative stress and promoting collagen formation, which strengthens skin and connective tissues as a barrier against pathogens.
- **Selenium**: Found in Brazil nuts, eggs, and fish, selenium is a trace mineral that enhances antioxidant activity and supports thyroid health, which influences immune function. Sufficient selenium levels help the body adapt to stress and infection.

6. Building Resilience Through Fasting and Intermittent Caloric Restriction

Periods of fasting or caloric restriction can enhance resilience by triggering cellular processes that promote longevity and stress resistance. These processes include autophagy, where cells clear out damaged proteins and recycle components, improving cellular health.

- **Intermittent Fasting (IF)**: IF involves alternating between periods of eating and fasting. This eating pattern has been shown to improve metabolic health, increase insulin sensitivity, and reduce inflammation. By periodically fasting, the body "resets" its metabolism, which supports resilience against metabolic diseases.
- **Caloric Restriction**: Long-term caloric restriction, when done moderately, has been associated with increased lifespan and improved stress resilience. By reducing overall caloric intake, the body conserves energy and enhances repair mechanisms.

7. Hormonal Balance

Hormones, including cortisol, insulin, and thyroid hormones, play a significant role in resilience. A nutrient-dense diet helps maintain hormone balance, which is essential for coping with stress, managing energy, and maintaining immunity.

- **Blood Sugar Control**: Keeping blood sugar levels stable by reducing refined carbs and processed foods prevents energy crashes and supports insulin sensitivity. Stable blood sugar levels reduce the risk of insulin resistance, which can compromise metabolic health.

- **Cortisol Regulation**: Cortisol, the body's primary stress hormone, can be regulated through lifestyle practices such as meditation, exercise, and balanced sleep. Foods high in magnesium, like leafy greens and nuts, also support cortisol management.
- **Thyroid Health**: Iodine, selenium, and zinc are critical for thyroid function. A balanced thyroid ensures that metabolic processes run smoothly, supporting resilience and energy stability.

8. Environmental Toxins and Detoxification Support

In modern society, exposure to environmental toxins—such as pesticides, heavy metals, and plastic residues—is nearly unavoidable. Nutritional resilience includes supporting the body's detoxification pathways to mitigate the effects of these toxins.

- **Liver-Supporting Foods**: The liver is the primary organ for detoxification. Foods like cruciferous vegetables (broccoli, Brussels sprouts) and garlic support liver enzymes that process toxins.
- **Hydration**: Drinking enough water is essential for flushing toxins from the body. Proper hydration supports kidney function, helping to eliminate metabolic waste products.
- **Antioxidant Support**: Antioxidants neutralize free radicals generated by toxin exposure. Foods rich in vitamin C, vitamin E, and polyphenols provide this support, reducing oxidative stress on cells.

9. Practical Strategies for Building Nutritional Resilience

Developing a resilient diet requires intention and balance. Here are practical steps to help foster nutritional resilience:

1. **Emphasize Whole Foods**: Whole, unprocessed foods provide essential nutrients without added sugars or inflammatory ingredients.
2. **Practice Intermittent Fasting**: Integrating fasting or time-restricted eating can improve metabolic flexibility and cellular resilience.
3. **Incorporate Adaptogens and Anti-Inflammatory Foods**: Foods that support hormone balance and reduce

inflammation, such as fatty fish, dark berries, and turmeric, enhance resilience.

4. **Focus on Gut Health**: Include prebiotic and probiotic foods to support the microbiome, which strengthens both immune and stress resilience.

5. **Manage Stress**: Chronic stress is a significant threat to resilience. Activities like mindfulness, moderate exercise, and quality sleep improve the body's ability to manage stress.

Creating a Foundation for Long-Term Health

Nutritional resilience is about preparing the body for both expected and unexpected stressors. By fostering metabolic flexibility, supporting gut health, incorporating antioxidants, and balancing hormones, individuals can enhance their capacity to thrive in the face of modern challenges. This approach goes beyond survival, offering a proactive way to build a strong foundation for lasting health and vitality.

The Role of Seasonal Eating and Natural Food Cycles

Seasonal eating is the practice of consuming foods that are naturally harvested during their peak growing season. This concept aligns with how humans traditionally ate before the advent of refrigeration and global food transportation, which made it possible to access nearly any food at any time. The practice of eating with the seasons not only offers nutritional and environmental benefits but also reconnects individuals with natural food cycles that promote balance in both the body and the ecosystem.

This chapter explores the benefits of seasonal eating, the science behind natural food cycles, and how these practices can support health, sustainability, and metabolic balance.

1. The History and Origins of Seasonal Eating

Historically, people ate according to what was available in their immediate environment. Before modern agriculture and food distribution, there was no choice but to rely on the foods that were in season. In tropical regions, a variety of fruits and vegetables were available year-round, while in colder climates, people relied on preserved or stored foods like root vegetables, grains, and meats during winter months.

Seasonal eating was not just a necessity but also influenced by cultural and spiritual practices. For example:

- **Agricultural Festivals**: Many cultures celebrated harvest festivals that aligned with seasonal crop yields, such as Thanksgiving in North America and the rice harvest festivals in Asia.
- **Food Preservation**: Techniques like pickling, fermenting, and drying allowed people to store foods during off-seasons, creating a natural rhythm of abundance and scarcity that guided dietary habits.

This rhythm created a natural balance that promoted metabolic health and aligned with the body's changing needs throughout the year.

2. Nutritional Benefits of Seasonal Eating

Eating seasonally has significant benefits for nutrient intake. Foods harvested in their peak season are often richer in vitamins, minerals, and antioxidants than those grown out of season. Modern research shows that produce harvested at peak ripeness has a higher nutritional value due to more sunlight exposure and natural ripening processes.

- **Increased Nutrient Density**: Seasonal foods, especially locally sourced, are typically fresher and retain more nutrients. For example, tomatoes grown in the summer have more vitamin C and lycopene than those grown in hothouses during winter.
- **Enhanced Antioxidant Content**: Many fruits and vegetables develop antioxidants in response to environmental stressors. Seasonal produce has higher concentrations of these compounds, which protect cells from oxidative damage.
- **Reduced Need for Preservatives**: Foods that are in season and locally sourced do not need extensive preservation, which can lead to a fresher and less processed diet.
-

3. Aligning with the Body's Natural Cycles

Just as nature goes through cycles, human biology operates in rhythms that change throughout the year. Seasonal eating aligns with these natural cycles, which can support the body's ability to adapt to varying environmental demands. Seasonal foods may also naturally supply nutrients that match our body's needs at different times of the year.

- **Spring and Summer**: In warmer months, nature provides an abundance of light, fresh produce like leafy greens, berries, and cucumbers. These foods are typically lower in calories and higher in water content, helping to keep the body hydrated and support detoxification, as the body is naturally more active and outdoors.
- **Autumn**: As the weather cools, root vegetables, squashes, and tubers become available. These foods provide the complex carbohydrates and energy needed to prepare the body for winter.
- **Winter**: Foods like root vegetables, hearty greens (e.g., kale, cabbage), and animal products are in season and provide the denser nutrients and calories that help sustain energy levels in colder weather.

By consuming foods that naturally thrive in each season, individuals can help balance their body's needs with environmental conditions, supporting metabolic health, immunity, and energy.

4. Environmental Benefits of Seasonal and Local Eating

In addition to personal health benefits, seasonal eating is also environmentally sustainable. It reduces the carbon footprint associated with importing out-of-season foods and supports local farming practices that rely less on artificial growing conditions and chemical inputs.

- **Reduced Carbon Emissions**: Foods grown and consumed locally in their season require less transportation, reducing greenhouse gas emissions.
- **Less Resource-Intensive Farming**: Seasonal crops require fewer resources like water, artificial lighting, and chemical

fertilizers compared to those grown out of season. This promotes healthier soil and reduces environmental stress.
- **Biodiversity**: Supporting local farms that practice crop rotation and seasonal growing helps preserve biodiversity, as it reduces the demand for monoculture crops that deplete soil nutrients and increase susceptibility to pests.

5. Practical Guidelines for Seasonal Eating

Incorporating seasonal eating into modern life may seem challenging, but with a few simple steps, it can become a sustainable practice that supports health and the environment.

- **Shopping at Farmers' Markets**: Local markets typically offer foods that are in season and grown locally, providing a reliable way to access seasonal produce.
- **Growing a Home Garden**: Growing your own seasonal fruits and vegetables, even on a small scale, can help align with natural food cycles and deepen your connection to the process.
- **Meal Planning with Seasonal Foods**: Planning meals around what is seasonally available encourages diversity in the diet and introduces new flavors and nutrients.
- **Preserving Seasonal Produce**: Techniques like canning, freezing, and fermenting allow you to enjoy seasonal produce throughout the year, minimizing waste and ensuring nutrient availability.

6. Seasonal Eating in Different Climates

The types of seasonal foods vary greatly depending on climate. Understanding your regional climate and local growing season can guide your approach to seasonal eating.

- **Tropical Climates**: In tropical areas, a variety of fruits (like bananas, mangoes, and papayas) and vegetables grow year-round. However, even in the tropics, there are natural cycles and peak seasons for certain crops.
- **Temperate Climates**: In regions with four seasons, diets often shift from fresh greens and berries in the summer to root vegetables, apples, and squashes in the fall and winter. In these climates, winter foods like hardy greens and stored root vegetables provide nutrients and calories for the colder months.

- **Cold and Mountainous Regions**: In colder regions, winter diets may be more reliant on stored grains, legumes, dried foods, and preserved meats. Fresh produce is minimal in the winter, but stored and fermented foods ensure nutrient availability.

7. Case Studies: Seasonal Eating in Traditional Diets

Several traditional diets provide examples of the benefits of seasonal eating. Cultures that rely on local food sources tend to reflect the natural cycles of their environments.

- **Mediterranean Diet**: The Mediterranean diet is rich in seasonal fruits, vegetables, grains, and seafood, supporting health and longevity. This diet naturally varies with the seasons, featuring abundant greens, tomatoes, and seafood in the summer and hearty legumes and root vegetables in the winter.
- **Japanese Diet**: Japanese cuisine emphasizes seasonal produce and regional foods, from fresh fish and vegetables in the summer to root vegetables and miso soup in winter. The concept of "shun" (seasonal peak) is a central element in Japanese food culture, focusing on foods at their best flavor and nutritional content.
- **Nordic Diet**: In Scandinavia, diets traditionally include seasonal root vegetables, fish, and fermented foods. The Nordic diet prioritizes local and seasonal foods, including seasonal berries, cabbage, and cold-water fish, which support health in colder climates.

8. How Seasonal Eating Supports Gut Health

Seasonal eating can benefit gut health by increasing dietary variety, which in turn supports a diverse microbiome. The human gut thrives on variety, and consuming a wide range of seasonal foods can introduce different fiber types and nutrients that feed beneficial bacteria.

- **Microbial Diversity**: Diverse fiber sources from seasonal vegetables, fruits, and grains contribute to a balanced microbiome. Each fiber type feeds different bacteria in the gut, promoting overall gut health.

- **Prebiotic Foods**: Foods like asparagus, leeks, and onions, often harvested in spring and early summer, are rich in prebiotics, which nourish beneficial gut bacteria.
- **Fermented Foods and Gut Health**: Seasonal practices like fermenting cabbage into sauerkraut or cucumbers into pickles provide probiotics that support digestion and immunity, especially beneficial in colder months.

9. Adapting Seasonal Eating in a Modern World

In modern society, where foods from around the world are available year-round, adopting seasonal eating may require deliberate choices. Here are some tips for making seasonal eating work in a modern context:

- **Explore Local Food Subscription Services**: Many communities offer farm-to-table services or seasonal produce boxes that deliver fresh, local food to your doorstep.
- **Educate Yourself on Seasonal Produce Calendars**: Research seasonal produce calendars for your region to learn what is naturally available throughout the year.
- **Flexibility and Moderation**: While seasonal eating has many benefits, it is important to remain flexible. Occasional out-of-season foods can still be part of a healthy diet, especially if they are nutrient-dense and unprocessed.

10. Potential Health Implications of Non-Seasonal Eating

Research indicates that consuming non-seasonal foods may disrupt metabolic rhythms, as modern diets often include year-round access to high-sugar fruits and refined grains that weren't naturally available in past eras. Non-seasonal eating can lead to:

- **Insulin Resistance**: Constant access to sugary fruits and refined carbohydrates may contribute to blood sugar imbalances and insulin resistance.
- **Increased Caloric Intake**: The lack of natural scarcity and overabundance of calorie-dense foods can contribute to overeating, weight gain, and obesity.
- **Disruption of Natural Rhythms**: Eating patterns that don't align with seasonal food availability can potentially disrupt circadian rhythms, affecting sleep, digestion, and mood.
-

Reconnecting with Natural Cycles for Health and Sustainability

Seasonal eating is more than a dietary choice; it's a way to align with the natural rhythms that our ancestors followed for millennia. By consuming foods at their nutritional peak, supporting local ecosystems, and promoting dietary variety, individuals can enhance their health, reduce environmental impact, and foster a deeper connection to the earth. Reintroducing seasonal eating into modern life offers a path toward nutritional resilience, metabolic balance, and a sustainable future.

Adaptogens and Ancient Remedies in Modern Nutrition

Adaptogens and ancient remedies have been used for centuries to help the body adapt to stress, enhance vitality, and support immune function. As modern lifestyles introduce more stressors—be they physical, mental, or environmental—interest in these traditional remedies has grown. Adaptogens, in particular, are natural substances that help stabilize the body's physiological processes and promote homeostasis, making them valuable tools in the realm of nutrition.

In this chapter, we'll explore the science behind adaptogens, the most commonly used ancient remedies, and how incorporating these plants, herbs, and practices can support health, balance, and resilience.

1. Understanding Adaptogens and Their Role in Stress Adaptation

Adaptogens are a unique category of herbs and plants that help the body resist stress, whether it's from physical exertion, mental demands, or environmental toxins. Unlike stimulants, which temporarily boost energy, adaptogens support the body's own resilience without creating dependency or exhausting its resources.

Adaptogens work by influencing the hypothalamic-pituitary-adrenal (HPA) axis, a system responsible for regulating the stress response. They balance cortisol levels, improve energy, and support immunity, helping the body adapt to stressors in a balanced way.

- **How Adaptogens Work**: By modulating the stress response, adaptogens improve energy levels, increase mental clarity, and support immune resilience. They don't forcefully alter body systems but rather help them adapt to change, restoring balance rather than overstimulation.

- **Broad-Spectrum Benefits**: Because adaptogens work at a foundational level, they offer a range of health benefits, from improving focus and endurance to reducing inflammation and enhancing recovery.

2. Key Adaptogens and Their Health Benefits

There are numerous adaptogenic herbs, each with specific effects on the body. Here are some of the most well-known and widely used adaptogens in traditional and modern medicine:

Ashwagandha

Origin: Ashwagandha (Withania somnifera) is an herb commonly used in Ayurvedic medicine.

Benefits: Known for its calming and balancing effects, ashwagandha helps reduce cortisol levels, improve sleep, and enhance mental clarity. It is often recommended for managing stress and improving stamina. Studies have shown that ashwagandha can reduce symptoms of anxiety, support muscle growth, and even improve sexual health.

Modern Applications: Ashwagandha is frequently used in supplements and adaptogenic blends aimed at stress relief and energy support.

Rhodiola Rosea

Origin: Rhodiola is a flowering herb that grows in cold, mountainous regions of Europe and Asia.

Benefits: Known for boosting physical endurance, mental clarity, and resilience against fatigue, rhodiola is a powerful adaptogen for those experiencing high physical or mental stress. It has been studied for its effects on reducing anxiety and supporting endurance.

Modern Applications: Rhodiola is often found in supplements that target cognitive performance, stress relief, and athletic recovery.

Holy Basil (Tulsi)

Origin: Holy basil is another Ayurvedic herb revered in traditional Indian medicine.

Benefits: Holy basil has both adaptogenic and anti-inflammatory properties, making it effective for managing stress, improving digestion, and supporting immune health. It is also known for its anti-anxiety effects and ability to enhance mood.

Modern Applications: Holy basil is commonly found in teas and supplements that target mental clarity and emotional balance.

Reishi Mushroom

Origin: Reishi is a medicinal mushroom that has been used in traditional Chinese medicine for thousands of years.

Benefits: Often called the "mushroom of immortality," reishi supports immune function, reduces inflammation, and promotes relaxation. It is especially useful for those seeking immune resilience and restful sleep.

Modern Applications: Reishi can be found in powders, capsules, and teas aimed at promoting sleep, immune health, and longevity.

Ginseng (Panax Ginseng)

Origin: Ginseng is native to East Asia and has been used in traditional medicine across China, Korea, and Japan.

Benefits: Ginseng is a well-known energy booster and is thought to improve cognitive performance, physical endurance, and immune function. It's particularly useful for those experiencing fatigue and weakened immunity.

Modern Applications: Ginseng is commonly included in energy supplements, teas, and immune support products.

3. How Ancient Remedies Complement Modern Nutrition

Ancient remedies encompass a broader range of practices and natural substances, from herbal concoctions to fermented foods, each of which supports health in unique ways. These remedies align closely with adaptogens and are increasingly popular in functional medicine and holistic health.

Turmeric and Curcumin

- **Traditional Use**: Turmeric has long been used in Ayurvedic and traditional Chinese medicine for its anti-inflammatory properties.
- **Benefits**: Curcumin, the active compound in turmeric, reduces inflammation and supports joint health, digestive health, and overall resilience.
- **Modern Applications**: Curcumin supplements are widely used for managing inflammation, arthritis, and even cognitive health.

Ginger

- **Traditional Use**: Ginger is a common remedy in Ayurvedic, Chinese, and Middle Eastern medicine for digestive health.
- **Benefits**: Known for its anti-inflammatory and anti-nausea effects, ginger aids digestion, reduces inflammation, and supports immune health.
- **Modern Applications**: Ginger is popular in teas, supplements, and even as an anti-nausea remedy for those undergoing chemotherapy.

Garlic

- **Traditional Use**: Used globally as a natural antibiotic, garlic has been a staple in traditional medicine for fighting infections.
- **Benefits**: Garlic has strong anti-inflammatory and immune-supporting properties. It also supports cardiovascular health by reducing blood pressure and cholesterol.
- **Modern Applications**: Garlic supplements are widely used for immune support and heart health.

4. Scientific Support for Adaptogens and Ancient Remedies

Recent research has validated many of the benefits attributed to adaptogens and ancient remedies. Here are a few examples of how modern science supports these traditional practices:

- **Stress Reduction and Adaptogens**: Studies on ashwagandha and rhodiola show significant reductions in cortisol levels, reduced symptoms of anxiety, and improved cognitive function.
- **Anti-Inflammatory Effects of Turmeric**: Numerous studies have documented curcumin's anti-inflammatory effects, which are beneficial for arthritis, digestive health, and even mood disorders.
- **Immune Support from Reishi and Garlic**: Reishi mushrooms contain beta-glucans, compounds known to enhance immune response. Garlic's immune-boosting effects have been confirmed in studies showing reduced cold symptoms and improved resistance to infection.

These findings affirm the relevance of adaptogens and ancient remedies in modern wellness, particularly as people face increasing stress and inflammation-related health issues.

5. Incorporating Adaptogens and Ancient Remedies into Daily Life

Integrating adaptogens and ancient remedies into daily routines is easier than ever, thanks to modern supplements, teas, and wellness products. Here are a few practical ways to start:

- **Adaptogenic Blends**: Many health brands offer adaptogenic blends, combining herbs like ashwagandha, reishi, and rhodiola for a balanced, holistic approach to stress management.
- **Cooking with Spices**: Cooking with turmeric, ginger, garlic, and other beneficial spices adds flavor while providing health benefits. These spices can be incorporated into soups, teas, and marinades.
- **Tea Rituals**: Drinking teas that include holy basil, reishi, or ginseng supports relaxation and resilience. Teas are a gentle way to introduce adaptogens into the body, particularly in the evening or during times of high stress.

6. Safety and Precautions with Adaptogens

While adaptogens and ancient remedies offer many benefits, it is important to use them responsibly. Here are a few guidelines:

- **Consult with a Healthcare Provider**: Individuals with medical conditions, especially those on medication, should consult with a healthcare provider before using adaptogens, as some herbs can interact with medications.
- **Start Slowly**: Adaptogens are best introduced gradually. Some people may experience mild side effects, such as digestive upset or mild anxiety, which usually subside as the body adapts.
- **Rotate Adaptogens**: To prevent tolerance or dependence, it's beneficial to rotate adaptogens rather than taking a single herb daily for long periods. Rotating allows the body to benefit from different properties while reducing potential risks.

7. The Future of Adaptogens in Functional Medicine

As adaptogens and ancient remedies gain popularity, their role in functional medicine and holistic wellness is expanding. Functional medicine practitioners often include adaptogens as part of a comprehensive treatment plan, targeting specific needs like adrenal support, immune resilience, and cognitive enhancement. As research continues, adaptogens may also be integrated into conventional medicine for stress-related disorders, inflammation, and immune support.

The rise of adaptogens reflects a broader movement towards holistic wellness, where health is supported by addressing underlying imbalances rather than only treating symptoms. This shift highlights the relevance of traditional practices in addressing the demands of modern life.

Integrating Ancient Wisdom for Modern Resilience

Adaptogens and ancient remedies offer a bridge between traditional wisdom and modern wellness, providing tools to strengthen resilience, manage stress, and support long-term health. By incorporating these powerful plants and herbs into a balanced diet, individuals can enhance their ability to navigate life's challenges without compromising their well-being. Adaptogens remind us of the deep connection between nutrition and healing, and they encourage us to consider health as a dynamic, holistic journey.

Environmental Nutrition: How Soil Health Impacts Nutritional Quality

The connection between soil health and human nutrition is a vital yet often overlooked aspect of our food system. Healthy, nutrient-rich soil is the foundation of nutritious crops, yet modern agricultural practices have increasingly depleted soil health, impacting the quality and nutrient density of our food. Environmental nutrition explores how the health of our soil and the methods we use to cultivate it directly influence the nutritional value of the foods we eat.

This chapter delves into the importance of soil health, the consequences of conventional agricultural practices, and how regenerative and organic farming can improve soil quality and, by extension, human health.

1. Understanding Soil Health and Its Role in Nutrition

Soil is a complex ecosystem that teems with life and is home to countless microorganisms, fungi, and insects. This living community interacts to break down organic matter, release nutrients, and support plant growth. Soil health is defined by its structure, organic matter content, microbial activity, and nutrient availability, all of which contribute to plant health and crop yield.

Nutrient-Rich Soil and Nutrient-Dense Food

When soil is rich in minerals and organic matter, plants can absorb a wider array of nutrients, leading to more nutrient-dense food. Essential minerals such as calcium, magnesium, zinc, and iron originate in the soil, and the healthier the soil, the more these minerals are available for plants to uptake. Nutrient-rich soil also supports plant immune systems, making crops more resilient to disease and reducing the need for chemical interventions.

The Soil Microbiome

Similar to the human gut microbiome, the soil microbiome plays an integral role in nutrient cycling and plant health. Microorganisms in the soil help break down organic matter, fix nitrogen, and release nutrients, making them accessible to plants. Without a diverse microbiome, soil loses its fertility, and plants suffer from nutrient deficiencies, which ultimately impacts the nutrient content of our food.

2. The Impact of Conventional Farming on Soil Health

While conventional farming practices have increased food production, they have also led to soil degradation, reduced biodiversity, and nutrient depletion in the soil. Here are some of the ways that industrial agriculture negatively impacts soil health:

Monocropping

Monocropping, the practice of growing a single crop repeatedly on the same land, depletes the soil of specific nutrients and disrupts the natural balance of the soil ecosystem. For example, continuous corn or soybean farming can strip the soil of nitrogen and other essential nutrients, requiring synthetic fertilizers to compensate.

Synthetic Fertilizers and Chemical Pesticides

While synthetic fertilizers add essential nutrients like nitrogen, phosphorus, and potassium, they lack the diversity of nutrients found in organic matter and disrupt the soil microbiome. Chemical pesticides and herbicides kill both harmful and beneficial organisms in the soil, reducing biodiversity and weakening the soil's resilience. Over time, this dependency on synthetic inputs creates a cycle of degradation, as the soil becomes increasingly reliant on external chemicals to sustain crop growth.

Soil Erosion and Tillage

Frequent tilling, or turning the soil, can break down soil structure, releasing carbon dioxide into the atmosphere and reducing soil organic matter. Tillage also disrupts fungal networks and earthworms, which play essential roles in maintaining soil health. Soil erosion, accelerated by tilling and lack of plant cover, removes the nutrient-rich topsoil layer, further reducing the soil's capacity to nourish crops.

3. How Soil Degradation Affects Human Health

The decline in soil health has direct implications for human nutrition. Over the past several decades, studies have shown that the nutrient content of fruits, vegetables, and grains has declined, likely due to soil depletion and changes in agricultural practices. Crops grown in nutrient-poor soil are less likely to contain the vitamins and minerals essential for human health, which can contribute to nutrient deficiencies even in individuals consuming a diverse diet.

Loss of Micronutrients

Crops grown in depleted soil are often lower in micronutrients such as zinc, iron, magnesium, and selenium. These nutrients are critical for immune function, bone health, and cellular processes, and deficiencies can lead to a range of health issues, including anemia, weakened immunity, and poor cognitive function.

Reduced Phytochemical Content

Soil health not only affects mineral content but also influences phytochemical levels in plants. Phytochemicals, such as polyphenols and flavonoids, are antioxidant compounds that help protect plants from environmental stressors. Plants grown in healthy soil with diverse microbial communities are typically richer in phytochemicals, which in turn offer anti-inflammatory and antioxidant benefits to humans.

4. Regenerative Agriculture: A Solution to Soil Degradation

Regenerative agriculture is an approach to farming that focuses on restoring soil health, increasing biodiversity, and improving the environment. By promoting practices that build organic matter and enhance soil structure, regenerative agriculture supports nutrient-dense food production and helps sequester carbon, which mitigates climate change. Here are some key practices within regenerative agriculture:

Cover Cropping

Cover crops, such as clover, legumes, and grasses, are planted to cover the soil when the main crops are not in season. Cover cropping prevents erosion, improves soil organic matter, and supports the soil microbiome. Certain cover crops can also fix nitrogen from the air, reducing the need for synthetic fertilizers.

Crop Rotation

Rotating different types of crops on the same land over time helps maintain soil fertility and reduces pest and disease buildup. By alternating between nitrogen-fixing crops, such as legumes, and other crops, farmers can replenish soil nutrients naturally.

Composting and Organic Amendments

Adding compost and organic amendments, such as manure and green waste, returns essential nutrients to the soil. Organic matter feeds soil microbes, improves soil structure, and increases water retention, which is especially valuable in regions prone to drought.

Reducing or Eliminating Tillage

No-till or reduced-till farming practices protect soil structure, preserving carbon and enhancing microbial communities. These practices help maintain the integrity of the soil, making it more resilient to erosion and nutrient loss.

5. Organic Farming and Its Role in Soil Health

Organic farming emphasizes natural inputs and prohibits synthetic pesticides and fertilizers, making it a beneficial practice for soil health. Organic farms typically use compost, cover crops, and crop rotation to build soil fertility, which supports biodiversity and promotes nutrient-dense food production.

Soil Fertility and Organic Matter

Organic matter in the soil helps retain moisture, provides nutrients to plants, and fosters beneficial microbial communities. Organic farming practices, which avoid synthetic chemicals, allow for a more balanced soil microbiome, resulting in healthier crops.

Long-Term Sustainability

By prioritizing soil health, organic farming contributes to long-term agricultural sustainability. Unlike conventional methods that degrade soil over time, organic farming builds soil fertility, making it a viable option for future generations.

6. Benefits of Nutrient-Dense Food from Healthy Soil

When soil health is prioritized, the resulting food is more nutrient-dense, offering numerous health benefits. Nutrient-dense foods support immune function, reduce inflammation, and improve overall well-being. Consuming these foods reduces the risk of chronic diseases linked to nutrient deficiencies, such as cardiovascular disease, diabetes, and osteoporosis.

Enhanced Immune Function

Foods grown in nutrient-rich soil contain higher levels of vitamins and minerals essential for immune health, such as zinc, selenium, and vitamin C. These nutrients strengthen the body's defenses against infections and support recovery from illness.

Improved Mental Health and Cognitive Function

Nutrients like magnesium, iron, and B vitamins are crucial for brain function and mental health. Nutrient-dense produce from healthy soil provides these essential nutrients, which support mood, cognitive function, and resilience to stress.

7. Consumer Choices and Supporting Soil Health

Consumers play a vital role in supporting soil health by making informed food choices. Here are some ways individuals can promote soil health and contribute to sustainable food systems:

Choosing Organic and Regenerative Foods

Supporting organic and regenerative farms by purchasing their products encourages practices that prioritize soil health and reduce environmental impact. Look for certifications such as USDA Organic, Regenerative Organic, and other labels that indicate sustainable practices.

Local and Seasonal Eating

Buying local, seasonal produce often means supporting smaller farms that use more sustainable practices. Local food is fresher and more likely to be grown in nutrient-rich soil, as it hasn't traveled long distances or been stored for extended periods.

Composting and Reducing Food Waste

Composting food scraps returns organic matter to the soil, reducing waste and contributing to soil fertility. By composting, individuals can contribute to the cycle of nutrient renewal and reduce reliance on synthetic fertilizers.

8. The Future of Soil Health and Human Nutrition

Addressing soil degradation is essential for ensuring a nutritious food supply for future generations. As awareness grows about the connection between soil health and human nutrition, there is an increasing movement towards adopting sustainable farming practices.

Agroecology and Community Farming

Agroecology integrates ecological principles into agricultural practices, promoting biodiversity, natural pest control, and crop diversity. Community-supported agriculture (CSA) and urban farms are examples of agroecological practices that bring consumers closer to the source of their food, fostering a greater understanding of soil health.

Education and Policy Changes

Government and educational institutions have a role in promoting soil health through research, subsidies for sustainable practices, and public awareness campaigns. Policies that support regenerative farming can create an agricultural system that produces more nutrient-dense food and preserves the environment.

The Path to Nutrient-Rich, Sustainable Diets

The connection between soil health and human nutrition cannot be overstated. As the foundation of our food system, healthy soil ensures that crops are rich in the vitamins, minerals, and phytochemicals essential for human health. By supporting practices that restore and maintain soil health, we can contribute to a food system that nourishes both people and the planet. Embracing environmental nutrition allows us to make choices that align with our health needs and support the long-term sustainability of our food resources.

Future Trends in Nutrition: Precision Nutrition and Personalized Health

In recent years, the field of nutrition has evolved from one-size-fits-all guidelines to more individualized approaches, acknowledging that every person's nutritional needs are unique. Precision nutrition, also known as personalized nutrition, tailors dietary recommendations based on individual factors like genetics, lifestyle, and metabolic responses. This emerging trend leverages advancements in technology, genomics, and data analytics to optimize health outcomes and disease prevention.

In this chapter, we'll explore how precision nutrition and personalized health are reshaping the future of nutrition, the technologies driving these changes, and how individuals can benefit from customized dietary plans tailored to their unique needs.

1. What is Precision Nutrition?

Precision nutrition is a scientific approach that recognizes the variability in people's responses to food and nutrition interventions. It takes into account factors such as genetics, microbiome composition, metabolic rate, and lifestyle to develop dietary recommendations that optimize health on an individual basis. Unlike traditional nutritional advice, which is generalized for the entire population, precision nutrition aims to provide specific guidance that caters to the needs of each person.

- **Personalized Diet Plans**: Precision nutrition provides diet plans based on unique genetic, biological, and lifestyle factors. For instance, a person with a genetic predisposition to insulin resistance may benefit from a low-carbohydrate diet, while someone with high antioxidant needs may be encouraged to eat more fruits and vegetables.
- **Optimizing Health Outcomes**: By tailoring nutrition to individual characteristics, precision nutrition can improve health outcomes, prevent diseases, and enhance quality of life. Studies suggest that personalized diets are more

effective than standard dietary interventions in achieving weight loss, reducing inflammation, and managing blood sugar.

2. The Science Behind Precision Nutrition

The scientific foundation of precision nutrition lies in understanding how various biological factors influence nutrient needs and metabolic responses. Here are some key elements that form the basis of precision nutrition:

Genomics and Nutrigenomics

Nutrigenomics studies the interaction between nutrition and genes, helping researchers understand how genetic variations impact nutrient requirements and responses to different diets.

Genetic Variants and Diet: Certain genetic variants influence how well a person metabolizes nutrients. For instance, some individuals have a variation that reduces their ability to process folic acid, making them more prone to folate deficiency. Nutrigenomics allows for dietary adjustments based on these specific needs.

Epigenetics and Lifestyle Influence: Epigenetics refers to changes in gene expression caused by environmental factors like diet, exercise, and stress. Precision nutrition considers how lifestyle choices impact gene expression, providing strategies to positively influence genetic predispositions.

The Microbiome's Role in Nutrition

The gut microbiome, composed of trillions of bacteria, plays a crucial role in digestion, immunity, and metabolic health. Precision nutrition examines an individual's microbiome composition to tailor dietary recommendations that support gut health.

Microbiome Diversity: A diverse microbiome is associated with better health outcomes, and precision nutrition can identify foods that promote beneficial bacteria. For example, prebiotic foods like garlic and onions nourish good bacteria, while probiotics found in fermented foods enhance gut diversity.

Microbiome and Metabolic Health: Certain gut bacteria are linked to metabolic conditions like obesity and diabetes. Personalized nutrition can target these imbalances by recommending specific fibers or fermented foods that support a healthy microbiome and improve metabolic health.

Biomarkers and Metabolic Testing

Biomarkers, such as blood glucose, cholesterol levels, and inflammatory markers, provide measurable data about an individual's metabolic health. By analyzing these biomarkers, precision nutritionists can tailor dietary plans that address specific health concerns.

Blood Sugar Response: People respond differently to the same foods, and precision nutrition can use blood glucose monitoring to design diets that minimize blood sugar spikes. This is especially beneficial for managing conditions like diabetes and insulin resistance.

Lipid Profiles: Individuals with specific cholesterol markers or high triglycerides may require dietary adjustments, such as increasing omega-3 intake or reducing saturated fats, to manage cardiovascular risk.

3. Technologies Enabling Precision Nutrition

The rise of precision nutrition is fueled by advancements in technology that allow for in-depth analysis of individual health data. These technologies make it possible to create highly specific dietary plans that are tailored to each person's unique biological makeup.

Genetic Testing

Companies like 23andMe and AncestryDNA offer genetic testing services that provide insight into genetic predispositions related to nutrition. Genetic testing can reveal everything from lactose intolerance to predispositions for conditions like celiac disease, which can be factored into personalized dietary recommendations.

Nutritional Genomics Reports: Many companies now provide reports that include dietary insights based on genetic information, allowing individuals to understand how their genes affect their nutrition and metabolism.

Disease Prevention: Genetic testing can identify risks for diseases like cardiovascular disease and diabetes, allowing for early dietary interventions that may reduce the risk of these conditions.

Wearable Health Devices

Wearable devices, such as Fitbit, Apple Watch, and continuous glucose monitors (CGMs), track real-time health metrics like heart rate, activity levels, and blood glucose. These devices empower individuals to monitor their responses to food and adjust their diet accordingly.

Continuous Glucose Monitoring (CGM): CGMs track blood glucose levels throughout the day, providing insights into how different foods affect blood sugar. This data is valuable for creating a diet that stabilizes blood sugar and improves energy levels.

Fitness Trackers: Wearables that monitor activity and sleep patterns help individuals understand their caloric and nutrient needs based on lifestyle factors, optimizing diet for physical and mental well-being.

AI and Machine Learning

Artificial intelligence (AI) and machine learning algorithms are revolutionizing precision nutrition by analyzing vast amounts of health data to identify patterns and provide tailored recommendations.

Predictive Dietary Modeling: AI can predict how an individual will respond to certain foods based on data such as genetics, microbiome composition, and metabolic biomarkers. This modeling allows for more precise dietary interventions.

Personalized Meal Planning: Machine learning can help create meal plans that cater to specific goals, such as weight loss or muscle gain, by analyzing individual preferences, allergies, and dietary restrictions.

Enhanced Health Outcomes

Personalized diets are more effective at addressing individual health issues than generalized dietary guidelines. Studies have shown that precision nutrition can improve outcomes in weight management, blood sugar control, and mental health, among other areas.

Weight Management: A personalized diet that considers genetics, microbiome, and metabolic rate can optimize weight loss and maintenance, making it more sustainable.

Chronic Disease Prevention: Precision nutrition can reduce the risk of diseases like heart disease and type 2 diabetes by addressing specific dietary and lifestyle factors that influence these conditions.

Improved Dietary Adherence

Tailoring dietary recommendations to individual preferences and needs makes it easier to adhere to a healthy diet over the long term. Precision nutrition considers food preferences, cultural factors, and lifestyle constraints, which increases the likelihood of success.

Increased Nutritional Awareness

Precision nutrition encourages a deeper understanding of how food choices affect health, promoting mindfulness about diet and lifestyle. This awareness fosters healthier eating habits and empowers individuals to make informed choices that support their well-being.

The Future of Precision Nutrition

As technology advances, precision nutrition is expected to become more accessible, affordable, and effective. Future trends include integrating AI with wearable devices, expanding research on the microbiome, and making personalized health a standard part of healthcare.

Integrating AI with Wearables and Smart Kitchens

AI-powered wearable devices and smart kitchen appliances that monitor dietary intake, nutrient levels, and metabolic responses are likely to become more common. This integration will allow for real-time dietary adjustments and offer a seamless experience for users.

Microbiome Research and Probiotics

Ongoing research into the microbiome will provide deeper insights into how gut bacteria influence nutrition. This may lead to more precise recommendations for probiotic and prebiotic intake, further personalizing diet for optimal gut health.

Wider Adoption in Healthcare

Precision nutrition has the potential to become a standard component of healthcare, where doctors and dietitians use personalized data to guide treatment plans. This shift could transform healthcare from reactive to proactive, with nutrition playing a preventive role.

A New Era of Personalized Health

Precision nutrition represents a shift toward individualized dietary guidance that optimizes health outcomes based on each person's unique biology. By considering factors like genetics, lifestyle, and microbiome composition, precision nutrition offers a tailored approach to health that is more effective than generalized dietary recommendations. As this field continues to evolve, precision nutrition has the potential to empower individuals to take control of their health and create a future where diet is a powerful tool for disease prevention, longevity, and overall well-being.

The Intersection of Nutrition and Mental Health: Food for the Mind

The link between nutrition and mental health is increasingly recognized as a critical component of overall well-being. While traditional mental health treatments have largely focused on therapy and medication, new research suggests that diet plays a significant role in mood regulation, cognitive function, and resilience to stress. This chapter explores how certain foods and nutrients influence the brain, the role of gut health in mental wellness, and practical dietary strategies to support mental health.

1. The Role of Nutrition in Brain Function

The brain is a highly active organ, using up to 20% of the body's energy. Its functioning relies on a steady supply of nutrients, including vitamins, minerals, amino acids, and essential fats, which support neurotransmitter synthesis, neural protection, and cognitive health. Poor nutrition can lead to deficiencies that impair brain function, potentially resulting in mood disorders, cognitive decline, and increased vulnerability to stress.

Essential Nutrients for Mental Health

Certain nutrients are particularly important for mental health due to their roles in neurotransmitter production, energy metabolism, and cellular repair:

Omega-3 Fatty Acids: Found in fish, flaxseed, and walnuts, omega-3 fatty acids are essential for brain health. They support cell membrane integrity and play a key role in reducing inflammation, which is linked to depression and anxiety.

B Vitamins: B vitamins, especially B6, B12, and folate, are involved in producing serotonin, dopamine, and other neurotransmitters that influence mood. Deficiencies in these vitamins are associated with depression, fatigue, and cognitive decline.

Magnesium: Magnesium, found in leafy greens, nuts, and seeds, plays a role in stress response and relaxation. Low magnesium levels are linked to anxiety and irritability, and supplementation can improve symptoms of stress-related disorders.

Vitamin D: Often called the "sunshine vitamin," vitamin D is crucial for mood regulation. Low levels are associated with seasonal affective disorder (SAD) and depression, particularly in regions with limited sunlight exposure.

2. Gut Health and the Gut-Brain Connection

The gut and brain are closely connected through what is known as the gut-brain axis. This bidirectional communication system involves the nervous system, immune system, and gut microbiota, all of which influence mood, cognition, and stress response. Emerging research shows that gut health is vital to mental health, and that imbalances in gut bacteria can contribute to mood disorders.

The Microbiome's Role in Mental Health

The gut microbiome—the trillions of bacteria residing in the intestines—produces neurotransmitters like serotonin, dopamine, and

GABA, which regulate mood, anxiety, and sleep. About 90% of the body's serotonin, often referred to as the "feel-good hormone," is produced in the gut.

Dysbiosis and Mood Disorders: Dysbiosis, or an imbalance in gut bacteria, is linked to anxiety, depression, and even autism. When harmful bacteria outnumber beneficial ones, it can lead to inflammation, which affects the brain and contributes to mood disorders.

Probiotics and Mental Health: Probiotic-rich foods like yogurt, kefir, and fermented vegetables can support mental health by enhancing gut microbiota diversity. Studies have shown that probiotics can reduce symptoms of anxiety and depression, likely by improving gut health and reducing inflammation.

3. Inflammation and Mental Health

Chronic inflammation is a common feature in conditions like depression, anxiety, and Alzheimer's disease. While inflammation is a natural immune response, prolonged inflammation can damage cells and tissues, including those in the brain. Diet plays a crucial role in either promoting or reducing inflammation, making it an essential component of mental health management.

Anti-Inflammatory Diets and Brain Health

Dietary patterns that reduce inflammation, such as the Mediterranean and anti-inflammatory diets, have been associated with lower rates of depression and cognitive decline.

Mediterranean Diet: Rich in fruits, vegetables, whole grains, and fats, the Mediterranean diet reduces inflammation and is associated with a lower risk of depression. The diet's high content of antioxidants and omega-3s supports brain health by protecting neurons from oxidative stress.

Foods to Avoid: Processed foods high in sugar, refined carbohydrates, and unhealthy fats promote inflammation and can worsen mental health. Studies suggest that diets high in trans fats and sugar may impair cognitive function and increase depressive symptoms.

4. Blood Sugar Stability and Mood Regulation

Blood sugar imbalances can significantly impact mood, energy levels, and mental clarity. Fluctuations in blood sugar can lead to irritability, anxiety, and fatigue, commonly known as "hangry" symptoms. A diet that stabilizes blood sugar helps to maintain steady energy and mood, reducing the risk of mood swings and irritability.

Low-Glycemic Diets and Mental Health

Low-glycemic diets, which avoid sudden spikes in blood sugar, support mental health by providing a steady supply of glucose to the brain.

Complex Carbohydrates: Foods like whole grains, legumes, and vegetables provide slow-releasing energy that stabilizes blood sugar. Complex carbs also promote serotonin production, which can enhance mood.

Healthy Fats and Proteins: Including healthy fats and proteins in meals slows digestion, leading to sustained energy and fewer blood sugar crashes. Fatty fish, nuts, and lean meats are excellent sources of these nutrients and support both mood and cognition.

5. The Impact of Diet on Neurotransmitter Production

Neurotransmitters are chemicals that transmit signals between nerve cells in the brain, influencing mood, motivation, and cognitive function. Many neurotransmitters are synthesized from nutrients found in food, which means that diet has a direct effect on brain chemistry and mood.

Serotonin and Tryptophan

Serotonin, a neurotransmitter associated with feelings of happiness, is synthesized from tryptophan, an amino acid found in foods like turkey, eggs, and tofu. Diets rich in tryptophan can support serotonin production and improve mood.

Tryptophan-Rich Foods: Incorporating foods high in tryptophan may increase serotonin levels, promoting relaxation and well-being.

Carbohydrates and Serotonin: Consuming carbohydrates helps tryptophan enter the brain, supporting serotonin production. This is why some people crave carbs when feeling down—they may be unconsciously seeking a serotonin boost.

Dopamine and Tyrosine

Dopamine, a neurotransmitter linked to motivation and reward, is synthesized from tyrosine, an amino acid found in foods like chicken, fish, and dairy.

Tyrosine-Rich Foods: Including tyrosine-rich foods supports dopamine production, which can improve focus, motivation, and mood. A balanced intake of protein is crucial for maintaining healthy dopamine levels.

Exercise and Dopamine: Physical activity can boost dopamine levels, further enhancing mood and mental well-being.

6. Specific Diets and Mental Health Benefits

Certain dietary patterns have been linked to better mental health outcomes, particularly for mood disorders and cognitive decline. Here are a few diets that show promise in supporting mental health:

Mediterranean Diet

The Mediterranean diet, rich in vegetables, fruits, whole grains, and healthy fats, has been widely studied for its positive effects on mental health. The high intake of omega-3s, antioxidants, and fiber reduces inflammation, improves gut health, and supports cognitive function.

Ketogenic Diet

The ketogenic diet is high in fats, moderate in protein, and low in carbohydrates, leading the body to produce ketones for energy. Ketones have neuroprotective effects and may reduce symptoms of anxiety and depression by stabilizing blood sugar and reducing inflammation.

- **Ketones as Brain Fuel**: Ketones provide a stable source of energy for the brain, which may improve mental clarity and focus. Research suggests that a ketogenic diet may be beneficial for those with mood disorders, especially where traditional treatments have been ineffective.

- **Anti-Inflammatory Effects**: The ketogenic diet's emphasis on fats, especially omega-3s, supports anti-inflammatory processes that can benefit the brain.

Anti-Inflammatory Diet

The anti-inflammatory diet includes foods like berries, leafy greens, nuts, seeds, and fatty fish, all of which help reduce inflammation. This diet supports brain health and can help alleviate symptoms of depression and anxiety.

The Future of Nutritional Psychiatry

Nutritional psychiatry, an emerging field of mental health research, focuses on the impact of diet on mood and cognition. As evidence grows, dietary interventions may become a standard part of mental health treatment, particularly for conditions like depression, anxiety, and even neurodegenerative diseases. Researchers are exploring how targeted nutrition can reduce symptoms and improve the efficacy of traditional treatments.

Personalized Diet Plans for Mental Health

Personalized nutrition, based on genetics, microbiome composition, and biomarkers, is gaining traction in mental health care. Personalized diets can help address specific deficiencies, optimize nutrient intake, and improve mood, potentially reducing the need for medication. This approach is promising for treatment-resistant patients, as it considers individual variability in how people respond to food.

Integrating Nutrition with Traditional Therapies

Many mental health practitioners are beginning to incorporate nutritional counseling alongside therapy and medication, recognizing that diet can either support or hinder mental well-being. In the future, mental health care may include comprehensive dietary assessments and recommendations to support a holistic treatment approach.

Key Takeaways: Nutrition as a Pillar of Mental Health

The connection between nutrition and mental health is complex and multi-faceted, involving everything from brain function and neurotransmitter production to gut health and inflammation. As research continues to reveal how diet affects mood and cognitive function, it becomes clear that a nutrient-rich, anti-inflammatory diet can support mental well-being. Here are the key points to remember:

Brain Health Requires Nutrients: Essential nutrients like omega-3s, B vitamins, and magnesium play a central role in brain function and mood regulation.

Gut-Brain Axis: A healthy gut supports mental health through the production of neurotransmitters and the reduction of inflammation, emphasizing the importance of gut-friendly foods.

Inflammation and Mental Health: Chronic inflammation is linked to mood disorders, making an anti-inflammatory diet a valuable strategy for mental wellness.

Blood Sugar Stability: Maintaining stable blood sugar through a balanced diet supports consistent energy and mood, reducing irritability and fatigue.

Personalized Approaches: As the field of nutritional psychiatry grows, personalized diets based on individual health profiles may offer new options for mental health support.

Eating for Mental Wellness

The food we eat has a powerful impact on mental health, influencing everything from energy levels and mood stability to resilience against stress. By prioritizing nutrient-dense, anti-inflammatory foods and fostering gut health, individuals can support both their physical and mental well-being. The future of mental health care may well lie in a combination of nutrition and traditional therapy, providing a holistic approach that empowers individuals to achieve optimal wellness in mind and body.

The Ethics of Food Choices: Health, Sustainability, and Animal Welfare

In recent years, ethical considerations in food choices have gained significant attention as consumers become more aware of the impact their diets have on health, the environment, and animal welfare. This chapter explores how ethical eating encompasses more than just personal health—it's about choosing foods that support a sustainable planet, humane treatment of animals, and social responsibility. By making mindful food choices, individuals can contribute to a healthier world while supporting their own well-being.

Sustainable Agriculture: Regenerative agriculture, which focuses on soil health, crop diversity, and minimal chemical inputs, sequesters carbon in the soil and reduces greenhouse gases. Choosing foods grown with sustainable methods can contribute to mitigating climate change.

Land Use and Deforestation

Deforestation for agriculture, particularly for cattle ranching and soy and palm oil production, is a major driver of biodiversity loss and carbon emissions. Ethically minded consumers can choose foods that do not contribute to deforestation or that are certified by organizations promoting sustainable land use.

Choosing Certified Products: Look for products certified by organizations like the Rainforest Alliance or Fair Trade, which support sustainable land practices. These certifications help ensure that the products do not contribute to deforestation and have a lower environmental impact.

Avoiding Palm Oil and Non-Sustainable Soy: Opting for products that use alternative oils or certified sustainable soy can reduce the demand for land-intensive crops and help preserve rainforests.

Supporting Local Economies

Buying locally produced foods supports farmers, reduces transportation emissions, and keeps money within local communities. This can contribute to food security, create jobs, and strengthen local economies.

- **Community-Supported Agriculture (CSA)**: CSAs allow consumers to buy a share of a local farm's harvest, providing financial support to farmers while delivering fresh, seasonal produce to consumers.

- **Farmers' Markets**: Shopping at farmers' markets promotes local food systems and gives consumers direct access to information about how their food was produced, ensuring greater transparency.

6. Ethical Food Choices and Personal Health

Ethical food choices are not only beneficial for the environment and society but can also enhance personal health. Diets that prioritize whole, sustainably sourced foods tend to be rich in nutrients and low in processed ingredients, supporting overall well-being.

Nutrient-Dense Foods

Foods that are grown sustainably and humanely, such as organic vegetables, pasture-raised meats, and seasonal produce, are often more nutrient-dense than conventionally produced alternatives. This nutrient density supports immune health, reduces inflammation, and promotes longevity.

Chapter 13 What is Healthy? And what is NOT

Most of us are familiar with the outdated food pyramid, a once-common guide that encouraged daily servings of grains as the base of a "healthy" diet. However, nutritional science has evolved, and so has our understanding of what truly supports optimal health. Rather than following rigid guidelines or simply filling up on carbohydrates, we now know that the quality, source, and nutrient profile of food are essential factors that can influence everything from metabolic health to cognitive function and longevity.

In this chapter, I'll outline foods according to a hierarchy from the healthiest options—those that provide the most nutrition with minimal health risks—to the least healthy options, which are often detrimental to health when consumed regularly. This updated hierarchy emphasizes foods in their natural or minimally processed states, prioritizing nutrient density, bioavailability, and the degree to which they align with our body's needs.

Also keep in mind that it's not necessarily a "ranking" but an overall guide to help choose foods that you can eat more or less of at your determination.

The hierarchy begins with high-quality animal products, such as grass-fed and grass-finished meats, organ meats, and eggs. These are followed by other meats and poultry, which, although slightly different in nutrient profile, are still nutrient-dense. As we progress through this list, you'll find foods like raw dairy, fermented foods, and certain vegetables and fruits, each with unique benefits. Toward the end, we touch on whole grains, which offer some nutritional value but can also contain antinutrients that affect mineral absorption. Finally, at the very bottom of the hierarchy, we find trans fats—highly processed and chemically altered fats that should be avoided for optimal health.

By understanding where different foods fall on this hierarchy, we can make informed dietary choices that prioritize quality over quantity, focusing on the foods that provide the highest health benefits. This new framework isn't just about filling up; it's about fueling our bodies with foods that support our biological needs, while limiting those that do more harm than good.

Most Healthy to Most Unhealthy

1. Grass Fed and Grass Finished Red Meat, Organ Meats, Eggs
2. Other Meats, Chicken, Other Poultry, Pork
3. Dairy, Raw Milk, Raw Cheese
4. Fermented Foods
5. Some vegetables and fruits
6. Whole grains, Bread, Pasta, Rice, Tortillas, Starchy Carbohydrates
7. Trans Fats

The Crème of the Crop: Foods at the Pinnacle of Nutritional Health

At the very top of the hierarchy lie the crème of the crop—foods that pack the most powerful nutritional punch with minimal drawbacks. These foods, including grass-fed and grass-finished red meats, organ meats, and eggs, are the most nutrient-dense, bioavailable sources of vitamins, minerals, and essential fatty acids available. Their placement at the top isn't based on any fad or trend; rather, it's rooted in science and our evolutionary biology. These foods align with what our bodies are designed to thrive on, offering complete proteins, crucial micronutrients, and healthy fats in a form that is easy for our bodies to absorb and utilize.

Grass-Fed and Grass-Finished Red Meat: Unlike conventionally raised meats, grass-fed and grass-finished beef comes from animals that graze on pasture their entire lives, resulting in meat that is richer in omega-3 fatty acids, CLA (conjugated linoleic acid), and antioxidants. These nutrients support cardiovascular health, reduce inflammation, and help maintain a healthy balance of fats in the body.

Organ Meats: Often referred to as "nature's multivitamin," organ meats like liver, heart, and kidneys offer an impressive concentration of essential nutrients. Liver, for instance, is a top source of bioavailable vitamin A, iron, and B vitamins. These nutrients play a critical role in everything from immune function to cognitive health, making organ meats invaluable for supporting overall well-being.

311

Eggs: Eggs, particularly those from pasture-raised hens, are incredibly nutrient-dense and contain a wealth of health-promoting nutrients. Rich in high-quality protein, choline (which supports brain function), and healthy fats, eggs are also a rare source of natural vitamin D. Their versatility and accessibility make them an ideal addition to almost any diet.

The crème of the crop foods aren't just about filling you up—they're about fueling your body with the most bioavailable, nutrient-dense sources possible. When included regularly in the diet, these foods provide the building blocks needed for optimal health, energy, and longevity.

Good For You: Chicken, Poultry, Pork, and Other Meats

While grass-fed red meats and organ meats hold the top spot in terms of nutrient density and bioavailability, the second tier features other animal proteins like chicken, poultry, pork, and various meats that provide valuable nutrients and high-quality protein but with slight differences in their health benefits. These meats are versatile and widely available, making them essential parts of a balanced diet. While they don't contain the same concentration of omega-3 fatty acids as grass-fed beef, they still deliver essential nutrients, vitamins, and amino acids that support muscle growth, metabolic function, and immune health.

Chicken and Poultry: Chicken and other poultry (like turkey and duck) are excellent sources of lean protein, low in saturated fat, and rich in B vitamins (particularly niacin and B6), which support energy production and brain health. White meat, found in chicken breasts, is particularly low in fat, making it a good option for those looking to reduce calorie intake while maintaining high protein levels. Dark meat, found in the thighs and drumsticks, provides higher levels of iron and zinc, which are crucial for immune health and red blood cell production. For the best nutritional profile, choosing pasture-raised or organic poultry can further enhance the quality of the meat.

Pork: Pork, often referred to as "the other white meat," is a rich source of thiamine, an essential vitamin that plays a vital role in energy metabolism and nerve function. Cuts like pork tenderloin and loin chops are relatively lean, while cuts like bacon and pork belly are higher in fat. Opting for pasture-raised pork when possible can provide a better balance of fats, including a modest amount of omega-3s compared to conventionally raised pork. Pork also contains zinc, selenium, and B vitamins, all of which are crucial for immune support and cellular repair.

Other Meats (Lamb, Goat, Bison): This category includes meats like lamb, goat, and bison, each offering a unique nutrient profile. Lamb and bison, especially when grass-fed, are particularly nutrient-dense, providing iron, zinc, B vitamins, and a slightly higher concentration of omega-3 fatty acids compared to conventional meats. Goat meat, a staple in many cuisines worldwide, is leaner than beef and often lower in cholesterol, making it an excellent option for those seeking variety without added fat. These meats are rich in high-quality protein and amino acids, supporting muscle repair, immune function, and overall health.

Butter and Ghee: Butter, especially when made from the milk of grass-fed cows, is rich in fat-soluble vitamins and CLA, which can reduce inflammation and improve immune response. Ghee, a clarified form of butter, is lactose-free and has a high smoke point, making it an excellent choice for cooking. Both butter and ghee provide healthy fats that support brain health, hormone production, and the absorption of fat-soluble vitamins.

Nutritional Benefits and Considerations

- **Protein Quality:** All meats in this tier provide complete proteins, meaning they contain all essential amino acids necessary for muscle repair, tissue health, and metabolic processes. This makes them especially beneficial for individuals looking to support an active lifestyle.
- **Micronutrient Diversity:** Chicken, pork, and other meats contribute important micronutrients such as iron, zinc, and B vitamins that support various bodily functions, including immune health, energy production, and cognitive function.
- **Fat Profile Differences:** Unlike grass-fed beef, which is richer in omega-3s, these meats generally contain a higher ratio of omega-6 fatty acids. While omega-6 fats are essential, a balanced intake relative to omega-3s is ideal for maintaining a healthy inflammatory response. Choosing pasture-raised or free-range options when available can slightly improve the omega-3 content.
-

Cooking and Pairing Tips

For optimal health benefits, consider preparing these meats in ways that retain their nutrients without adding unnecessary calories. Grilling, baking, or lightly sautéing with healthy oils like olive or avocado oil can preserve flavor and nutrient quality. Pairing these meats with fiber-rich vegetables and antioxidant-dense spices (like turmeric or garlic) can further enhance the meal's nutritional value, supporting digestion and nutrient absorption.

OK for Some: Dairy – Raw Milk, Raw Cheese, and Nutrient-Dense Dairy Products

In the third tier of the hierarchy, we find dairy products, particularly those in their raw, unprocessed forms. Raw milk, raw cheese, and other minimally processed dairy offer a rich array of nutrients, including essential vitamins, minerals, healthy fats, and bioavailable proteins. For those who can tolerate dairy, these foods provide significant health benefits and contribute to bone health, immune support, and muscle repair. However, quality and source matter greatly when it comes to dairy, as processing can diminish nutritional value and add unnecessary additives.

Raw, unpasteurized dairy is prized for retaining natural enzymes, probiotics, and vitamins often lost in conventional dairy processing. The enzymes and beneficial bacteria found in raw dairy can enhance digestion and nutrient absorption, making these products not only nutritious but also supportive of gut health.

Raw Milk: Raw milk is milk in its most natural state, free from pasteurization and homogenization. This milk retains valuable enzymes like lactase, which helps break down lactose and can make it easier to digest for those who may struggle with lactose intolerance. Raw milk is also a rich source of fat-soluble vitamins (A, D, E, and K2), essential for bone health, immune function, and cellular growth. Additionally, raw milk offers high-quality protein, calcium, and healthy fats that promote overall health. When choosing raw milk, sourcing from grass-fed, pasture-raised cows is ideal, as it can contain higher levels of omega-3 fatty acids and CLA (conjugated linoleic acid), beneficial for metabolic health.

Raw Cheese: Raw, unpasteurized cheese retains live enzymes and beneficial bacteria, contributing to a healthy gut microbiome and supporting digestive health. Raw cheese is also rich in calcium, protein, and B vitamins, particularly B12, which is crucial for energy production and nervous system health. Because it is aged, raw cheese is often lower in lactose than milk, making it easier for those with lactose sensitivities to tolerate. Like raw milk, cheese from grass-fed animals provides a better balance of omega-3 to omega-6 fatty acids and includes a natural source of vitamin K2, which is important for cardiovascular and bone health.

Yogurt and Kefir: Fermented dairy products like yogurt and kefir are excellent sources of probiotics, which support gut health and immune function. Yogurt and kefir provide high-quality protein, calcium, and various B vitamins while also helping to promote a healthy digestive system. The fermentation process increases the bioavailability of certain nutrients, making them easier to absorb. Opting for unsweetened, full-fat versions and ideally those made from raw milk ensures minimal processing and maximum health benefits.

Nutritional Benefits and Considerations

Bioavailability of Nutrients: Dairy products are rich in bioavailable calcium, which is essential for bone density and muscle function. They also provide magnesium, potassium, and phosphorus, all of which contribute to cellular health and fluid balance.

Healthy Fats and Protein: Full-fat dairy products contain healthy fats that aid in vitamin absorption and provide lasting satiety. Dairy proteins, like casein and whey, are complete proteins, containing all essential amino acids needed for muscle growth and repair.

Probiotics and Digestive Health: Fermented dairy products, like raw yogurt and kefir, are natural sources of probiotics that help balance the gut microbiome, improve digestion, and support the immune system. These probiotics can be especially beneficial in maintaining gut health, which is closely linked to mental and metabolic health.

Choosing the Best Dairy Options

When selecting dairy, quality is paramount. The benefits of raw milk and raw cheese come from their unprocessed nature, which preserves natural enzymes, probiotics, and nutrients. Conventional dairy products are often pasteurized, which kills beneficial bacteria, and homogenized, which alters the fat structure. These processes can reduce the nutritional value of dairy and, in some cases, make it harder for individuals to digest.

For those without access to raw dairy, choosing organic, grass-fed, and minimally processed dairy options can provide similar benefits. Grass-fed dairy products contain higher levels of beneficial fats, like omega-3 fatty acids, and more vitamin K2, which supports cardiovascular health.

Addressing Lactose Intolerance and Sensitivity

For individuals sensitive to lactose, fermented dairy products (like yogurt and kefir) or aged cheeses are often better tolerated, as they contain lower levels of lactose. Ghee, which is lactose- and casein-free, is another excellent alternative for those sensitive to dairy. Additionally, raw dairy may be more easily digested by some due to its natural lactase content, which aids in breaking down lactose.

Practical Tips for Including Dairy in the Diet

Opt for Full-Fat Options: Full-fat dairy is less processed than low-fat alternatives and provides the full range of natural vitamins and healthy fats.

Add Fermented Dairy to Meals: Incorporating fermented dairy products like kefir or yogurt into smoothies, breakfasts, or snacks can support gut health and provide a balanced source of protein, fat, and carbohydrates.

Use Butter and Ghee for Cooking: Butter and ghee are excellent for cooking at medium to high temperatures due to their stability and high smoke points. They also add a rich flavor to dishes, making them a versatile addition to savory recipes.

Conclusion: The Nutritional Power of Quality Dairy

Dairy products, particularly in their raw, unprocessed forms, offer a wealth of health benefits and fit well into a nutrient-dense diet. From supporting bone density and digestive health to providing high-quality protein and essential vitamins, dairy holds a unique place in the hierarchy of healthiest foods. For those who can tolerate dairy, raw milk, raw cheese, and fermented dairy products are valuable sources of nutrients that contribute to overall health. However, sourcing high-quality, minimally processed options is essential to unlocking the full potential of dairy's nutritional benefits.

By selecting quality dairy products and incorporating them into meals mindfully, individuals can enjoy the benefits of dairy without the downsides often associated with conventional, heavily processed options.

Good For Your Gut: Fermented Foods

Fermented foods hold a unique place in the hierarchy due to their powerful benefits for gut health. Through the natural fermentation process, these foods develop beneficial bacteria (probiotics) that can improve digestion, support immune function, and enhance nutrient absorption. Fermentation also often enhances the flavor, shelf life, and nutritional value of the foods, making them a valuable addition to any diet.

Examples of Fermented Foods

Fermented foods come in a variety of forms, flavors, and cultural traditions. Here are some common and widely enjoyed options:

Sauerkraut: A traditional German dish of fermented cabbage, sauerkraut is rich in probiotics and high in fiber, supporting digestion and gut health.

Kimchi: A Korean staple, kimchi is a spicy, fermented cabbage dish often made with garlic, ginger, and chili flakes. It's loaded with probiotics and antioxidants that promote immune health.

Yogurt: Perhaps the most widely recognized fermented food, yogurt is made from fermented milk and contains live bacteria cultures. Full-fat, unsweetened yogurt provides beneficial probiotics and protein.

Kefir: A fermented milk drink similar to yogurt but with a thinner consistency, kefir is rich in a wider variety of probiotic strains. It's often better tolerated by those with lactose sensitivities.

Miso: A Japanese fermented soybean paste, miso is commonly used in soups and sauces. It provides probiotics along with protein, vitamins, and minerals.

Tempeh: A fermented soybean product from Indonesia, tempeh has a firm texture and is high in protein, fiber, and probiotics. It's a versatile addition to many dishes.

- **Kombucha:** A slightly tangy, effervescent tea, kombucha is fermented with a symbiotic culture of bacteria and yeast (SCOBY). It provides probiotics and antioxidants, supporting gut health and hydration.
- **Natto:** A traditional Japanese food made from fermented soybeans, natto is an acquired taste but is extremely rich in probiotics and vitamin K2, beneficial for heart and bone health.

Benefits of Fermented Foods for Gut Health

Fermented foods are particularly beneficial for gut health due to their high probiotic content. Probiotics are beneficial bacteria that can help restore the natural balance of microorganisms in the gut, which is essential for a well-functioning digestive system. Here's how fermented foods support a healthy gut:

Improved Digestion: The beneficial bacteria in fermented foods help break down food, making it easier to digest and absorb nutrients. They can also alleviate digestive discomfort and reduce symptoms of bloating and gas.

Enhanced Nutrient Absorption: Fermentation increases the bioavailability of nutrients, meaning that the body can absorb them more easily. For example, fermented dairy products like yogurt and kefir enhance calcium absorption.

Support for Gut Flora Diversity: A diverse microbiome is linked to better health outcomes. Fermented foods help introduce a wide variety of beneficial bacteria strains, which support a balanced gut environment.

Reduction of Antinutrients: Fermentation can reduce antinutrients (like phytates in grains and legumes), which otherwise inhibit the absorption of minerals like zinc and iron. By reducing these compounds, fermented foods make nutrients more accessible to the body.

The Importance of Maintaining a Healthy Gut

A healthy gut goes far beyond digestion. In fact, the gut is sometimes referred to as the "second brain" due to its close connection with overall health and its impact on various bodily systems, especially the immune system. Approximately 70-80% of the body's immune cells reside in the gut, meaning that a healthy gut is essential for a well-functioning immune response. Here's why maintaining a healthy gut is so critical:

Supports the Immune System: The gut microbiome, a diverse community of bacteria, plays a central role in modulating the immune system. Beneficial bacteria in the gut help train immune cells to recognize and respond to harmful pathogens without overreacting to harmless substances, reducing the risk of chronic inflammation.

Protects Against Pathogens: A balanced gut microbiome acts as a barrier against harmful bacteria and viruses. The beneficial bacteria in fermented foods can outcompete potentially harmful microbes, keeping the digestive system and immune system strong.

Reduces Inflammation: Chronic inflammation is linked to many diseases, from autoimmune disorders to cardiovascular issues. A healthy gut microbiome helps regulate inflammation in the body, lowering the risk of inflammatory conditions.

Enhances Mental Health and Cognitive Function: Research has shown that gut health is closely connected to mental well-being, as the gut microbiome influences neurotransmitter production and communication between the gut and brain. This means that a healthy gut can positively impact mood, stress levels, and cognitive function.

Practical Tips for Incorporating Fermented Foods

Adding fermented foods to your diet is a simple and effective way to support gut health and the immune system. Here are some tips for making fermented foods a regular part of your meals:

Start Slowly: If you're new to fermented foods, introduce them gradually to give your body time to adjust. Begin with small servings and increase the amount as your gut gets used to the additional probiotics.

Opt for Unpasteurized Products: Many store-bought fermented foods are pasteurized, which kills beneficial bacteria. Choose raw, unpasteurized versions for the highest probiotic content.

Incorporate a Variety: Eating a range of fermented foods, like yogurt, sauerkraut, and kefir, provides a diverse spectrum of probiotic strains, which can better support the gut microbiome.

Use as Condiments or Sides: Fermented foods make excellent condiments or side dishes. For example, add a spoonful of sauerkraut or kimchi to meals, use yogurt as a base for smoothies, or enjoy a glass of kombucha as a refreshing drink.

Fermented Foods as a Pillar of Gut Health

Fermented foods offer unique and powerful benefits for gut health, digestion, and the immune system. By incorporating these nutrient-rich, probiotic-packed foods into your diet, you're not only supporting your digestive health but also bolstering your body's natural defenses. As part of the food hierarchy, fermented foods play an essential role in maintaining a balanced, resilient microbiome, which is fundamental for overall health and well-being.

OK For Some: Vegetables and Fruits – Separating Nutrient-Dense Choices from Potential Risks

Vegetables and fruits often come to mind as "health foods," but not all are created equal. Some plant foods offer impressive health benefits, while others contain natural compounds that may interfere with nutrient absorption or even irritate the digestive system. In particular, fruits commonly thought of as vegetables—such as cucumbers, squash, and avocados—tend to be nutrient-dense and low in natural sugars, making them more compatible with a healthy diet than many other fruits and vegetables. By understanding the differences in nutrient density, phytochemicals, and the potential pitfalls of high-fructose fruits, we can make informed choices about which plant foods to consume regularly and which to enjoy in moderation.

Distinguishing Fruits Commonly Thought of as Vegetables

Fruits like cucumbers, squash, avocados, and tomatoes are botanically classified as fruits but are often used in savory dishes and thought of as vegetables. These fruits are generally low in sugar and provide a range of vitamins, minerals, and fiber with minimal impact on blood sugar. Here's a closer look at some of these unique plant foods:

Cucumbers and Squash: Both cucumbers and summer squash (like zucchini) are low in calories and carbohydrates, making them ideal for low-carb diets. They are also rich in water, which helps with hydration, and provide small amounts of vitamins A and C.

Avocados: Avocados are exceptionally nutrient-dense, offering healthy monounsaturated fats, fiber, and high levels of potassium. Their low sugar content and high nutrient density make them one of the healthiest plant foods available.

Tomatoes: Although higher in sugar than some vegetables, tomatoes contain lycopene, a powerful antioxidant associated with heart health and cancer prevention. Cooking tomatoes increases the bioavailability of lycopene, making cooked tomatoes particularly beneficial.

These "vegetable-like" fruits are often better options than traditional fruits due to their nutrient density, low sugar content, and overall health benefits.

Nutrient Concerns in Vegetables: Lectins, Oxalates, and Bioavailability

While vegetables can be rich in vitamins, minerals, and fiber, certain compounds within them—such as lectins and oxalates—can pose challenges to nutrient absorption and digestion. Here's a breakdown of these compounds and their potential impact:

Lectins: Lectins are proteins found in legumes, grains, and some vegetables (particularly nightshades like tomatoes and peppers). In their raw form, lectins can bind to cell membranes, which can lead to digestive irritation and impair nutrient absorption. Cooking or fermenting foods with lectins can reduce their levels, making them safer to consume. However, individuals with sensitivities to lectins may benefit from minimizing high-lectin vegetables.

Oxalates: Oxalates are naturally occurring compounds found in foods like spinach, beets, and rhubarb. They can bind to calcium in the digestive tract, reducing the bioavailability of this mineral and, in some cases, leading to kidney stones. People prone to kidney issues or calcium deficiencies may benefit from avoiding high-oxalate vegetables or consuming them in moderation.

Phytochemicals and Bioavailability: Vegetables contain beneficial phytochemicals—such as polyphenols, flavonoids, and carotenoids—that have antioxidant and anti-inflammatory properties. However, some phytochemicals are more bioavailable when cooked, while others are better absorbed raw. For example, the lycopene in tomatoes becomes more bioavailable when cooked, while vitamin C in bell peppers is most potent when raw.

By being mindful of lectins, oxalates, and the bioavailability of specific nutrients, we can choose vegetables that offer the most benefit without the drawbacks.

The Downside of High-Fructose Fruits

Fruits can be rich in vitamins, fiber, and antioxidants, however many of them contain high levels of fructose, a type of sugar that can contribute to metabolic issues when consumed in large amounts. Here are a few key points to consider when it comes to fruit consumption:

Fructose and Metabolic Health: Unlike glucose, which can be used by nearly all cells in the body, fructose is primarily processed by the liver. High intake of fructose can lead to fat accumulation in the liver, contributing to non-alcoholic fatty liver disease (NAFLD) and insulin resistance over time. Even though fruits contain fiber, which can moderate blood sugar spikes, high-fructose fruits (such as grapes, mangoes, and bananas) can still pose a risk when consumed frequently.

Seasonal Availability: Historically, fruits were only available seasonally, meaning they were consumed in smaller, infrequent amounts. Today, fruits are available year-round due to global agriculture and refrigeration, which can encourage overconsumption and result in high fructose intake throughout the year.

Genetic Modification and Selective Breeding: Many modern fruits have been selectively bred to be larger, sweeter, and longer-lasting, often at the expense of nutrient density. For example, wild apples were once small, fibrous, and far less sweet compared to the large, sugary varieties available today. These modified fruits contain more sugar than their wild counterparts and can contribute to sugar cravings and blood sugar imbalances.

A Bit More on Fructose

Fructose is a simple sugar found naturally in fruits and honey, has become a significant public health concern due to its prevalence in processed foods, especially in the form of high-fructose corn syrup (HFCS) and table sugar (sucrose, which is 50% fructose). While small amounts of naturally occurring fructose in whole foods are generally safe, the high levels of added fructose in modern diets pose several health risks. Here are key reasons why fructose is considered dangerous in excess:

Unique Metabolic Pathway and Liver Overload: Unlike glucose, which can be used by virtually all cells in the body for energy, fructose is primarily metabolized in the liver. When large amounts of fructose are consumed, the liver is forced to process it rapidly, which can lead to an overload. This overload pushes the liver to convert fructose into fat, some of which is stored in the liver itself, contributing to non-alcoholic fatty liver disease (NAFLD). Excessive fat in the liver can impair its function, increase insulin resistance, and promote inflammation.

Insulin Resistance and Metabolic Syndrome: Fructose doesn't stimulate insulin secretion the way glucose does, nor does it prompt the release of leptin, the hormone responsible for satiety. As a result, fructose can lead to overeating and weight gain because it doesn't signal fullness as effectively as other sugars. Over time, high fructose intake can contribute to insulin resistance, a condition where the body's cells become less responsive to insulin. Insulin resistance is a core feature of metabolic syndrome and is closely linked to type 2 diabetes, obesity, and cardiovascular disease.

Increased Fat Storage and Obesity: Fructose promotes fat storage more than glucose does. When consumed in high amounts, fructose enhances the production of triglycerides and very low-density lipoprotein (VLDL) particles, which circulate in the bloodstream and deposit fat in tissues. This increase in circulating fats raises the risk of obesity and visceral fat accumulation, a type of fat associated with increased risk of metabolic diseases, including heart disease.

Elevated Uric Acid Levels: Fructose metabolism increases the production of uric acid, a waste product that, when elevated, can contribute to gout and kidney stones. Uric acid also plays a role in the development of hypertension (high blood pressure) by inhibiting nitric oxide, a molecule that helps blood vessels relax. Elevated uric acid can therefore impair blood flow and increase cardiovascular risks.

Oxidative Stress and Inflammation: Excessive fructose consumption is linked to increased oxidative stress, as it produces byproducts that can damage cells and tissues. Fructose metabolism generates more reactive oxygen species (ROS) than glucose metabolism, which can lead to oxidative damage within cells. This oxidative stress is associated with chronic inflammation, a risk factor for several diseases, including heart disease, diabetes, and cancer.

Impaired Gut Health: High fructose intake, particularly from processed foods, can disrupt the gut microbiome and lead to gut permeability, often referred to as "leaky gut." An imbalance in the gut microbiota may increase susceptibility to inflammation, metabolic dysfunction, and immune-related diseases. Additionally, some people have difficulty absorbing fructose, leading to gastrointestinal symptoms such as bloating, gas, and abdominal pain.

Addictive Properties: Fructose has been shown to stimulate reward centers in the brain in a similar way to addictive substances, potentially leading to cravings and overconsumption. The lack of satiety signals combined with the pleasurable response to fructose makes it easy for people to overeat foods high in fructose, contributing to a cycle of poor eating habits and obesity.

Increased Risk of Cardiovascular Disease: Through its effects on insulin resistance, inflammation, lipid metabolism, and hypertension, excessive fructose intake has been associated with an increased risk of cardiovascular disease. The rise in triglycerides, LDL cholesterol, and blood pressure due to fructose can all damage cardiovascular health over time.

While small amounts of fructose in whole fruits pose minimal risk, the high levels of added fructose in processed foods can lead to **serious** health consequences. The unique metabolic pathway of fructose strains the liver, promotes fat storage, drives inflammation, and impairs metabolic health, all of which contribute to the development of chronic diseases. Reducing added fructose intake and focusing on whole foods can help mitigate these risks and support long-term health.

For these reasons, it may be wise to consume high-fructose fruits more sparingly and choose those that are lower in fructose and high in fiber, such as berries, which provide a range of nutrients with a lower glycemic impact.

Benefits of Certain Vegetables and Low-Sugar Fruits

While it's essential to be mindful of sugar content and antinutrients, certain vegetables and low-sugar fruits can still be valuable additions to a balanced diet. These options provide essential vitamins, minerals, and antioxidants that support overall health with minimal risk of negative effects:

Leafy Greens (e.g., Spinach, Kale, Swiss Chard): Leafy greens are rich in fiber, vitamins A, C, K, and folate. They support heart health, eye health, and immune function. For those concerned about oxalates, rotating greens (e.g., mixing in romaine or arugula) can help manage intake.

Cruciferous Vegetables (e.g., Broccoli, Cauliflower, Brussels Sprouts): Cruciferous vegetables are high in fiber, vitamins, and sulfur-containing compounds that support liver detoxification. Cooking these vegetables can reduce their goitrogen content, which may interfere with thyroid function if eaten in excess.

Berries (e.g., Blueberries, Raspberries, Strawberries): Berries are some of the lowest-sugar fruits and are high in fiber, vitamins, and antioxidants. They provide anti-inflammatory benefits and have a low impact on blood sugar, making them a good choice for regular consumption.

Bell Peppers: High in vitamin C, antioxidants, and fiber, bell peppers are a versatile, low-sugar vegetable that can support immune health and reduce oxidative stress.

Practical Tips for Consuming Vegetables and Fruits

To maximize the benefits of vegetables and fruits while minimizing potential downsides, here are some practical tips:

Cook Certain Vegetables: Cooking vegetables like spinach, kale, and broccoli can reduce their levels of oxalates and goitrogens, making them easier to digest and enhancing nutrient absorption.

Rotate High-Oxalate Vegetables: Rather than consuming high-oxalate vegetables daily, rotate them with lower-oxalate options to prevent excessive accumulation of oxalates in the body.

Prioritize Low-Sugar Fruits: Focus on low-sugar, high-fiber fruits like berries and limit high-fructose fruits like bananas and mangoes. This helps reduce fructose intake and supports metabolic health.

Choose Seasonal and Local Options: Whenever possible, select seasonal, local fruits and vegetables, which are often fresher and less likely to have been genetically modified or heavily treated with chemicals.

Experiment with Fermented Vegetables: Fermented options like kimchi, sauerkraut, and pickled vegetables offer probiotic benefits that can support gut health while delivering fiber and nutrients.

Vegetables and Fruits in Moderation for Optimal Health

While vegetables and fruits can offer valuable nutrients, it's essential to choose wisely and consider the impact of antinutrients, sugar content, and nutrient bioavailability. Low-sugar, nutrient-dense fruits and carefully selected vegetables can be healthy additions to the diet, while others, particularly high-fructose fruits and high-lectin vegetables, may be better enjoyed in moderation. By prioritizing quality, seasonal availability, and nutrient density, we can make vegetables and fruits a beneficial part of a balanced diet without compromising on health.

Not Great: Whole Grains, Pasta, Rice, Bread, and Tortillas – A Nutritional Misstep?

Whole grains and carbohydrate-rich foods, such as pasta, rice, bread, and tortillas, have long been promoted as foundational to a balanced diet. However, emerging science, along with an understanding of human physiology and metabolic health, has challenged the role of these foods in optimal nutrition. While whole grains and similar foods provide some nutrients, they also come with drawbacks that can negatively impact metabolic health, weight management, and overall well-being. In this section, we'll explore why carbohydrates are not "essential" in the diet, how the Randle Cycle sheds light on their metabolic impact, and the reasons to consider minimizing or avoiding these foods for better health.

The Myth of "Essential Carbohydrates"

One of the most persistent myths in nutrition is that carbohydrates are essential for health. Unlike fats and proteins, which provide essential fatty acids and amino acids respectively, carbohydrates do not contain any "essential" nutrients. In fact, the human body can create glucose, the simple sugar that fuels cells—from non-carbohydrate sources through a process called *gluconeogenesis*. This means that while carbohydrates can provide energy, they are not required for survival or optimal health.

Proteins and Fats as Essential Nutrients: Proteins provide amino acids necessary for tissue repair, immune function, and hormone production, while fats supply essential fatty acids needed for brain health, cellular structure, and hormone synthesis. Carbohydrates, by contrast, do not provide any unique, irreplaceable nutrients.

Carbohydrate Energy as Non-Essential: Since the body can convert proteins and fats into glucose as needed, carbohydrates are not a mandatory source of energy. The liver and kidneys can synthesize sufficient glucose to meet the body's needs, particularly for tissues like the brain that prefer glucose for energy.

The Randle Cycle and Carbohydrate Metabolism

The Randle Cycle, also known as the glucose-fatty acid cycle, is a metabolic mechanism that helps explain how the body chooses to burn carbohydrates or fats as fuel. This cycle highlights why a diet high in carbohydrates can be detrimental, especially in combination with dietary fats.

Understanding the Randle Cycle: When carbohydrate intake is high, the body prioritizes glucose as its primary energy source and suppresses fat oxidation. This occurs because glucose metabolism inhibits fatty acid metabolism, causing fat to be stored rather than burned for energy. On the other hand, when carbohydrate intake is low, the body readily uses fats for energy, resulting in better metabolic flexibility and less fat storage.

Implications for Metabolic Health: Constantly fueling the body with carbohydrates can overload glucose metabolism, contributing to insulin resistance and fat accumulation over time. The Randle Cycle suggests that high-carb diets disrupt the body's natural ability to switch between burning glucose and fat, leading to metabolic inefficiency. This can increase the risk of obesity, type 2 diabetes, and other metabolic diseases.

Drawbacks of Whole Grains and Processed Carbohydrate-Rich Foods

Whole grains and other starchy foods, such as rice, pasta, and bread, are often viewed as nutrient-dense options, yet they come with significant drawbacks:

High Glycemic Index and Blood Sugar Spikes: Carbohydrate-rich foods, even whole grains, can cause rapid increases in blood sugar and insulin levels. Over time, these spikes strain the pancreas and lead to insulin resistance, which is a precursor to type 2 diabetes and other metabolic disorders. Foods like white rice, pasta, and bread have particularly high glycemic indices, causing blood sugar levels to rise sharply.

Presence of Antinutrients: Whole grains contain antinutrients, such as phytic acid, that bind to minerals (like iron, zinc, and magnesium) and inhibit their absorption. This can lead to nutrient deficiencies, particularly in diets heavily reliant on grains. Phytates can reduce the bioavailability of key nutrients, making it harder for the body to access essential vitamins and minerals.

Gut Irritation and Inflammation: Grains, especially those containing gluten (such as wheat), can cause digestive issues and inflammation in certain individuals. Gluten can be difficult to digest and may cause gut permeability or "leaky gut" in susceptible people, which can lead to autoimmune conditions and chronic inflammation. Other grains, while gluten-free, may still irritate the gut lining and cause bloating or discomfort.

Limited Nutritional Value Relative to Caloric Content: While whole grains contain fiber and some B vitamins, they lack the dense concentration of nutrients found in animal products, vegetables, and fruits. Most whole grains are primarily a source of starch and offer few unique nutrients relative to the calories they provide.

Potential to Drive Overeating and Cravings: Carbohydrates can trigger cravings and promote overeating due to their rapid digestion and impact on blood sugar. When blood sugar spikes and then crashes after consuming high-carb foods, it can lead to feelings of hunger and encourage further snacking, creating a cycle that promotes excessive caloric intake.

Specific Types of Carbohydrate-Rich Foods and Their Effects

Pasta and Bread: Processed grains, like those in pasta and bread, have a higher glycemic load and are often stripped of fiber and nutrients. White bread and refined pasta are quickly absorbed, leading to rapid blood sugar spikes that can contribute to metabolic dysregulation.

Rice: White rice, in particular, is a highly refined carbohydrate with minimal fiber. Although brown rice retains more nutrients, it also contains higher levels of phytic acid, which can inhibit mineral absorption. Both forms of rice are calorie-dense with limited nutritional benefits relative to other food groups.

Whole Grains (e.g., Oats, Barley, Quinoa): Whole grains offer more fiber and micronutrients than refined grains, but they still contain antinutrients like phytates that can hinder mineral absorption. The high carbohydrate content of these foods makes them less ideal for individuals aiming for metabolic health or those seeking to avoid insulin spikes.

Tortillas: While corn tortillas provide some fiber and iron, they are still primarily starch-heavy. Flour tortillas, on the other hand, are often made with refined flour and contain added fats, which makes them a higher-calorie option with little nutritional value.

Alternatives to High-Carbohydrate Grains and Starches

For those looking to reduce carbohydrate intake and avoid the negative effects of grains and starches, there are numerous alternatives that can provide better nutritional value without the drawbacks:

- **Vegetable-Based Substitutes:** Foods like cauliflower rice, zucchini noodles, and lettuce wraps can replace grains while providing fiber, vitamins, and fewer calories.
- **Nut and Seed Flours:** Almond flour, coconut flour, and flaxseed meal are lower in carbohydrates and higher in protein and healthy fats, making them good alternatives for baking and cooking.
- **Fiber-Rich, Low-Glycemic Carbs:** If including some carbohydrates, focus on non-starchy vegetables, berries, and low-sugar fruits. These options provide fiber, vitamins, and antioxidants with minimal impact on blood sugar.

Practical Tips for Reducing Carbohydrate Intake

If you're looking to reduce or avoid grains and other starchy foods, here are a few tips:

- **Experiment with Low-Carb Cooking**: Use low-carb vegetables and flours as substitutes in traditional dishes. For example, cauliflower rice can replace rice in stir-fries, and zucchini noodles are a great alternative to pasta.
- **Limit Carb Intake to Evening Meals:** If you do include carbohydrates, having them later in the day can improve insulin sensitivity and may help reduce post-meal blood sugar spikes.
- **Focus on Protein and Fat for Satiety:** Eating meals rich in protein and healthy fats promotes longer-lasting satiety and reduces the likelihood of cravings.

Whole Grains and Starches – Not Essential, Often Detrimental

Whole grains, pastas, rice, bread, and tortillas, while common in the modern diet, are not essential for health and come with notable drawbacks. The Randle Cycle demonstrates how high carbohydrate intake can disrupt metabolic health, while antinutrients, blood sugar spikes, and digestive issues further complicate their benefits. By limiting or avoiding these foods and focusing on more nutrient-dense options, individuals can support better metabolic health, avoid insulin resistance, and reduce the risk of chronic diseases associated with carbohydrate-heavy diets.

Final Tier: Trans Fats, Processed Foods, and the "Worst of the Worst"

At the bottom of the hierarchy, we find foods that offer little to no nutritional value and come with significant health risks: trans fats, heavily processed foods, and foods that combine refined carbohydrates with unhealthy fats. These items are often calorie-dense, nutrient-poor, and engineered for taste and convenience, making them easy to overconsume and difficult for the body to process effectively. Regular consumption of these foods is linked to increased risk of chronic diseases, such as cardiovascular disease, obesity, type 2 diabetes, and even certain cancers. This tier includes the most dangerous foods that can contribute to metabolic dysfunction, inflammation, and long-term health complications.

Trans Fats: Artificial Fats with Dangerous Consequences

Trans fats, also known as partially hydrogenated oils, are chemically altered fats that are used in processed foods to improve shelf life and texture. While they were once common in margarine, baked goods, and fast foods, research has shown that they are extremely harmful to health. Many countries have now restricted or banned trans fats due to their role in increasing bad cholesterol (LDL), lowering good cholesterol (HDL), and promoting inflammation.

- **Impact on Heart Health:** Trans fats are directly linked to an increased risk of heart disease. They raise LDL cholesterol levels, which contributes to plaque buildup in the arteries, while simultaneously lowering HDL cholesterol, which normally helps clear cholesterol from the bloodstream. This combination increases the likelihood of heart attacks and strokes.
- **Inflammation and Cellular Damage:** Trans fats contribute to systemic inflammation, which is linked to chronic diseases such as arthritis, diabetes, and cancer. Inflammation can weaken the immune system, accelerate aging, and damage cells and tissues.
- **Examples of Foods with Trans Fats:** Although trans fats are being phased out, they are still found in certain processed foods, especially in some snack foods, baked goods, frozen pizza, and fried foods. Foods labeled as containing "partially hydrogenated oils" are likely to contain trans fats.
-

Highly Processed Foods: The Hidden Risks of Convenience

Processed foods are foods that have been altered from their natural state through the addition of preservatives, artificial colors, flavors, and other additives. These items are often engineered to be hyper-palatable, meaning they are designed to be incredibly flavorful and addictive. Processed foods are typically low in nutrients, high in calories, and contain a host of artificial ingredients that can be harmful to health over time.

- **Lack of Nutritional Value:** Processed foods are often stripped of natural nutrients during manufacturing and enriched with synthetic vitamins and minerals. However, synthetic nutrients are not as bioavailable as those found in whole foods, meaning they are not absorbed as effectively by the body.
- **Additives and Artificial Ingredients:** Many processed foods contain preservatives, artificial colors, and flavor enhancers like monosodium glutamate (MSG), which can contribute to food sensitivities and even trigger inflammatory responses in some individuals.
- **Increased Risk of Chronic Diseases:** Diets high in processed foods are associated with higher rates of obesity, diabetes, and cardiovascular disease. Processed foods are often high in added sugars, unhealthy fats, and refined grains, all of which contribute to insulin resistance and metabolic issues.
- **Examples of Processed Foods:** This category includes items like chips, cookies, candy, sugary breakfast cereals, instant noodles, soda, and many frozen or packaged meals. These foods are typically high in empty calories, meaning they provide little to no nutritional value beyond energy.

The Toxic Combination: High-Carb and High-Fat Foods

One of the most dangerous combinations in modern diets is foods that are high in both refined carbohydrates and unhealthy fats. This combination is relatively rare in nature, but it is common in processed foods, where sugars, refined grains, and trans fats or vegetable oils are mixed together to create calorie-dense, palatable foods that promote overeating. When carbohydrates and fats are consumed together in excess, they overwhelm the body's ability to efficiently metabolize either macronutrient, leading to fat storage, blood sugar spikes, and eventual insulin resistance.

- **The Randle Cycle Revisited:** The Randle Cycle, which dictates whether the body burns carbs or fats for energy, cannot efficiently handle high-carb and high-fat foods simultaneously. The body prioritizes glucose (from carbs) for immediate energy and stores the fat for later. This creates a cycle of blood sugar spikes followed by crashes, promoting further hunger and fat storage.
- **Insulin Resistance and Fat Accumulation:** Constantly consuming foods that are high in both carbs and fats contributes to insulin resistance, as the body becomes overwhelmed by the energy load and cannot process it effectively. Insulin resistance is a precursor to type 2 diabetes, obesity, and metabolic syndrome.
- **Examples of High-Carb, High-Fat Foods:** Foods that combine refined carbs and unhealthy fats include items like donuts, French fries, pizza, ice cream, pastries, and many fast-food meals. These foods are engineered to be addictive and calorie-dense, making them easy to overconsume while offering little nutritional benefit.

Sugar-Sweetened Beverages: Empty Calories and Metabolic Havoc

Although not a food, sugar-sweetened beverages like soda, energy drinks, and sweetened teas deserve a mention due to their detrimental impact on health. These drinks are high in added sugars and provide no nutritional value, yet they contribute to rapid blood sugar spikes, insulin resistance, and fat accumulation.

Fructose and Fatty Liver Disease: Many sugary drinks are sweetened with high-fructose corn syrup, which is metabolized primarily in the liver. Excessive fructose intake can lead to non-alcoholic fatty liver disease (NAFLD), a condition that is increasingly common in populations consuming high amounts of sugar-sweetened beverages.

Increased Risk of Obesity and Type 2 Diabetes: Regular consumption of sugary drinks is strongly linked to obesity and type 2 diabetes. These beverages provide liquid calories that are quickly absorbed, causing rapid spikes in blood sugar and insulin and promoting fat storage.

Examples of Sugar-Sweetened Beverages: In addition to sodas and energy drinks, sweetened teas, flavored coffee drinks, sports drinks, and fruit juices with added sugar all contribute to metabolic disturbances and should be minimized or avoided for optimal health.

Practical Tips for Avoiding the Worst of the Worst

Eliminating or significantly reducing these dangerous foods is one of the most effective ways to improve health and reduce the risk of chronic diseases. Here are some practical tips:

Read Labels Carefully: Look for terms like "partially hydrogenated oils" or "hydrogenated fats," which indicate the presence of trans fats. Also, avoid foods with a long list of artificial ingredients, additives, or preservatives.

Choose Whole Foods Over Packaged Options: The closer a food is to its natural state, the healthier it tends to be. Opt for fresh fruits, vegetables, meat proteins, and fats over packaged and processed options.

Limit Sugar Intake: Avoid sugary beverages and choose water, herbal teas, or unsweetened beverages. If you need sweetness, opt for naturally low-sugar options like infused water or tea with lemon.

Focus on Single-Ingredient Foods: A good rule of thumb is to prioritize foods that contain a single ingredient, such as "almonds," "broccoli," or "salmon." These whole foods do not contain hidden sugars, unhealthy fats, or artificial additives.

Minimizing or Eliminating the Bottom Tier for Health

Trans fats, processed foods, and the dangerous combination of refined carbs and fats represent the bottom tier of the food hierarchy for good reason. These foods are not only nutritionally void but also actively harmful, contributing to chronic inflammation, metabolic dysfunction, and a range of diseases. Unlike natural, unprocessed fats—such as those found in high-quality meats, dairy, and eggs—trans fats are chemically altered and toxic, leading to cardiovascular damage and other health issues. Similarly, the idea that we need to limit ourselves to "lean" proteins is based on outdated myths, as whole, nutrient-dense proteins with natural fats provide vital nutrients in a balanced form that our bodies are designed to utilize.

Creating Homemade Trans Fats

Reheating certain oils, especially those high in polyunsaturated fats like vegetable oils, can unintentionally create harmful trans fats. Trans fats, notorious for their link to inflammation and heart disease, form when oils are repeatedly heated, causing a chemical transformation known as partial hydrogenation. This process changes the structure of some natural "cis" fatty acids into "trans" configurations, which alters their behavior in the body and makes them potentially harmful.

How Reheating Leads to Trans Fat Formation

Polyunsaturated oils, such as soybean, corn, and sunflower oils, contain multiple double bonds in their molecular structure, which makes them chemically unstable under high heat. When these oils are exposed to repeated heating—common in deep frying or when reusing cooking oil—some of these double bonds shift into "trans" forms, creating trans fats. These changes often occur when oils are overheated or heated to their smoke point, where they begin to break down, releasing free radicals and other harmful byproducts alongside trans fats.

Health Risks of Trans Fats and Oxidative Compounds

Trans fats created from reheated oils pose multiple health risks:

- **Promotion of Inflammation**: Trans fats can integrate into cell membranes, disrupting normal cellular function and promoting inflammatory responses in the body. Chronic inflammation is a root cause of many diseases, including heart disease, diabetes, and certain cancers.
- **LDL Cholesterol and Oxidation**: Trans fats have been shown to raise levels of LDL cholesterol; however, the true risk is their contribution to the oxidation of small, dense LDL particles. These oxidized particles can lead to arterial damage and contribute to atherosclerosis, a major factor in cardiovascular disease. LDL itself is merely a transport protein, but small, oxidized particles within it are more likely to cause harm.
- **Insulin Resistance and Metabolic Dysfunction**: Trans fats are also associated with insulin resistance. Regular consumption of foods fried in reheated oils, which may

335

contain trans fats, can impair insulin sensitivity, increasing the risk of metabolic disorders like type 2 diabetes.

The Role of Oxidative Byproducts from Reheating

Beyond trans fats, reheated oils produce other harmful compounds:

- **Free Radicals**: Repeatedly heated oils generate free radicals—unstable molecules that cause oxidative damage in the body. These free radicals can damage cellular components, including DNA, proteins, and lipids, accelerating aging and contributing to chronic diseases.
- **Toxic Byproducts**: Compounds such as aldehydes and acrolein, produced when oils are heated past their smoke point, can have neurotoxic and carcinogenic effects. Prolonged exposure to these compounds may increase the risk of neurological diseases and cancer.

Choosing Stable Oils for Cooking

To minimize the formation of trans fats and other harmful byproducts when cooking:

1. **Use Heat-Stable Fats**: Opt for saturated and monounsaturated fats, such as coconut oil, ghee, lard, or tallow, which are more resistant to heat. These fats have fewer double bonds, making them less likely to break down or form trans fats when heated.
2. **Avoid Reheating and Reusing Oils**: Each time oil is reheated, it becomes more chemically unstable. Limit the reuse of cooking oils, especially for frying, and avoid overheating oils to their smoke point.
3. **Opt for Lower Heat Cooking Methods**: Methods like baking, steaming, or sautéing at lower temperatures reduce the risk of forming trans fats and other toxic byproducts, preserving both the nutritional quality of the oil and your health.

By choosing the right fats and avoiding repeated high-heat cooking, you can reduce the potential for harmful trans fats in your diet and support a healthier approach to cooking.

To protect long-term health and metabolic resilience, focusing on whole, nutrient-dense foods—such as unprocessed meats, high-quality dairy, natural fats, and low-sugar fruits and vegetables—is key. By avoiding the calorie-dense, nutrient-poor foods of this final tier and choosing foods that align with our biological needs, we can achieve a diet that supports vitality, longevity, and true health. This hierarchy is a reminder to fuel our bodies with real, unprocessed nourishment, not artificial, engineered products that ultimately compromise well-being.

This is a big topic for many, and I've saved it for last because, once you understand and apply the rest of the material, this concept will naturally fall into place. As I mentioned, if you're focused on weight loss, it may indicate an underlying metabolic imbalance. Shows like *The Biggest Loser* often promote outdated approaches, restricting calories and pushing extreme exercise. There are two major issues with this: first, weight lost in this way is very often regained; second, rapid fat loss can leave you with sagging skin. By following a natural approach that includes periodic fasting, autophagy can help the body gradually break down excess skin, supporting a healthier and more sustainable transformation.

What causes weight GAIN?

Generations of consuming processed foods and sugar have had a profound impact on human health, contributing significantly to weight gain and the widespread development of insulin resistance. Processed foods, which are often stripped of essential nutrients and loaded with refined carbohydrates, unhealthy fats, and added sugars, have become a staple in modern diets. These foods cause rapid spikes in blood sugar levels, triggering an overproduction of insulin. Over time, the constant demand on the pancreas to produce insulin leads to insulin resistance, a condition where cells become less responsive to insulin's effects, leaving excess glucose in the bloodstream. This cycle perpetuates fat storage, particularly around the abdominal area, and paves the way for metabolic disorders such as type 2 diabetes.

The rise of processed foods parallels the sharp increase in obesity and related metabolic diseases. Unlike whole, nutrient-dense foods that support satiety and balanced blood sugar levels, processed foods are designed to be hyper-palatable, leading to overconsumption. Coupled with a sedentary lifestyle, the chronic intake of sugary snacks, sugary beverages, and refined grains overwhelms the body's ability to maintain metabolic balance. This dietary shift has not only impacted individual health but has also created generational consequences, as children inherit the habits and metabolic vulnerabilities of their parents. To reverse these trends, there is an urgent need to prioritize whole, unprocessed foods and educate future generations about the dangers of processed food consumption and the benefits of balanced, nutrient-dense diets.

Weight gain is closely linked to the body's response to insulin, a hormone that regulates blood sugar and fat storage. When we eat carbohydrates, our digestive system breaks them down into glucose, a form of sugar. This increase in blood glucose triggers the pancreas to release insulin, signaling cells to absorb glucose for immediate energy. However, when we consume more glucose than the body immediately needs—especially from processed or high-carb foods—insulin directs the excess to be stored as fat, typically in adipose tissue.

Over time, high and frequent carbohydrate intake can lead to a condition known as insulin resistance. In this state, cells become less responsive to insulin's signals, requiring the pancreas to produce more insulin to manage blood sugar levels. This elevated insulin level, or hyperinsulinemia, promotes continuous fat storage and makes it harder for the body to access stored fat for energy. Essentially, insulin resistance traps the body in a cycle of fat accumulation because insulin actively prevents the breakdown of fat while promoting its storage.

As insulin resistance worsens, blood sugar remains elevated for longer periods, which not only perpetuates weight gain but can also lead to further metabolic issues such as type 2 diabetes. The constant signaling for fat storage, coupled with decreased fat utilization, drives weight gain and makes weight loss increasingly difficult without addressing the underlying insulin resistance. Reducing carbohydrate intake and managing insulin levels can help reverse this process, allowing the body to more efficiently use stored fat for energy and break free from the cycle of weight gain.

"No Amount of Evidence Will Ever Convince an Idiot"

Don't listen to stupid advice. The "calories in, calories out" (CICO) model, which suggests that weight loss or gain is simply a matter of eating fewer calories than one burns, falls short because it overlooks how our baseline metabolism adjusts in response to calorie intake. When we restrict calories significantly, our bodies interpret this as a potential threat to survival. In response, metabolism slows down to conserve energy, meaning we burn fewer calories at rest. This adaptive response, known as metabolic adaptation or adaptive thermogenesis, is one reason many people experience plateaus during weight loss or regain weight after a diet.

The health and fitness world is full of stupid advice, here are some examples of particularly misguided or "stupid" advice that can do more harm than good:

Stupid Advice in Health and Fitness

"Calories In, Calories Out Is All That Matters"
This oversimplification ignores the hormonal and metabolic effects of different foods. Not all calories are created equal—calories from processed foods and sugar spike insulin and drive fat storage, while calories from fats and proteins promote satiety and metabolic balance. Focusing solely on calorie counting overlooks the root causes of weight gain and metabolic dysfunction.

"Carbs Are Necessary for Energy"
This is one of the biggest myths perpetuated by traditional nutrition advice. The Randall cycle and modern research show that the body can efficiently run on fats and ketones for fuel. There are no essential carbohydrates, and many health issues stem from the overconsumption of carbs, particularly refined ones.

"Eat 6 Small Meals a Day"
Constant eating prevents the body from ever tapping into its fat stores, keeping insulin levels elevated throughout the day. This advice disrupts the natural fasting and feeding cycles our ancestors followed, which were crucial for maintaining metabolic health.

"Eat a Low-Fat Diet"
This outdated advice has led to decades of metabolic dysfunction. Fat is essential for hormone production, brain health, and overall well-being. Replacing fat with sugar and processed carbs, as promoted during the low-fat craze, has fueled the rise of obesity, diabetes, and heart disease.

"Just Do More Cardio to Lose Weight"
Endless cardio sessions do little to address the root cause of weight gain: insulin resistance. Overtraining with cardio can also elevate stress hormones like cortisol, leading to muscle loss and fat storage. Strength training and addressing diet are far more effective for fat loss and overall health.

"Detox Teas and Cleanses Will Fix Everything"
The idea that you need a tea or juice cleanse to "detox" is pure marketing. Your liver and kidneys already handle detoxification naturally. Many of these products are glorified laxatives that can cause dehydration and electrolyte imbalances, offering nothing more than temporary water weight loss.

"If You're Not Sweating, You're Not Working Hard Enough"
Sweat is not an indicator of calorie burn or workout effectiveness. Low-sweat activities like walking or weightlifting can be just as beneficial—if not more—than grueling sweat sessions, especially for building strength and metabolic health.

"BMI Accurately Reflects Health"
BMI is an outdated and overly simplistic tool. It doesn't account for muscle mass, fat distribution, or metabolic health. Many lean individuals with high BMI are metabolically healthy, while those with normal BMI can have serious underlying health issues, like visceral fat or insulin resistance.

"Cheat Days Are Necessary for Progress"
This advice can sabotage metabolic health by encouraging people to binge on harmful foods. Regular "cheat days" often lead to insulin spikes, cravings, and a reversal of progress. Sustainable dietary changes, not indulgent cheat days, are key to long-term success.

"Supplements Can Replace Real Food"
While some supplements can be helpful, relying on them as a substitute for nutrient-dense whole foods is a mistake. Many supplements are poorly absorbed, and nothing compares to the bioavailability and nutrient profile of high-quality meats and animal-based fats.

"Watch your Cholesterol" – Outdated.

Furthermore, this approach ignores the hormonal responses to different types of food. For example, a calorie of sugar will affect the body differently than a calorie of protein or fat, largely due to insulin response. High insulin levels, triggered by carbohydrate-rich foods, promote fat storage rather than fat burning, which is why insulin resistance often leads to weight gain. Hormones like leptin and ghrelin, which regulate hunger and satiety, also adjust with calorie restriction, often increasing hunger signals and decreasing fullness signals, making it challenging to sustain a low-calorie diet over time.

In reality, sustainable weight management requires more than just reducing calorie intake. It involves addressing metabolic health, managing insulin levels, and supporting a balanced hormonal environment that allows the body to utilize stored fat effectively rather than continually adjusting to conserve energy. This means that focusing on nutrient quality, meal timing, and metabolic flexibility may be more effective strategies for long-term weight and health management than simply adhering to CICO.

So what is the best way to lose FAT?

One effective way to lose fat is by focusing on nutrient-dense foods that support metabolic health and *minimize insulin spikes*. The carnivore diet, which emphasizes eating animal-based foods like meat, fish, eggs, and organ meats, is one approach that can help with this. By eliminating carbohydrates and focusing on high-protein, high-fat foods, the carnivore diet keeps insulin levels low, encouraging the body to use stored fat for energy. Additionally, it's rich in essential nutrients and can reduce inflammation, often a factor in weight gain and metabolic dysfunction. For those who thrive on animal-based nutrition, the carnivore diet can be an effective and straightforward way to lose fat while potentially improving overall health.

Whats the SECOND-best way?

Once again, I am realistic that most of you will not sustain a carnivore diet, so I would like to offer a solution for the second-best option, and much more sustainable. I do have to mention that I absolutely detest the term "keto" because it has become a buzzword associated with fad diets. However, the ketogenic diet is a scientifically backed and powerful approach to weight loss that aligns closely with ancestral macronutrient consumption. By drastically reducing carbohydrate intake, typically to fewer than 20 grams per day, the ketogenic diet encourages the body to enter a state called ketosis, where it primarily burns fat for fuel. This approach emphasizes moderate protein and high fat consumption, which not only stabilizes blood sugar levels but also minimizes insulin production. By reducing insulin spikes, the body is better able to access and utilize stored fat, making this a highly effective strategy for sustainable weight management and metabolic health.

The Basics of the Ketogenic Diet

The primary goal of the ketogenic diet is to shift the body from using glucose (derived from carbs) as its main energy source to using ketones, which are produced when the body burns fat. With only 20 grams of carbs per day—a small amount compared to the 200–300 grams typically consumed on a standard diet—the body quickly exhausts its glucose stores. In response, the liver begins breaking down fatty acids into ketones, which are then used as the primary fuel source for the brain, muscles, and other organs.

Why 20 Grams of Carbs?

The 20-gram daily limit is strategic because it's low enough to ensure the body consistently stays in ketosis, a state where fat is used instead of carbs for energy. This number can vary slightly from person to person, but it is generally low enough to keep insulin levels steady, prevent blood sugar spikes, and force the body to rely on fat for energy. By keeping carbohydrate intake extremely low, the body avoids the insulin response that would otherwise trigger fat storage.

Benefits of the Ketogenic Diet for Fat Loss

1. **Promotes Fat Burning**: When carbs are restricted, the body is compelled to burn stored fat for fuel, which naturally leads to weight loss. Ketosis promotes fat loss without causing muscle loss, as the body preserves lean muscle to support metabolic function.
2. **Reduces Hunger and Cravings**: The high-fat content of the ketogenic diet, along with moderate protein intake, promotes satiety. Fats and proteins are digested slowly, so you stay fuller longer, reducing the need to snack and eat extra calories throughout the day.
3. **Stabilizes Blood Sugar and Insulin Levels**: By minimizing carbs, the ketogenic diet keeps insulin levels low and stable. Stable insulin levels prevent the body from entering a "storage mode," which is ideal for losing fat. This is particularly helpful for individuals with insulin resistance, metabolic syndrome, or type 2 diabetes.
4. **Encourages Hormonal Balance**: Many hormones that regulate hunger, metabolism, and fat storage—like insulin, ghrelin, and leptin—respond positively to the ketogenic diet. This hormonal balance makes it easier to maintain a calorie deficit and lose weight over time.

The Science Behind Ketosis and Fat Loss

In ketosis, the body undergoes metabolic changes that favor fat burning over fat storage. Normally, carbohydrates provide a quick source of energy that can easily be stored as fat if it isn't burned immediately. When carbohydrates are minimized to around 20 grams per day, the body is essentially deprived of its preferred energy source. This "carb shortage" triggers the liver to produce ketones from stored fat to fuel the body. The result is that fat stores are steadily used up for energy.

A Typical Day on a Ketogenic Diet with Fewer than 20 Grams of Carbs

Following a ketogenic diet may seem challenging at first, especially with such a low carb intake, but it can be satisfying once you become accustomed to it. Here's what a sample day might look like:

- **Breakfast**: Eggs cooked in butter with avocado slices
- **Lunch**: Grilled chicken salad with leafy greens, olive oil, and a few slices of cucumber
- **Snack**: Small portion of cheese or a handful of nuts
- **Dinner**: Steak with sautéed spinach and a side of broccoli cooked in olive oil

Note: I would limit the amount of spinach you consume because of the ridiculously high oxalate content, but cooking will reduce it a little.

This way of eating not only keeps carbs under 20 grams but also provides a rich source of healthy fats and moderate protein, which are key to staying in ketosis.

Practical Tips for Starting and Maintaining a Ketogenic Diet

1. **Track Your Macros**: To stay under 20 grams of carbs, it's important to track your macronutrient intake, at least initially. Many apps can help monitor your carbs, fats, and proteins to ensure you're staying within your ketogenic targets.
2. **Prioritize Whole Foods**: Processed foods often contain hidden sugars and carbs that can throw you out of ketosis. Sticking to whole, unprocessed foods like meats, fish, eggs,

non-starchy vegetables, and healthy fats is crucial for success on the ketogenic diet.

3. **Stay Hydrated**: The ketogenic diet has a diuretic effect, meaning your body may flush out more water and electrolytes than usual. Drinking plenty of water and replenishing electrolytes (sodium, potassium, magnesium) helps prevent symptoms of the "keto flu," such as fatigue and headaches.

4. **Allow Your Body to Adapt**: It may take a few days to enter ketosis, and during this transition, you might experience symptoms as your body adjusts to burning fat instead of glucose. Once adapted, many people report feeling more energized and focused.

5. **Incorporate Fasting**: Intermittent fasting pairs well with the ketogenic diet, as it can help deepen ketosis and enhance fat burning. Skipping breakfast, for instance, allows the body to spend more time in a fasted state, increasing the reliance on fat for energy.

How the Ketogenic lifestyle Differs from Other Diets

The ketogenic diet stands out because it addresses weight loss from a metabolic and hormonal perspective, rather than just focusing on calorie restriction. Unlike typical calorie-cutting diets, which can slow metabolism and lead to hunger, keto maintains metabolic health by stabilizing blood sugar and insulin levels. This approach makes it easier to sustain weight loss without constant hunger or cravings, a common challenge in conventional dieting.

Long-Term Considerations

While the ketogenic diet can be highly effective for fat loss, it's important to listen to your body and assess your long-term goals. Some people find that after reaching their target weight, they can maintain their results with a modified low-carb diet that allows for slightly higher carbohydrate intake. This flexibility can help make keto a sustainable, lifestyle-friendly approach to maintaining a healthy weight. Pay attention to inflammatory markers and ask your primary physician for blood labs to maintain control.

In summary, a ketogenic diet that minimizes carbs to under 20 grams a day can be a powerful tool for fat loss. By focusing on high-fat, moderate-protein foods and cutting out carbs, the body enters ketosis, a metabolic state that favors burning fat over storing it. This approach, combined with the diet's ability to control hunger and stabilize insulin, makes the ketogenic life one of the most effective ways to lose weight and improve metabolic health.

Combining a ketogenic diet with intermittent fasting (IF) is a highly effective approach for weight loss and metabolic health. Both strategies work synergistically to promote fat burning, stabilize insulin levels, and support overall health, but they each function in unique ways. While the ketogenic diet shifts the body into ketosis by limiting carbohydrates and encouraging fat for fuel, intermittent fasting maximizes the time spent in fat-burning mode by extending the fasting window between meals.

The Benefits of Combining the Ketogenic Diet and IF

Enhanced Ketosis: The ketogenic diet already promotes ketosis by restricting carbs, but IF can deepen this state. During fasting periods, insulin levels naturally drop, and the body's reliance on stored fat for energy increases. With both the ketogenic diet and IF, you can reach and sustain ketosis more efficiently, leading to faster and more consistent fat loss.

Increased Fat-Burning Efficiency: IF extends the time the body spends in a fasted state, which allows for greater fat-burning periods. Since the body is already adapted to using fat as fuel on a ketogenic diet, fasting can accelerate fat metabolism, as it does not need to switch from burning carbs to burning fat.

Hormone Optimization: Both the ketogenic diet and IF contribute to hormonal balance, which is crucial for weight management. Lower insulin levels help reduce fat storage, while increased sensitivity to insulin makes the body more effective at using energy. Fasting also promotes the release of human growth hormone (HGH), which supports muscle preservation and boosts metabolism.

Reduced Appetite and Cravings: The ketogenic diet and IF naturally suppress appetite by promoting satiety and reducing hunger hormones. The high-fat content of meals within a ketogenic diet provides longer-lasting fullness, while fasting reduces ghrelin (the hunger hormone) levels over time, making it easier to maintain a calorie deficit without constant cravings.

Improved Metabolic Flexibility: By combining the ketogenic diet with IF, the body becomes more efficient at switching between energy sources, such as stored fat and ketones, without experiencing the energy crashes associated with carbohydrate reliance. This flexibility leads to more stable energy levels throughout the day, increased mental clarity, and a reduced dependency on frequent meals.

How to Implement the Ketogenic Diet and IF Together

To start combining keto and intermittent fasting, consider these steps:

Begin with Ketosis First: If you're new to both the ketogenic diet and IF, it's often helpful to start with the ketogenic diet for a couple of weeks. This gives your body time to adapt to burning fat and entering ketosis, making it easier to handle extended fasting periods without feeling fatigued or hungry.

Ease into IF with a 16:8 Schedule: Once you're comfortable with the ketogenic diet, begin with a 16:8 fasting schedule, where you fast for 16 hours and eat during an 8-hour window. For example, you might have your first meal at noon and finish eating by 8 PM. As you become accustomed to fasting, you can adjust to longer fasting windows if desired.

Focus on Nutrient-Dense Ketogenic Meals: During your eating window, consume high-quality, nutrient-dense foods to support energy and satiety. Foods like fatty cuts of meat, eggs, avocados, and leafy greens provide essential nutrients while keeping you in ketosis.

Stay Hydrated and Mindful of Electrolytes: Fasting and ketosis both increase fluid loss, so drinking plenty of water and replenishing electrolytes (sodium, potassium, magnesium) is essential. This will help prevent dehydration and reduce symptoms of the "keto flu" that can occur with electrolyte imbalance.

Experiment with Extended Fasts if Desired: After adapting to a ketogenic diet and shorter fasting windows, some people find success with longer fasts, such as 24-hour fasts once a week or even 48-hour fasts. These extended fasts allow for deeper ketosis and can boost autophagy, the body's process of cleaning out damaged cells, which can promote both health and weight loss.

What a Typical Day Might Look Like on Keto and IF

Here's an example of how you might structure a day combining low-carb ketosis with a 16:8 fasting window:

- **8 AM - 12 PM (Fasting Period)**: Drink water, black coffee, or herbal tea to stay hydrated and support mental clarity during the fast.
- **12 PM (First Meal)**: Break your fast with a keto-friendly meal, such as scrambled eggs with avocado and a side of leafy greens.
- **3 PM (Snack)**: Have a small, high-fat snack like a handful of macadamia nuts or cheese to maintain energy and satiety.
- **7 PM (Final Meal)**: Enjoy a satisfying dinner with protein (like salmon or steak), low-carb vegetables, and a healthy fat source like olive oil or butter.

Potential Challenges and Tips for Success

Combining the ketogenic lifestyle and IF can be challenging at first, especially for those who are new to low-carb eating or extended fasting. Here are a few tips to overcome common hurdles:

- **Listen to Your Body**: Transitioning to ketogenic life and IF can take time, and it's essential to listen to your body's signals. Start slowly and gradually increase fasting windows as you adapt to both.
- **Avoid Processed Foods**: While it may be tempting to fill your eating window with "keto friendly" processed snacks, focusing on whole foods will provide more nutrients, support satiety, and improve overall health outcomes.
- **Plan Your Meals**: Meal planning can help ensure you're getting enough calories, protein, and fat during your eating window. This is crucial to avoid feeling deprived or overeating after your fast.
- **Be Patient with Adaptation**: It can take a few weeks to adapt fully to ketosis and IF. Fatigue or mild hunger may occur initially, but they typically diminish as your body becomes accustomed to burning fat for fuel.

Long-Term Benefits of the Ketogenic Lifestyle and IF for Weight Loss and Health

Combining the ketogenic diet with intermittent fasting can be a sustainable, long-term approach to weight management and metabolic health. This combination helps maintain lean muscle mass, reduces inflammation, and supports steady energy levels. Over time, many people experience improved mental clarity, enhanced focus, and better overall metabolic flexibility.

This approach is particularly effective for those struggling with insulin resistance, as it can reset the body's response to insulin and reduce the need for frequent meals or snacks. By combining these two strategies, individuals can achieve greater control over their metabolism, promote sustainable fat loss, and improve health markers beyond weight loss, such as blood sugar regulation, lipid profiles, and inflammatory markers.

One Meal a Day (OMAD): An Advanced Step in Combining Ketogenesis with Intermittent Fasting

One Meal a Day (OMAD) is an advanced form of intermittent fasting where you consume all of your daily calories in a single meal, typically within a one-hour window, and fast for the remaining 23 hours. When combined with a ketogenic diet, OMAD can provide a powerful boost to weight loss and metabolic health. For those who have adapted to both the ketogenic diet and intermittent fasting, OMAD can be a natural progression that offers even deeper ketosis, enhanced fat-burning, and simplified eating routines.

Benefits of OMAD on a Ketogenic Diet

Maximized Ketosis and Fat Burning: With an extended fasting period of 23 hours, the body remains in ketosis for a longer duration. This prolonged state helps burn through fat stores efficiently, as there's minimal insulin secretion throughout the day. Ketogenesis already supports fat burning, and OMAD amplifies this process by extending the fasting window.

Simplified Meal Planning: OMAD requires planning just one meal a day, making it ideal for those who want a minimalist approach to eating. This simplicity can reduce food-related decisions, save time on meal prep, and reduce overall stress around food choices.

Enhanced Autophagy: Extended fasting periods stimulate autophagy, a cellular process that clears out damaged cells and regenerates new, healthier cells. Autophagy is associated with various health benefits, including reduced inflammation, improved longevity, and better immune function. The combination of ketosis and OMAD promotes autophagy more effectively than shorter fasting windows.

Improved Insulin Sensitivity: OMAD on a ketogenic diet keeps insulin levels low for most of the day, giving the body a break from insulin spikes and allowing cells to become more sensitive to insulin. This is especially beneficial for individuals with insulin resistance or type 2 diabetes, as it helps the body process carbohydrates and sugars more effectively over time.

Mental Clarity and Focus: Many people report heightened focus and mental clarity when doing OMAD, particularly on a ketogenic diet. Fasting for extended periods reduces the body's reliance on glucose, and the brain benefits from ketones as a steady energy source, resulting in more sustained focus throughout the day.

What to Eat on OMAD with the Ketogenic Diet

When eating only once a day, it's crucial to make that meal as nutrient-dense as possible to meet daily nutritional needs. An OMAD meal on ketosis should ideally include:

High-Quality Protein: Aim for protein-rich foods like steak, salmon, chicken, or eggs. Protein helps preserve muscle mass, which is important for metabolic health, especially during fasting.

Healthy Fats: Incorporate fats from sources like avocado, olive oil, butter, and fatty cuts of meat to ensure you're getting enough calories and staying in ketosis. Healthy fats provide sustained energy and satiety.

Low-Carb Vegetables: Include nutrient-dense, low-carb vegetables like leafy greens, broccoli, cauliflower, and zucchini. These vegetables provide fiber, vitamins, and minerals that support digestion and overall health.

Electrolytes and Hydration: Given the extended fasting period, it's essential to prioritize electrolytes. Foods rich in potassium and magnesium, or supplements if necessary, help maintain electrolyte balance and prevent dehydration.

A Sample OMAD Meal on The Ketogenic Diet

An example of a nutrient-dense OMAD meal could look like this:

- **Main Dish**: Grilled ribeye steak or baked salmon (protein and healthy fats)
- **Side Dish**: Large salad with mixed greens, avocado, cucumbers, and a drizzle of olive oil and vinegar
- **Additional Fats**: A handful of olives, a slice of full-fat cheese, or a small portion of nuts like macadamias for extra fats and flavor
- **Optional Drink**: Bone broth for added minerals and electrolytes

Tips for Success with OMAD on The Ketogenic Diet

1. **Ease into OMAD**: If you're new to OMAD, start by gradually reducing your eating window from 8 hours to 4 hours, eventually progressing to one meal a day. This will help your body adapt to a longer fasting period.
2. **Stay Hydrated**: Drink plenty of water throughout the day to stay hydrated, especially during the fasting hours. You may also drink black coffee, tea, or electrolyte drinks (without sugar) to help curb hunger and support hydration.
3. **Listen to Your Body**: While OMAD is effective, it's essential to listen to your body. Some people thrive on OMAD, while others may feel fatigued or overly hungry. If OMAD doesn't feel sustainable, consider returning to a shorter fasting window, like 16:8.
4. **Prioritize Nutrient Density**: Since you're eating only once, focus on high-quality, nutrient-dense foods to ensure you're meeting your body's daily requirements. Avoid processed foods and low-nutrient options.
5. **Monitor Electrolytes**: Extended fasting can lead to electrolyte imbalances, so make sure you're getting enough sodium, potassium, and magnesium. You may consider using an electrolyte supplement or adding salt to your water.

Long-Term Considerations for OMAD and The Ketogenic Diet

One of the things I have heard about the people who fear the one meal a day plan is that they are accustomed to eating 3 times a day and they get hungry at breakfast and/or lunch. This will be mitigated after a few days because your hunger hormone ghrelin will not be triggered by circadian rhythm after a short time. It gets easier. OMAD can be an excellent tool for weight loss and metabolic health, but it may not be ideal for everyone as a long-term lifestyle. For some, OMAD may work best as an occasional strategy—such as once or twice a week—to enhance fat burning and stimulate autophagy. Others may find it sustainable for longer periods. It's essential to assess your energy levels, mood, and overall health to decide if OMAD is a long-term fit.

By combining OMAD with the ketogenic diet, you're leveraging the power of both ketosis and fasting to maximize fat loss, improve metabolic health, and simplify your daily routine. As with any dietary approach, customization and listening to your body's needs are key to long-term success.

Prolonged Fasting Once a Month: Harnessing the Benefits of Autophagy

Prolonged fasting—fasting for 24 to 72 hours or longer—is a powerful strategy for enhancing health and metabolic function, especially when practiced on a monthly basis. Unlike shorter fasting windows, prolonged fasting pushes the body into a deeper state of ketosis and triggers significant levels of autophagy, a cellular cleanup process with profound benefits for health and longevity. Monthly prolonged fasting can be a highly effective addition to a ketogenic or intermittent fasting lifestyle, as it amplifies the effects of regular fasting while providing unique health benefits.

What is Autophagy and Why Is It Important?

Autophagy is the body's natural process of cellular recycling, where old or damaged cells are broken down, and the resulting components are reused to form new, healthy cells. This process becomes particularly active during prolonged fasting because, in the absence of food, the body begins to prioritize survival by clearing out dysfunctional or unnecessary cells, which provides energy and promotes optimal cellular function. Autophagy is associated with a range of health benefits, including reduced inflammation, improved

352

immune function, and even a lower risk of diseases like cancer and neurodegenerative disorders.

Key Benefits of Prolonged Fasting and Autophagy

Enhanced Cellular Repair: Autophagy removes damaged cells, reducing the accumulation of cellular "waste" that can contribute to aging and disease. This cleanup process is crucial for maintaining healthy tissues and organs over time, as it helps repair damaged cells and optimize cellular function.

Reduced Inflammation: Prolonged fasting triggers autophagy and reduces inflammation by clearing out inflammatory markers and proteins that contribute to chronic illnesses. This reduction in inflammation can help improve symptoms in conditions such as arthritis, cardiovascular disease, and autoimmune disorders.

Boosted Immune Function: By clearing out old and dysfunctional immune cells, autophagy encourages the production of new, more effective immune cells. Prolonged fasting, therefore, supports a healthier, more resilient immune system, helping the body respond better to infections and illnesses.

Improved Insulin Sensitivity and Metabolic Health: Extended fasting improves insulin sensitivity by giving the body an extended break from insulin production, allowing cells to become more responsive to insulin. This increased sensitivity helps regulate blood sugar levels more effectively and is beneficial for those managing insulin resistance or type 2 diabetes.

Support for Healthy Aging: Autophagy's cell-recycling process has been linked to longevity and a lower risk of age-related diseases. By regularly engaging in prolonged fasting, you're promoting a slower aging process at the cellular level, which can reduce the likelihood of degenerative conditions.

Increased Growth Hormone Production: Prolonged fasting stimulates the release of human growth hormone (HGH), which supports muscle preservation, fat loss, and overall metabolic health. HGH plays a crucial role in tissue repair and recovery, which is essential during extended fasting.

How to Practice Prolonged Fasting Safely

To get started with prolonged fasting once a month, here are some guidelines to maximize benefits and ensure safety:

1. **Choose a Fasting Duration**: A common range for prolonged fasting is between 24 and 72 hours. Beginners may want to start with a 24-hour fast and gradually extend the duration as they become more comfortable. A 48-hour fast is a great target for experienced fasters looking to trigger deeper autophagy.
2. **Stay Hydrated**: During prolonged fasts, water intake is crucial to prevent dehydration. Adding electrolytes (sodium, potassium, magnesium) can help maintain balance and reduce symptoms like fatigue, headaches, or muscle cramps. Non-caloric beverages like black coffee or herbal tea can also support hydration.
3. **Listen to Your Body**: Fasting can be challenging, especially during the first few attempts. It's essential to listen to your body; if you feel weak, dizzy, or unwell, consider breaking the fast. Gradually building up to longer fasts is better than forcing an extended fast.
4. **Plan for Recovery**: After a prolonged fast, break your fast with a small, nutrient-dense meal to ease your digestive system back into eating. Bone broth, eggs, or a light salad with olive oil are gentle options for refeeding.
5. **Avoid Strenuous Activity**: During prolonged fasting, it's best to keep physical activity light, as the body is already in a stressed state from fasting. Walking, stretching, and meditation can support mental clarity and physical relaxation during your fast.

A Typical Monthly Prolonged Fasting Routine

A routine monthly 48-hour fast might look like this:

- **Day 1**: Finish your last meal in the evening, then begin fasting.
- **Day 2**: Hydrate throughout the day with water, herbal tea, or black coffee. Monitor how you feel and rest as needed.
- **Day 3**: Break your fast with a light, low carbohydrate meal to support gentle refeeding. It is important that you do not

introduce carbohydrates when breaking a prolonged fast because your insulin receptors will be extremely sensitive and may signal your body to store fat.

Practicing a prolonged fast monthly, in combination with a ketogenic or intermittent fasting regimen, offers the dual benefits of deep autophagy and sustainable fat loss. With each fast, the body strengthens its resilience, clears out damaged cells, and optimizes metabolic function, making it an effective way to support both weight management and long-term health.

Losing fat is a common goal for many, but true, lasting success comes from prioritizing overall health rather than focusing solely on the scale. When we emphasize nourishing our bodies, balancing hormones, and supporting natural processes like insulin sensitivity and metabolic function, the body finds its way back to a healthier baseline, or **homeostasis.**

This approach means choosing nutrient-dense, low-carb foods, practicing intermittent fasting, and incorporating longer fasts for deeper metabolic benefits like autophagy. By supporting health first—through balanced eating, regular movement, proper sleep, and managing stress—the body naturally shifts towards a healthy weight. Fat loss becomes a byproduct of achieving balance within the body, making it more sustainable and beneficial for long-term wellness.

Conclusion: A New Chapter in Health

As we reach the end of this journey through the myths, truths, and science behind health and nutrition, it's important to take a step back and see the bigger picture. The goal of this book was not just to challenge conventional thinking, but to empower you with the knowledge to make better choices for your health. By dissecting long-held misconceptions, exploring ancestral and scientifically backed dietary practices, and understanding the complex interplay of metabolic health, we have built a foundation that redefines what it means to truly thrive.

Our modern world often bombards us with conflicting information, dietary fads, and quick fixes that promise miraculous results but rarely deliver. The path forward requires discernment, patience, and a return to understanding the fundamentals of human physiology and nutrition. It's about embracing a lifestyle that aligns with our biology and evolution, fostering resilience and longevity. Remember that real health is not achieved overnight but through consistent, informed actions that honor your body's natural processes.

As you close this book, I encourage you to take these insights and apply them thoughtfully in your life. Share them with loved ones, question what you see in mainstream health narratives, and be an advocate for a more informed, evidence-based approach to well-being. Your journey to health is personal, yet connected to a broader movement that seeks truth, balance, and the betterment of society as a whole.

The future of health isn't just about surviving; it's about thriving with vitality and purpose. Let this book be the starting point for a deeper understanding and commitment to a "life well-lived". Together, we can shift perspectives and inspire a new chapter in health, rooted in truth, knowledge, and empowered choice.

Author Bio:

Steven Yutani holds a B.S. in Applied Nutritional Science and an M.S. in Medical Nutrition from Arizona State University (2025) and is a Corporate Medical Nutritionist. Steve also holds several certificates from Harvard Medical School on various health subjects. With over 5 years of experience in clinical nutrition, medical pathways research, Steven has worked to promote better health through diet. He has conducted research on lipidology, endocrinology, cardiology, and biochemistry. As a speaker at various conferences, Steven advocates for evidence-based dietary practices and the importance of nutrition in preventing chronic disease. He is also a member of the American Heart Association, furthering his commitment to advancing nutrition science.

Some of the Experts

In any exploration of health, nutrition, and metabolic science, it is essential to recognize the individuals whose groundbreaking work has shifted paradigms and influenced the conversation around these topics. This chapter highlights notable experts who have significantly contributed to our understanding of diet, metabolism, chronic diseases, and holistic health. Their research, clinical work, and advocacy have laid the foundation for a broader comprehension of how nutrition and lifestyle impact long-term wellness. Also, there are several publications associated with some of them I recommend each of them.

Dr. Jason Fung

Dr. Jason Fung, a nephrologist, has revolutionized the approach to type 2 diabetes and obesity through his work on intermittent fasting and low-carb diets. Known for his books *The Obesity Code* and *The Diabetes Code*, Dr. Fung argues that traditional treatments focusing on caloric restriction and medication miss the root causes of metabolic dysfunction.

Dr. Robert Lustig

An endocrinologist and researcher, Dr. Robert Lustig is renowned for his work on the toxic impact of sugar on the human body. His lectures and books, such as *Fat Chance*, and *Metabolical* have exposed the hidden dangers of processed foods and fructose, drawing attention to the metabolic pathways that contribute to obesity and chronic diseases.

Dr. Ken Berry

Dr. Ken Berry, a family physician and vocal advocate for the "Proper Human Diet," has garnered a large following through his teachings on low-carb, high-fat nutrition. His emphasis on ancestral eating patterns and elimination of processed foods has inspired countless individuals to reconsider mainstream dietary guidelines. He is the author of *Lies My Doctor Told Me*

Dr. Paul Saladino

Known for promoting the carnivore diet, Dr. Paul Saladino focuses on nutrient density and the idea of eliminating plant-based anti-nutrients. His book *The Carnivore Code* challenges conventional dietary wisdom and presents an argument for animal-based nutrition as an optimal human diet.

Dr. Pradip Jamnadas

Cardiologist Dr. Pradip Jamnadas has been a leading advocate for fasting and the reduction of processed carbohydrate intake. His educational videos and lectures stress the importance of metabolic health and the negative effects of chronic insulin exposure.

Dr. Philip Ovadia

Dr. Philip Ovadia is a cardiothoracic surgeon whose work centers on metabolic health as a preventative measure for heart disease. His book *Stay Off My Operating Table* emphasizes the power of diet and lifestyle changes in maintaining cardiovascular health.

Dave Feldman

A citizen scientist known for his research on cholesterol, Dave Feldman has challenged conventional understandings of lipid metabolism through his "lean mass hyper-responder" hypothesis. His work has provided valuable insights into how cholesterol functions in low-carb and ketogenic contexts.

Dr. Shawn Baker

A prominent figure in the carnivore movement, Dr. Shawn Baker advocates for an all-meat diet and its purported health benefits. His book *The Carnivore Diet* and personal clinical experiences offer an alternative view on nutrition, backed by testimonials and emerging research.

Dr. Stephen Sinatra

Dr. Stephen Sinatra, a cardiologist, has contributed significantly to the field with his research on cholesterol, CoQ10, and heart health. He has been a critic of the overprescription of statins and has promoted a more holistic view of cardiovascular care. He is the author of *The Great Cholesterol Myth* and *Metabolic Cardiology*.

Sally Norton

An expert in oxalate toxicity, Sally Norton has focused on educating the public about the potential dangers of consuming high-oxalate foods. Her work has been pivotal in helping people understand how certain plant compounds can contribute to health problems. *Toxic Superfoods*

Dr. Nadir Ali

A cardiologist and cholesterol expert, Dr. Nadir Ali has been vocal about the misconceptions surrounding cholesterol and its link to heart disease. He advocates for low-carb and high-fat diets as a means to improve metabolic health and prevent cardiovascular issues.

Dr. Bart Kay

Dr. Bart Kay is known for his critical approach to nutritional science and exercise physiology. He emphasizes evidence-based analysis and challenges popular health myths, advocating for a return to foundational principles in health and nutrition research.

Dr. David Perlmutter

A board-certified neurologist and author, Dr. David Perlmutter has pioneered the connection between diet and brain health. His influential books, such as *Drop Acid* and *Grain Brain*, delve into the adverse effects of high carbohydrate intake and chronic inflammation on cognitive function. Also, *Drop Acid* deals with the uric acid theory that I have addressed. His research emphasizes the critical role of nutrition in preventing neurological diseases and maintaining optimal brain health.

I would like to thank all those that helped me develop my knowledge for nutritional science and are concerned for the health of our youth.